Surgical Foundations: Essentials of Breast Surgery

Surgical Foundations: Essentials of Breast Surgery

Michael S. Sabel, MD, FACS
Associate Professor of Surgery
Division of Surgical Oncology
University of Michigan Comprehensive Cancer Center
Ann Arbor, Michigan

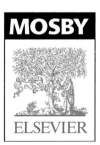

MOSBY

ELSEVIER

1600 John F. Kennedy Blvd.
Ste 1800
Philadelphia, PA 19103-2899

SURGICAL FOUNDATIONS: ESSENTIALS OF BREAST SURGERY   ISBN: 978-0-323-03758-7

Notice

Knowledge and best practice in this field are constantly changing. As new research and experience broaden our knowledge, changes in practice, treatment and drug therapy may become necessary or appropriate. Readers are advised to check the most current information provided (i) on procedures featured or (ii) by the manufacturer of each product to be administered, to verify the recommended dose or formula, the method and duration of administration, and contraindications. It is the responsibility of the practitioner, relying on their own experience and knowledge of the patient, to make diagnoses, to determine dosages and the best treatment for each individual patient, and to take all appropriate safety precautions. To the fullest extent of the law, neither the Publisher nor the Editor assumes any liability for any injury and/or damage to persons or property arising out of or related to any use of the material contained in this book.

The Publisher

Library of Congress Cataloging-in-Publication Data

Sabel, Michael S.
  Essentials of breast surgery / Michael S. Sabel. – 1st ed.
      p. ; cm. – (Surgical foundations)
  Includes bibliographical references and index.
  ISBN 978-0-323-03758-7 (alk. paper)
1. Breast–Cancer–Surgery. 2. Breast–Surgery. I. Title. II. Series: Surgical foundations.
  [DNLM: 1. Breast–surgery. 2. Breast Diseases–surgery. 3. Breast Neoplasms–therapy.
WP 910 S115e 2009]
  RD667.5.S23 2009
  616.99′449059–dc22

                                                                                        2009004600

Acquisitions Editor: Judith Fletcher
Developmental Editor: Martha Limbach
Project Manager: Mary Stermel
Design Direction: Steve Stave
Marketing Manager: Brenna Christensen

Printed in the United States of America

Last digit is the print number: 9 8 7 6 5 4 3 2 1

Dedication

To my wonderful wife, Janeel, who was extremely understanding when family time needed to be compromised, and to my beautiful children, Alex and Madison, although they weren't quite as understanding. Also, to my parents, Steven and Rhoda, who through their love and patience got me to the point where I can hopefully make them proud.

Preface

The management of both benign and malignant breast disease represents a major portion of a surgeon's responsibility, yet often comprises only a minor portion of their training. The diagnostic workup and treatment of breast disease is constantly changing and increasingly complex, making it extremely challenging for the surgical trainee or practicing general surgeon to keep up with changes in the field. Surgeons will see an extremely high volume of patients with complaints related to the breast, and it is imperative that they allay fears, palliate symptoms, and not miss diagnosing malignant disease. Surgeons must also identify patients at high risk of developing breast cancer so that appropriate screening and prophylactic measures may be considered. The management of malignant breast disease is increasingly multifaceted. The days of the surgeon seeing the patient, completing surgical therapy, and then referring the patient to other specialists have passed; today the surgeon needs to work in concert with radiologists, pathologists, medical and radiation oncologists, plastic surgeons, and other medical professionals to formulate an appropriate diagnostic and therapeutic plan. Multidisciplinary management of the breast cancer patient is critical and often guided by the surgeon even though surgery may not be the first modality employed.

Any surgeon dealing with breast disease is in need of a strong grasp of not only the anatomy and physiology of the breast, but the potential and limitations of breast imaging, benign and malignant breast histology, genetics, cancer biology, and an understanding of all treatment modalities such as radiation and systemic therapies. However, most textbooks on breast disease are meant for clinicians and researchers from multiple disciplines, containing extremely thorough reviews of the research, the evolution of treatment, and the randomized trials that led us to this point. This can be too confusing and overwhelming for the surgeon in training or the practicing general surgeon who must also focus on diseases outside of the breast. *Surgical Foundations: Essentials of Breast Surgery* captures the true essentials of the management of breast disease in an easily readable and absorbable format. The principles of multimodality therapy (chemotherapy, radiation therapy, hormonal therapy) are explained from a surgical perspective, as are the basics of breast anatomy and physiology, the diagnostic workup and management of benign breast disease, and risk stratification and reduction. Our goal is a textbook that surgery residents, surgical oncology fellows, and breast surgery fellows can utilize in training (and beyond) and that practicing general surgeons can use to enhance their management of breast disease. Easy to read, with a list of key topics to help focus the reader and a liberal use of tables, boxes, and figures to reinforce the information in each chapter, this textbook will hopefully be a useful resource to any surgeon responsible for the management of diseases of the breast, particularly breast cancer.

Contents

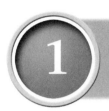
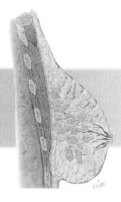

Anatomy and Physiology of the Breast

Key Points

- Know the development of the breast from intrauterine development through puberty.
- Describe the anatomy of the breast and the relationship of the breast to the chest wall and axilla.
- Understand the segmental distribution of the ductal-lobular units and the pathway of milk from the lobules to the nipple
- Name the muscles of the chest wall and axilla, their blood supply and innervation, and the impact of a nerve injury.
- Understand the arterial supply and venous and lymphatic drainage of the breast and how this impacts breast pathology and surgery.
- Describe the anatomy of the axilla, the boundaries of the "axillary pyramid," and the groupings of the lymph nodes in the axilla.
- Understand the hormones that can affect breast physiology and how lactation occurs.
- Know the changes that the breast undergoes during the menstrual cycle, during pregnancy, and after menopause.

Development of the Breast

The breast undergoes multiple changes throughout life, from intrauterine life to senescence. The development of the breast has several implications that impact the breast surgeon. These include not only developmental anomalies that the breast surgeon may face, but also the routine surgical approach to both benign and malignant disease. Although the majority of growth occurs with puberty, the development and differentiation of the breast are truly completed by the end of the first term of pregnancy. This is relevant to the development of cancer, because breast cancer risk is clearly and inversely related to the age at which pregnancy first occurs. It is possible that this is secondary to an increased risk of carcinogenesis when the pre-parity, undifferentiated, and proliferating mammary epithelium is exposed to carcinogens, as compared to the effect of these same carcinogens on the differentiated breast.

Embryology

Breast development takes place in several stages (Box 1–1). Essentially, the breast arises from a single ectodermal bud. At approximately the fifth to sixth week of fetal life, a *milk streak* develops as an ectodermal thickening, extending from the axilla to the pelvis. This is also referred to as the *galactic band*. By the ninth week, most of this has atrophied except for a mammary ridge in the pectoral region. It is here that a mass of basal cells proliferates to form the *nipple bud*. By the 12th week, squamous cells from the surface begin to invade the nipple bud. While the epithelial cells grow downward as mammary ducts, terminating in lobular buds, the mesenchymal cells differentiate into smooth muscle of the nipple and areola. The anlage of the lactiferous ducts invades the mesodermal connective tissue by 16 to 24 weeks.

The fact that the entire gland thus originates as a large dermal and subcutaneous organ from a single focus on the skin is relevant to the breast surgeon. One can think of the breasts as modified eccrine glands. This is pertinent to the lymphatic drainage, and has implications for lymphatic mapping and sentinel lymph node biopsy (see Chapter 13). Failure of some of these steps to take place can result in congenital abnormalities of the breast (Box 1–2). Most of these are quite rare; however, ectopic breast tissue may be found in 1% to 6% of individuals and is commonly encountered by the

BOX 1–1 STAGES OF EMBRYOLOGIC BREAST DEVELOPMENT

Ridge stage (<5-mm embryo)
Milk hill stage (7 to 8 weeks, 5- to 10-mm embryo)
  Thickening of the mammary anlage in the region of the thorax
  Regression of the remainder of the milk streak
Mammary disc stage (10-mm embryo)
  Invagination into the chest wall mesenchyme
Lobule stage (11- to 25-mm embryo)
  Tridimensional growth
Cone stage (10 to 14 weeks, 25- to 30-mm embryo)
  Flattening of the ridge
Budding stage (12 to 16 weeks, 30- to 70-mm embryo)
  Mesenchymal cells differentiate into smooth muscle of nipple and areola
  Epithelial buds develop
Indentation stage (70 mm to 10 cm)
Branching stage (16 weeks, 10-cm fetus)
  Epithelial buds branch into 15 to 25 strips of epithelium
  Differentiation of hair follicle, sebaceous gland, and sweat gland elements
  Apocrine glands develop to form Montgomery glands around the nipple
Canalization stage (20 to 32 weeks of gestation)
  First stage dependent on hormonal influences
  Placental sex hormones induce canalization of the branched epithelial tissues
End-vesicle stage (newborn)
  Development of lobuloalveolar structures containing colostrum

breast surgeon. Ectopic breast tissue is a result of a failure of the milk streak to completely atrophy. The ectopic tissue is usually located in the axilla, and women may present with complaints of a mass or pain in this area. Both benign fibrocystic changes and cancer can arise in this tissue.

During the second trimester, the breast continues to develop with the appearance of sweat glands, sebaceous glands, and apocrine glands, which will develop into the Montgomery glands around the nipple. The epithelial buds begin to branch into between 15 and 25 branches. Until this point, all of this has occurred independent of the placental sex hormones. In the third trimester, these hormones can enter the fetal circulation and stimulate

BOX 1–2 ABNORMAL BREAST DEVELOPMENT

Accessory Nipple (Polythelia)

Ectopic nipple tissue due to failure of complete regression of the milk streak

May occur anywhere from axilla to groin

Accessory Mammary Gland (Polymastia)

Accessory breast tissue due to failure of complete regression of the milk streak

Most often in axilla; may enlarge during pregnancy

Hypoplasia

Underdevelopment of the breast, which may be unilateral or bilateral with asymmetry

Poland's syndrome

Unilateral hypoplasia of the breast, thorax, and pectoralis muscles

Can also be associated with hand abnormalities (symbrachydactyly, hypoplasia of the middle phalanges, and central skin webbing)

Hyperplasia

Overdevelopment of the breast; may be unilateral or bilateral with asymmetry

Amazia

The nipple is present but there is no underlying breast tissue

Congenital Amastia

Absent breast and nipple

Acquired Amastia

Iatrogenic amastia due to excisional biopsy of the breast bud

Can also result from radiation or trauma (burn)

the branched epithelial tissues to canalize. The ends of these branches differentiate into lobuloalveolar structures that contain colostrum. This colostral milk is stimulated by the placental hormones and can be expressed for 4 to 7 days after birth, in both male and female newborns (often referred to as "witch's milk"). During these final weeks of development, the mammary gland mass increases fourfold and the nipple-areolar complex develops and becomes pigmented. Shortly after birth there is withdrawal of the placental hormones, causing colostral secretion to stop and involution of the breast.

After birth, mammary gland development does very little more other than keeping pace with the growth of the body. During early childhood, there is further canalizing and branching of the vesicles, but no significant changes will take place until puberty.

Development during Puberty

Under the influence of gonadotropin-releasing hormone from the hypothalamus, puberty begins in children between 8 and 12 years of age. This leads to the release of follicle-stimulating hormone (FSH) and luteinizing hormone (LH) from the pituitary gland, resulting in maturation of the ovarian follicles and the secretion of estrogens. As puberty begins, the circulating estrogen causes the ductal epithelium and surrounding stroma to grow. These ducts begin to extend into the superficial pectoral fascia and arborize within the supporting stroma to form collecting ducts and terminal duct lobular units. These ultimately form buds that precede further breast lobules. Surrounding the ducts, vascularity increases and connective tissues increase in volume and elasticity, replacing adipose tissue and providing support for the developing ducts (Fig. 1–1).

In addition to the development of pubic hair, breast budding is one of the first signs of adolescence in girls, along with the adolescent growth spurt, beginning anywhere between age 8 and 13 years. Although there are many ways one can define the stages of breast development from puberty to adulthood, the most commonly used system is the Tanner phases, which is based on the external appearance of the breast (Table 1–1). Approximately a year or 2 following menarche, the breasts acquire their mature structure (Tanner stage 5).

Anatomy of the Adult Breast

The adult breast sits atop the anterior chest wall (Fig. 1–2). Superiorly, the breast extends to the second intercostal space, while inferiorly it extends to the inframammary fold, located at the sixth or seventh intercostal space. The medial margin is at the lateral margin of the sternum, and the lateral margin sits at the midaxillary line. The shape of the breast is not spherical, but rather that of a teardrop, with an extension of breast tissue toward the axilla known as *the tail of Spence*. This is an important concept to keep in mind when performing a mastectomy (see Chapter 12: Surgical Management of Breast Cancer). These are the classic descriptions of the boundaries of the breast, but breast tissue can extend

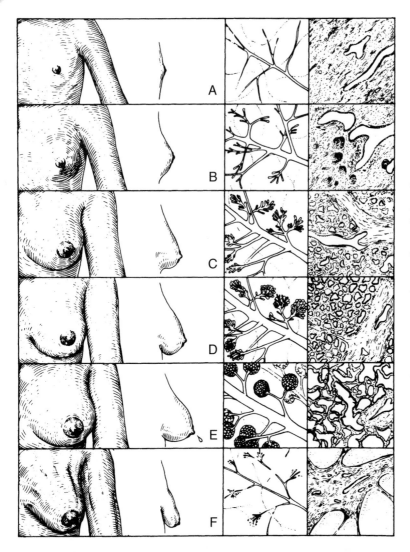

Figure 1-1. Schematic drawing illustrating mammary gland development. Anterior and lateral views of the breast are shown in columns 1 and 2. The microscopic appearances of the ducts and lobules are illustrated in columns 3 and 4, respectively. **A,** Prepubertal (childhood). **B,** Puberty. **C,** Mature (reproductive). **D,** Pregnancy. **E,** Lactation. **F,** Postmenopausal (senescent) state. (From Copeland EM III, Bland KI. The breast. In Sabiston DC Jr, ed. Essentials of surgery. Philadelphia: WB Saunders, 1987.)

TABLE 1-1 • Tanner Stages

Stage	Approximate Age	Description
Stage 1	Puberty	Preadolescent, with slight elevation of the papilla
Stage 2	11.1 ± 1.1 yr	Elevation of the breast and papilla as a small mound Increase in size of the areola
Stage 3	12.2 ± 1.1 yr	Further enlargement of the breast
Stage 4	13.1 ± 1.2 yr	The areola and papilla form a secondary mound above the breast
Stage 5	15.3 ± 1.7 yr	Areola recedes into the general contour of the breast

beyond these described boundaries. Ductal tissue can extend as high as the clavicle, beyond the inframammary fold, into the axilla, or beyond the border of the latissimus dorsi. The two breasts may be widely separated on the chest, or partially synthesized at the midline, although ducts do not communicate across the midline of the chest.

On average, the breast is 10 to 12 cm in diameter and 5 to 7 cm thick at its center. The contour of the breast is typically conelike with breast tissue projecting into the axilla as the axillary tail of Spence. The volume of the breast can range from 21 to 2000 mL, with an average of 400 mL. The volume fluctuates with the menstrual cycle (see later). The breast

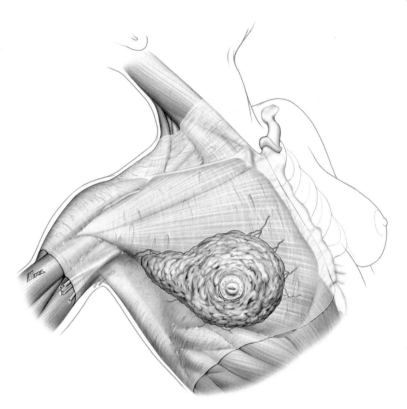

Figure 1–2. The breast tissue typically extends from the 2nd rib to the inframammary fold at the 6th or 7th rib, and from the lateral border of the sternum to the midaxillary line. The breast is teardrop shaped, with an extension of breast tissue extending into the axilla, known as the axillary tail or the tail of Spence. (From Bloom N, Beattie E, Harvery J. Atlas of cancer surgery. Philadelphia: Elsevier, 2000.)

is more conical in the nulliparous woman and more pendulous in women who have had children. The contour and volume of the breast, however, vary greatly among individuals, and may vary from left to right. More than half of women have volume differences of greater than 10% and more than one fourth of women have volume differences greater than 20%. These differences are typically not appreciated by most women.

The breast comprises three major structures: the skin, the subcutaneous tissue, and the fibroglandular breast tissue. The skin of the breast is thin and contains hair follicles, sebaceous glands, and eccrine sweat glands. The nipple-areolar complex is typically located over the fourth intercostal space (in the nonpendulous breast). Both the nipple and areola consist of a keratinizing stratified squamous epithelium with a dense basal melanin deposition, which accounts for the pigmentation. It can range from 15 to 60 mm in diameter. Within the nipple are multiple sensory nerve endings, including Ruffini-like bodies and end bulbs of Krause. Within the dermis are radially arranged smooth muscle fibers that contract with stimulation, hardening and elevating the nipple. The areola has hair follicles,

sebaceous glands, and sweat glands. At the periphery of the areola are the Morgagni tubercles, elevations formed by openings of the ducts of the Montgomery glands. These glands are a cross between sweat and mammary glands, and are capable of producing milk.

Underneath the skin is the subcutaneous fat, which contributes to the size of the breast and which fluctuates with the amount of total body fat. Beneath this is the superficial pectoral fascia (Fig. 1–3). The gland of the breast lies within the superficial fascia, with the anterior layer between the skin and the mammary gland, and the posterior layer between the gland and the fascia of the pectoralis major muscle. Connecting these two fascial layers are fibrous bands (Cooper suspensory ligaments). Cooper's ligaments help give the breast its shape and anchor the gland to the skin. They are particularly dense at the lower periphery of the breast, where they maintain the inframammary fold.

The breasts maintain mobility on the chest wall because of the retromammary bursa. Between the posterior layer of the superficial pectoral fascia and the pectoralis major muscle fascia is a cleft known as the *retromammary space*, or *retromammary bursa*. The deep surface

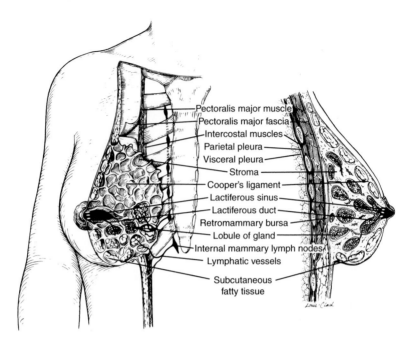

Pectoralis major muscle
Pectoralis major fascia
Intercostal muscles
Parietal pleura
Visceral pleura
Stroma
Cooper's ligament
Lactiferous sinus
Lactiferous duct
Retromammary bursa
Lobule of gland
Internal mammary lymph nodes
Lymphatic vessels
Subcutaneous
fatty tissue

Figure 1–3. Tangential and sagittal view of the breast. The breast lies in the superficial fascia just deep to the dermis, attached to the skin by the suspensory ligaments of Cooper. The retromammary bursa separates it from the investing fascia of the pectoralis major muscle. Cooper's ligaments form fibrosepta in the stroma that provide support for the breast parenchyma. From 15 to 20 lactiferous ducts extend from lobules comprised of glandular epithelium to openings located on the nipple. Subcutaneous fat and tissue are distributed around the lobules of the gland and account for much of its mass. (From Copeland EM III, Bland KI. The Breast, 3rd ed. Philadelphia: WB Saunders, 2004.)

of the breast rests on portions of the deep investing fasciae of the pectoralis major, serratus anterior, and external oblique muscles, as well as the upper extent of the rectus sheath. As the breast tissue develops through the layers of the superficial fascia, they remain relatively close to the skin. This is especially true at the nipple-areolar complex. These relationships are all important when performing a mastectomy.

The fibroglandular tissue, or parenchyma, of the breast, is divided into 15 to 20 segments that converge at the nipple in a radial arrangement (Fig. 1–4). These segments are not always evenly distributed around the breast. The upper half of the breast, particularly the upper outer quadrant, tends to contain more glandular tissue than does the remainder of the breast. Each segment contains a lobe made of 20 to 40 lobules, each consisting of 10 to 100 alveoli. Two-millimeter ducts drain each segment into subareolar lactiferous sinuses of 5 to 8 mm in diameter. Ten major collecting milk ducts then open at the nipple. The ductal-lobular unit is the biologically active unit of the breast. The epithelial lining of the lobule consists of superficial (luminal) A cells that

are involved in milk synthesis. The B cells (basal) have stem cell activity. Finally there are myoepithelial cells located around the alveoli and small excretory mild ducts between the inner aspect of the basement membrane and the tunica propria. These cells are not innervated, but rather are stimulated to contract by the hormones prolactin and oxytocin.

Muscular Anatomy of the Chest Wall

Underneath the breast lies the musculature of the chest wall and upper abdomen (Table 1–2). The pectoralis major muscle broadly originates over the medial half of the clavicle, lateral sternum, and sixth and seventh ribs, and then converges to an insertion point on the greater tubercle of the humerus. It is fan shaped and made of two divisions. The clavicular division originates from the clavicle. The costosternal division originates from the sternum and costal cartilages, and is the larger of the two divisions. When the deep pectoral fascia has been reflected laterally, the natural cleavage between the clavicular and costosternal portions of the pectorals major can be appreciated.

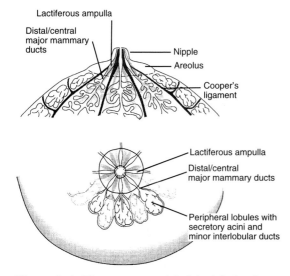

Figure 1–4. The secretory acini of the lobular tissue open into small intralobular ducts, which then drain into major lobar ducts. These ducts are organized into 16 to 18 lobular groupings separated by Cooper's ligaments. As they approach the nipple, they dilate into lactiferous ampullae, just below the nipple-areolar complex, before traversing the nipple. There may be as many as 18 openings at the apex of the nipple, although two major ducts may converge into one ampulla. (From Copeland EM III, Bland KI. The Breast, 3rd ed. Philadelphia: WB Saunders, 2004.)

Separation of this cleavage can provide access to the axillary fat pad. The pectoralis major acts primarily in flexion, adduction, and medial rotation of the arm at the shoulder joint (bringing the arm across the chest).

The cephalic vein runs along the upper lateral border of the pectoralis major muscle and sits between the pectoralis major and deltoid muscle (Fig. 1–5).

Underneath the pectoralis major muscle is the pectorals minor muscle, arising from the medial surfaces of the third, fourth, and fifth ribs and inserting as a tendon into the coracoid process of the scapula. The pectoralis minor helps depress the shoulder inferiorly. However, except for the loss of some mass on the anterior thoracic wall, no significant disability comes from the loss of the pectoralis minor muscle. The functional loss following division or removal of the pectoralis minor muscle is small and well tolerated. This should be kept in mind when performing an axillary dissection in a patient with clinically involved nodes, because division of the pectoralis minor results in minimal morbidity but does allow for a more extensive dissection of the high level II and level III axillary nodes.

The serratus anterior muscle arises from a series of digitations from the lateral aspect of

TABLE 1–2 • *Muscular Anatomy Relevant to Breast Surgery*

Muscle	Attachments	Innervation	Action
Pectoralis major	Clavicle, sternum, and costal cartilages 1 to 6 to the greater tubercle of the humerus	Medial and lateral pectoral nerves	Flexion, adduction, and medial rotation of the arm
Pectoralis minor	Ribs 2, 3, 4, and 5 to the coracoid process of the scapula	Medial pectoral nerve	Inferior depression of the shoulder
Serratus anterior	Ribs 1 to 8 to the anteromedial border of the scapula	Long thoracic nerve	Abduction and lateral rotation of the scapula, fixation of the scapula
Latissimus dorsi	Spinous processes T-6 to T-12, L-1 to L-5, sacrum, and lilac crest to the intertubercular groove of the humerus	Thoracodorsal nerve	Extension, adduction and medial rotation of the arm
Subscapularis	Scapula to the lesser tubercle of the humerus	Subscapular nerve	Medial rotation and adduction of the arm
Coracobrachialis	Coracoid process of the scapula to the medial humerus	Musculocutaneous nerve	Flexion and adduction of the arm
Subclavius	First rib of costochondral junction to the clavicle	Subclavian nerve	Depression of the clavicle
Rectus abdominis	Pubis to cartilage of ribs 5, 6, and 7	Intercostal nerves, iliohypogastric nerve, ilioinguinal nerve	Tension of the anterior abdomen, flexion of the vertebral column
External abdominis oblique	Ribs 5 to 12 to the linea alba, pubis, inguinal ligament, and iliac crest		Respiration, increased abdominal pressure (micturition, defecation)

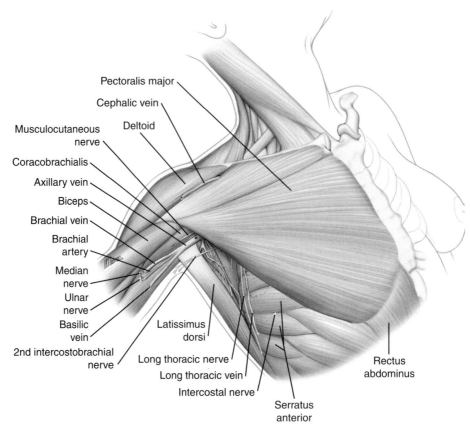

Figure 1–5. Muscular anatomy of the chest wall. (From Bloom N, Beattie E, Harvery J. Atlas of Cancer Surgery. Philadelphia: Elsevier, 2000.)

the upper eight ribs. It inserts into the vertebral border of the scapula on its costal surface and stabilizes the scapula on the chest wall. The functional deficit of losing function of the serratus anterior is an inability to raise the arm above the level of the shoulder. The serratus anterior is also important in stabilization of the scapula on the thorax, and an injury to the long thoracic nerve, which innervates the serratus anterior, can result in a "winged scapula."

The latissimus dorsi muscle has a wide origin from the spinous processes and supraspinous ligaments of the thoracic (7-12), lumbar, and sacral vertebrae. It inserts into a 2.5-cm insertion in the bicipital groove of the humerus. The narrow tendon of the latissimus dorsi forms the posterior axillary fold. The latissimus dorsi functions to extend, internally rotate, and adduct the humerus.

The subclavius muscle arises from the costochondral junction of the first rib. At the tendinous part of the lower border of this muscle, the clavipectoral fascia forms a well-developed band stretching from the coracoid process to the first costochondral junction. This costocoracoid ligament (the Halsted ligament) defines the point anatomically where the axillary vessels enter the thorax (under the clavicle, over the first rib).

These muscles also form a compartment between the chest wall and the arm, known as the *axilla*. This is of obvious importance to the breast surgeon because the axillary lymph nodes reside here. The nerves and vessels to some of these muscles run through the axilla, and can be injured during axillary dissection. The axilla is described in more detail later. One muscular abnormality that can occur in this region is the presence of the Langer axillary arch (Fig. 1–6). This represents a portion of the latissimus dorsi muscle that arises separately and crosses the base of the axilla superficially, passing deep to the pectoralis major muscle to the coracoid process. This band of tissue occurs in 7% of cases and can often cause confusion when performing an axillary dissection.

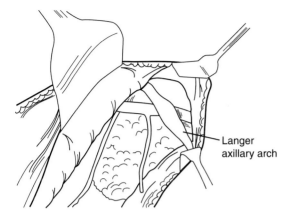

Figure 1–6. The Langer axillary arch is a portion of latissimus dorsi muscle that arises separately and crosses the axilla superficially before joining the coracoid process. This band of muscle can cause confusion during an axillary lymph node dissection.

The skeletal component of the thoracic wall consists of 12 thoracic vertebrae, 12 ribs and their costal cartilages, and the sternum. The intercostal spaces between the ribs are filled with the external, internal, and innermost or intimal intercostal muscles. The external intercostal muscles are the most superficial layer, running from the tubercles of the ribs toward the costochondral junction. The internal intercostal muscles run downward and posterior, from the sternum toward the angle of the ribs. The intercostal veins, arteries, and nerves pass in the plane that separates the internal intercostal muscle from the intimal layer.

Fascia of the Breast and Chest Wall

As stated earlier, the breast is enveloped by the superior pectoral fascia, with the anterior layer ventrally and a posterior layer dorsally. Connecting these two fascial layers are Cooper's suspensory ligaments, the fibrous bands that provide support of the breast. Above the breast, the superior pectoral fascia is continuous with the superficial cervical fascia. At the inferior aspect of the breast, the anterior and posterior layers of the superior pectoral fascia rejoin and are continuous with Camper's and Scarpa's superficial abdominal fascia at the inframammary fold.

The proximity of the breast parenchyma to the skin is of critical importance to the breast surgeon. The ducts and lobules of the breast extend to the anterior layer of the superficial fascia and extend directly to the nipple-areolar complex. Preserving the nipple areolar complex, as is done in a "subcutaneous mastectomy," will

leave breast tissue. For this reason the nipple-areolar complex is routinely removed with a mastectomy, although some surgeons have begun examining the possibility of preserving just the areola or the entire nipple-areolar complex (see Chapter 12). The anterior layer of the superior pectoral fascia may be absent in some patients; in others, only a few millimeters from the overlying dermis may be present. Raising a flap below the fascia will also leave residual breast tissue, which is often done when "thick flaps" are maintained.

Leaving residual breast tissue has important implications if a mastectomy is being performed to prevent either a recurrence (as in the case with invasive or intraductal cancer) or a primary cancer (as with a prophylactic mastectomy). It is important that the surgeon operate between the dermis and the superficial fascia. This not only minimizes residual breast tissue, but allows the surgeon to operate in an almost bloodless plane, leaving the blood vessels and lymphatics passing in the deeper layer of the superficial fascia undisturbed.

The deep pectoral fascia covers the pectoralis major muscle and is attached to the sternum and clavicle. Inferiorly it is continuous with the deep fascia of the abdominal wall. As with the superficial fascia, the ducts and lobules are in close proximity to the deep fascia, so the fascia should be removed with a mastectomy (or during a lumpectomy for a posterior tumor).

The clavipectoral fascia runs deep to the pectoralis major muscle and envelops the pectoralis minor muscle. Superiorly, this fascia thickens and attaches to the clavicle. Surgically, this is an important landmark because this fascia forms the "roof" of the axillary space; it is also known as the *axillary fascia*. This fascia covers the serratus anterior and envelops the axillary vessels, forming the vascular sheath. The fatty areolar tissue posterior to the clavipectoral fascia encompasses the large axillary lymphatics and axillary lymph nodes. When performing a sentinel lymph node biopsy, the surgeon needs to incise this fascia in order to reach the lymph nodes. When performing an axillary lymph node dissection, the flaps should be raised above this fascia.

Neural Anatomy of the Breast and Chest Wall

There are several motor and sensory nerves that the breast surgeon needs to be familiar with. Segmental thoracic nerves provide the cutaneous sensation to the breast via anterior and lateral perforating branches. The most sensitive portion of the breast is the nipple, which is innervated by branches of the fourth thoracic nerve. The surgeon should be aware that these nerves approach the nipple medially and laterally. For this reason, circumareolar incisions in the superior or inferior aspect of the nipple are less likely to disturb the nipple's sensory innervation.

The pectoralis major muscle is innervated by the *medial and lateral pectoral (anterior thoracic) nerves.* What is often confusing is that these names come from their origin from the medial and lateral cords of the brachial plexus, and not their position on the chest wall (Fig. 1–7). The *lateral* pectoral nerve actually innervates the *medial* portion of the pectoralis, and courses *medial* to the pectoralis minor muscle to reach its destination. The nerve passes over the first part of the axillary vein medial to the pectoralis minor muscle, and its branches pierce the clavipectoral fascia to enter the deep surface of the muscle. The pectoralis major muscle is mainly innervated by the lateral

pectoral nerve, as this innervates the clavicular and sternal origins of the pectoralis major muscle.

The *medial* pectoral nerve innervates the *lateral* portion of the muscle; the lower third and the costoabdominal insertions of the pectoralis major muscle. It courses lateral (or in some cases through) the pectoralis minor muscle (which it also innervates). By understanding the anatomy of the pectoral nerves, it is possible to perform an axillary lymph node dissection without sacrificing the innervation. If one of these nerves is cut, the denervated portions of the muscle become flaccid and atrophic.

The *long thoracic nerve* (also called the external respiratory nerve of Bell) innervates the serratus anterior muscle. Arising from the fifth, sixth, and seventh cervical nerves, it passes deep to the axillary artery and vein, staying close to each segment of the thoracic wall. As it passes caudally, it gives branches to each segment of the serratus anterior muscle. The long thoracic nerve is superficial to the deep fascia investing the serratus anterior. During an

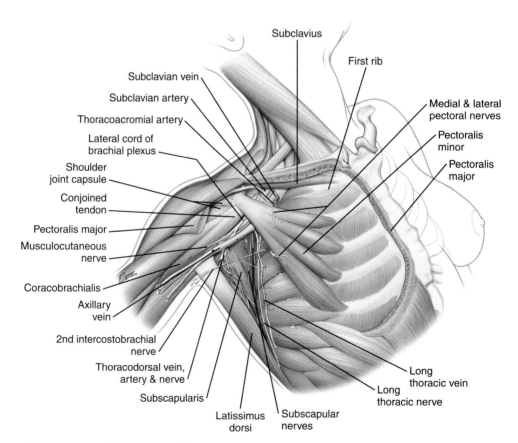

Figure 1–7. Neurovascular anatomy of the axilla. (From Bloom N, Beattie E, Harvery J. Atlas of Cancer Surgery. Philadelphia: Elsevier, 2000.)

axillary dissection, the nerve can be seen by stripping the fascia away from the serratus anterior. Dissection directly on top of the serratus anterior (between the muscle and superficial fascia) will be medial to the nerve, pulling it into the specimen and increasing the likelihood of injury. The result of this would be an inability to raise the arm above the level of the shoulder, as well as a winged scapula.

The *thoracodorsal nerve* innervates the latissimus dorsi muscle. It arises from the posterior cord of the brachial plexus, runs beneath or dorsal to the axillary vein along the posterior axillary wall, and passes through the fibrofatty tissue of the axilla to the upper portion of the muscle. Injury to this nerve denervates the latissimus dorsi, which weakens extension, internal rotation, and adduction of the humerus. Although this is extremely well tolerated by most patients, every attempt should be made to preserve the nerve during axillary dissection both to lessen functional loss and preserve the muscle for reconstructive purposes.

An important nerve to preserve during surgery is the nerve to the subscapularis muscle. This muscle passes between the subscapular fossa and the lesser tubercle of the humerus. It is seen at the posterior wall of the axilla, inferior to the axillary vein. The nerve sits on the upper anterior surface of the muscle and can be injured when dissecting the fascia from the muscle inferior to the vein. Injury to this nerve denervates the muscle, affecting medial rotation of the arm. As the muscle both stabilizes the humerus in the glenoid fossa and assists with flexion, extension, abduction, and adduction of the arm, palsy can produce significant morbidity.

The intercostobrachial nerve is a sensory nerve that runs through the axilla and innervates the skin of the axilla and upper medial aspect of the arm. The intercostobrachial nerve is the posterior ramus of the lateral perforating branch of the second intercostal nerve. It appears in the second intercostal space and courses anterior to the long thoracic nerve and thoracodorsal nerve. Often it divides early, giving the appearance of two nerves. It is important because the nerve is always exposed during an axillary dissection. Although many surgeons routinely divide this nerve, it is possible to dissect these nerves out and preserve them (see Chapter 13). The nerve typically innervates the upper arm, but can extend as far as the level of the elbow, so division can sometimes result in a significant area of numbness.

Vascular Anatomy

The breast is supplied by multiple sources (Fig. 1–8). Multiple muscle-perforating branches of the thoracoabdominal artery perforate the pectoralis major muscle to enter the breast. The inner quadrants also receive blood flow from the perforating branches of the internal mammary arteries. These penetrate each intercostal space and the pectoralis major muscle to reach the breast. The outer quadrants receive blood from branches of the lateral thoracic artery, which both penetrate and come around the pectoralis major. Additional blood supply comes from lateral cutaneous branches of the posterior intercostal arteries. All of these arteries connect with each other by collateral branches in both the breast and overlying skin. Overall, 60% of the breast is supplied by the internal mammary artery, 30% of the breast is supplied by the lateral thoracic artery, and 10% is supplied by minor contributions from the thoracoacromial, intercostals, subscapular, and thoracodorsal arteries.

The venous drainage does not completely follow the arterial supply. Rather, venous

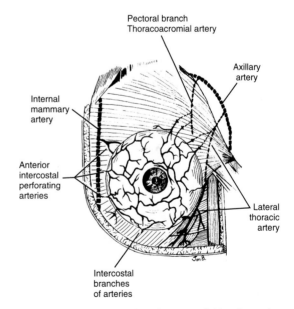

Figure 1–8. Arterial distribution of blood to the breast. The breast receives its blood supply via three major routes: (1) medially from anterior perforating intercostal branches off of the internal thoracic artery, (2) laterally from branches of the thoracoacromial trunk or lateral thoracic artery (both of which come off of the axillary artery), and (3) lateral cutaneous branches off of the intercostal arteries. (From Copeland EM III, Bland KI. The Breast, 3rd ed. Philadelphia: WB Saunders, 2004.)

drainage heads toward an anastomotic circle in the subcutaneous tissue beneath and around the areola. This plexus then drains centrifugally toward the periphery via large subcutaneous veins. These veins then travel with the arteries supplying the breast. When venous flow increases, as with lactation, these veins become more apparent.

Lymphatic Anatomy

The lymphatic drainage of the breast is through two sets of lymphatic vessels; the superficial (also known as subepithelial or subdermal) and the deep (Fig. 1–9). The subepithelial plexus of lymphatic vessels exists throughout the entire body surface. These vessels are valveless, allowing lymph to flow in any direction, although it does so sluggishly. The subepithelial plexus connects to subdermal lymphatic vessels by vertical lymphatics. The subdermal vessels do have valves. Thus lymph flows unidirectionally from the superficial to the deep plexus. In the breast, the subepithelial and subdermal plexuses are confluent with the subareolar plexus. Also draining into the subareolar plexus are the fine lymphatics of the lactiferous ducts and the lymphatics of the areola and nipple. It is because of these connections between the subareolar plexus and the subepithelial and

subdermal lymphatics that subareolar or periareolar injection of tracers during intraoperative lymphatic mapping and sentinel lymph node biopsy is possible.

From the deep lymphatics, the lymph flow moves centrifugally toward the axillary and internal mammary lymph nodes. Approximately 3% of the lymph from the breast goes to the IM chain, which can come from all quadrants of the breast, not just the inner quadrants. The internal mammary nodes (IMN) are found with the internal mammary artery and vein within the intercostal spaces at the sternal border, deep to the intercostal muscles and within the extrapleural fat. Most of the nodes are in the upper parasternal area (upper three interspaces); however, the number of nodes is variable and can extend as low as the fifth intercostal space and as high as the retroclavicular region. The other 97% of lymph flows to the axillary lymph nodes.

Anatomy of the Axilla

The anatomy of the axilla and axillary lymph nodes is obviously crucial to the breast surgeon. The axilla is typically thought of as a four-walled pyramid that sits between the upper arm and the chest (Fig. 1–10). The dome-shaped base of the pyramid is the armpit, made of the axillary fascia and the skin. The apex of the pyramid is an aperture that extends into the posterior triangle of the neck through the cervicoaxillary canal. This canal is

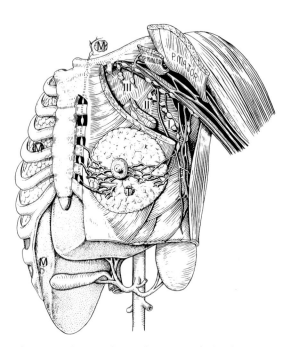

Figure 1–9. Lymphatic drainage of the breast. (From Copeland EM III, Bland KI. The Breast, 3rd ed. Philadelphia: WB Saunders, 2004.)

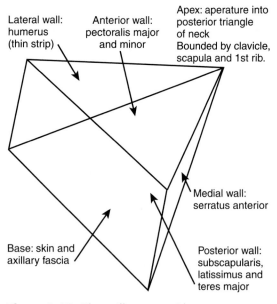

Lateral wall: humerus (thin strip)

Anterior wall: pectoralis major and minor

Apex: aperature into posterior triangle of neck
Bounded by clavicle, scapula and 1st rib.

Medial wall: serratus anterior

Base: skin and axillary fascia

Posterior wall: subscapularis, latissimus and teres major

Figure 1–10. The axillary pyramid.

bounded by the clavicle anteriorly, the scapula posteriorly, and the first rib medially. Almost all of the structures heading toward the upper extremity pass through the cervical axillary canal. This leaves the four walls. The anterior wall is the pectoralis major and minor muscles. The posterior wall is the subscapularis muscle (and to a lesser extent the teres major and latissimus dorsi muscles and tendons). The medial wall is the serratus anterior muscle. The lateral wall is a thin strip of humerus between the insertions of the muscles of the anterior and posterior walls.

Coming through the apex of the pyramid are the great vessels and nerves of the upper extremity, enclosed within a layer of fascia, the axillary sheath. The sheath is dense connective tissue extending from the neck, but gradually disappears as the nerves and vessels begin to branch. Throughout their course in the axilla, the axillary artery and vein are associated with the cords of the brachial plexus (medial, lateral, and posterior).

The axilla is enveloped in fascia. The most significant fascia is the clavipectoral fascia. This fascia extends from the clavicle toward the floor of the axilla (the axillary fascia). It encloses both the subclavius muscle and the pectoralis minor muscle. The upper portion of the clavipectoral fascia is known as the *costocoracoid membrane*. The lower portion is sometimes called the *suspensory ligament of the axilla* or the *coracoaxillary fascia*. A dense condensation of the clavipectoral fascia, extending from the medial end of the clavicle to the first rib, is known as *Halsted's ligament*. This ligament covers the subclavian artery and vein as they cross the first rib and is an important landmark when performing a level III axillary lymph node dissection.

Within the pyramid, in addition to the great vessels and nerves and their branches, are the axillary lymph nodes. We tend to group the lymph nodes by their anatomic location, having been arbitrarily divided into levels based on their relation to the pectoralis minor muscle. The level I lymph nodes lie lateral to the muscle, the level II nodes like directly beneath the muscle, and the level III nodes are medial to the medial border of the pectoralis minor. However, the lymph nodes are better categorized by several groups (Fig. 1–11):

- The lateral group, or axillary vein group, consists of four to six nodes that lie medial or posterior to the axillary vein. These lymph nodes receive most of the lymph draining from the upper extremity.

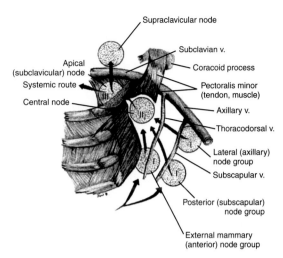

Figure 1–11. The major lymph node groups of the axilla. The Roman numerals indicate the three levels of the axillary nodes in relation to the pectoralis minor muscle. (From Copeland EM III, Bland KI. The Breast, 3rd ed. Philadelphia: WB Saunders, 2004.)

- The anterior group, or external mammary group, consists of four or five lymph nodes that lie along the lower border of the pectoralis minor muscle in association with the lateral thoracic vessels. These lymph nodes receive the major portion of the lymph draining from the breast.
- The posterior, or scapular, group consists of six or seven nodes that lie along the posterior wall of the axilla at the lateral border of the scapula. These nodes receive lymph primarily from the posterior neck and trunk.
- The central group consists of three or four lymph nodes that lie within the fat beneath the pectoralis minor muscle. These lymph nodes receive drainage from the lateral, anterior, and posterior groups.
- The subclavicular, or apical, nodes consist of 6 to 12 lymph nodes that sit at the apex of the axilla, superior to the pectoralis muscle and along the medial side of the axillary vein. These receive drainage from all of the other lymph node groups.
- The interpectoral nodes, or Rotter's nodes, consist of one to four nodes between the pectoralis major and minor muscles and drain into the central and subclavicular nodes) (Table 1–3).

Thus the level I lymph nodes, those nodes lateral or below the lower border of the pectoralis minor muscle, include the external mammary, axillary vein, and scapular lymph node groups. The level II lymph nodes, located deep

TABLE 1–3 • *Major Lymph Node Groups of the Axilla*

Group	Location	Nodes	Drainage From
Lateral (axillary vein)	Medial-posterior to axillary vein	4 to 6	Upper extremity
Anterior (external mammary)	Along lower border of pectoralis minor	4 to 5	Breast
Posterior (scapular)	Lateral border of scapula	6 to 7	Posterior neck/trunk
Central	Beneath pectoralis minor	3 to 4	Lateral, anterior, and posterior groups
Subclavicular (apical)	Apex of axilla	6 to 12	All other groups
Interpectoral (Rotter's)	Between pectoralis major and minor	1 to 4	

to the pectoralis minor muscle, include the central and some of the subclavicular lymph node groups. The remainder of the subclavicular lymph nodes are the level III lymph nodes, located medial to the pectoralis minor.

The locations of the axillary groups and the flow of the lymph are important in regard to metastatic dissemination of breast cancer. Typically there is unidirectional flow toward the regional lymph nodes; however, when the lymphatics are blocked by neoplasm, flow can reverse, leading to endolymphatic metastases of both the dermis and breast parenchyma. Therefore the presence of metastases in the regional nodes, which can obstruct the lymphatic vessels, will increase the likelihood of parenchymal metastases (manifesting as in breast recurrences) and dermal metastases (e.g., chest wall recurrences after mastectomy).

Physiology of the Breast

The purpose of the breast is milk production for the sustenance of the newborn. The secretory units of the breast are the alveoli, small saccules off of the lactiferous ducts. The growth of these secretory units and their production of milk is controlled by an intricate network of hormones. Fluctuation of these hormones and changes in their relative ratios cause several histologic changes in the breast, not just during pregnancy but also during the menstrual cycle. Changes occur in both the epithelium and the stroma and profoundly influence the morphology of the breast.

Hormones Affecting the Breast

See Table 1–4.

TABLE 1–4 • *Hormones Influencing Breast Development During Pregnancy*

Hormone	Effect During Development	Effect During Pregnancy and Lactation
Estrogen	Causes ductal growth during adolescence	Required for lobuloalveolar growth
Progesterone	Required for lobuloalveolar differentiation and growth	
Glucocorticoids	Contributes to ductal growth in puberty	Enhances lobuloalveolar growth Stimulus for lactation
Growth hormone	Contributes to ductal growth in puberty	Stimulus for lactation Maintains mammary epithelial cell survival
Insulin	Enhances growth of mammary epithelium Enhances ductal alveolar growth	
Prolactin	Contributes to ductal growth in puberty	Required for lactogenesis and maintenance of lactation
Human placental lactogen		Stimulates alveolar growth and lactogenesis
Thyroid hormones		Increases epithelial secretory response to prolactin
Oxytocin		Causes contraction of myoepithelial cells and milk ejection

Estrogen

Estrogen stimulates the growth of the breast at puberty. However, while development is dependent on estrogen, estrogen alone will have no effect. In the presence of other hormones, such as hydrocortisone, insulin, or growth hormone, it leads to growth of the ductal system.

Progesterone

Progesterone also stimulates breast growth at puberty, but unlike estrogen, which works primarily on the ducts, progesterone induces development of the terminal ducts and lobuloalveolar structures. As with estrogen, this response requires the presence of other hormones, specifically growth hormone and insulin.

Prolactin

Prolactin is produced by lactotrophs in the pituitary gland. Prolactin stimulates mammary growth and differentiation and ultimately milk production. The synthesis of prolactin is stimulated by a wide variety of hormones and neurotransmitters (Box 1–3). Thyrotropin releasing hormone (TRH) is the primary stimulator of prolactin secretion, dopamine is the primary inhibition. However, prolactin can also be produced by cells in the breast; thus prolactin can not only behave as a classic hormone, but also as a paracrine or autocrine factor. The extrapituitary prolactin is not regulated by TRH or dopamine but is controlled by progesterone.

Oxytocin

Oxytocin is a peptide hormone secreted by the pituitary gland. Oxytocin is released in response to a variety of stimuli. Suckling results in oxytocin release and may also be a conditioned reflex in response to an infant's cry. Oxytocin receptors are located on the myoepithelial cells located in the basement membrane of the alveoli and intralobular ducts. These receptors increase in number at parturition. When oxytocin binds to these receptors, contraction of the myoepithelial cells occurs.

Human Placental Lactogen

Human placental lactogen (hPL) is produced by the placenta and serum levels continue to rise throughout pregnancy. The major role of hPL is related to breast growth and differentiation during pregnancy. After delivery, the decrease in the serum concentration is rapid.

The Breast during the Menstrual Cycle

Follicular Phase

The follicular phase of the menstrual cycle is defined as the first day of menstruation until ovulation. It is initiated by a rise in follicle-stimulating hormone (FSH) levels at the first day of the cycle. This is triggered by a decrease in progesterone and estrogen (which act to inhibit FSH secretion). FSH stimulates the development of follicles and their secretion of estrogen (Fig. 1–12).

In the breast, the increased estrogen levels initiate cellular mitoses, RNA synthesis, increased nuclear density, and other changes within the epithelial cells. In addition, estrogen has a histamine-like effect on the mammary microcirculation. This leads to an increased blood flow to the breast in the 3 to 4 days before menstruation. The breast can increase in volume from 15 to 30 cm^3 due to both the increasing interlobular edema and the enhanced cellular proliferation.

Estrogen inhibits the secretion of FSH, and FSH levels decrease. Estrogen levels peak toward

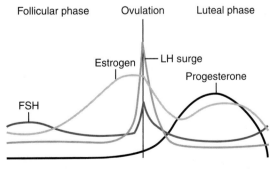

Figure 1–12. Changes in hormone levels with the menstrual cycle.

the end of the follicular phase of the menstrual cycle, which exerts a positive feedback on luteinizing hormone (LH). There is a dramatic pre-ovulatory LH surge at this point, which is required for ovulation. The LH causes the follicle to swell and rupture, with expulsion of the oocyte, and corona radiate into the peritoneal cavity and ultimately into the fallopian tube.

Luteal Phase

The luteal phase is initiated by the surge in LH. During the luteal phase, progesterone synthesis is maximum. The major effects of the LH surge are the conversion of granulose cells from primarily androgen-converting cells to predominantly progesterone-synthesizing cells. At this point there is increased progesterone secretion with some estrogen secretion.

In the breast, the progestogens trigger the mammary ducts to dilate and the alveolar epithelial cells to differentiate into secretory cells. The breast epithelial cell proliferation increases during the luteal phase of the menstrual cycle.

Menstruation

The high progesterone levels exert a negative feedback on GnRH, and as this decreases so does FSH and LH secretion. Ultimately there is a decrease in estrogen and progesterone levels, which removes the inhibition of FSH, which begins to rise once again to initiate the next menstrual cycle.

In the breast, the rapid decline in the circulating levels of estrogen and progesterone lead to a regression of the secretory activity of the epithelium. The tissue edema is reduced, with the minimum breast volume observed 5 to 7 days after menstruation.

The Breast after Menopause

Menopause typically occurs when a woman is in her late 40s and early 50s; it is associated with a variety of symptoms related to the loss of estrogen and progesterone. These include hot flashes, night sweats, mood disturbances and difficulty sleeping, and vaginal dryness.

The breasts will also undergo changes with menopause. The loss of hormonal stimulation produces a decrease in the absolute number of lobular units, as well as a diffuse atrophy of the residual lobular units. This results in a decrease in the glandular tissue, which is replaced with fatty tissue. This decrease in breast density makes it easier to detect breast cancer on mammography, which is why sensitivity increases with age. The duct system remains intact. The loose paralobular and intralobular connective tissue become progressively collagenized and less cellular. The loss of strength of the connective tissue results in an increase in size and sag to the breasts. However, these changes of atrophy are variable and incomplete. Some women in their 60s and 70s still have a lobular appearance similar to a premenopausal state.

We tend to associate fibrocystic disease with the menstrual cycle, matching the increase in pain and palpable masses to the changes in hormone levels. It would therefore seem logical that fibrocystic disease should resolve with menopause, but this is not always the case. For some women, the breasts can become more tender with menopause, with an increase in "lumpiness" or cysts.

The Breast during Pregnancy

It is not until pregnancy that the breast attains its maximum development. In the pregnant patient, there is marked growth of the ducts, lobules, and alveoli under the influence of luteal and placental sex steroids and prolactin. During the first 3 to 4 weeks of pregnancy, under the influence of estrogen, there is growth and branching of the ducts, as well as increased lobule formation. By the second month, the breasts have enlarged dramatically. The superficial veins dilate and there is increased pigmentation of the nipple-areolar complex. The breasts become tender and the nipples become sore. This can begin just a few weeks after conception.

Estrogen and progesterone prohibit the hypothalamus from producing prolactin-inhibiting factor (PIF). With this influence gone, prolactin is released and this continues progressively during pregnancy, although increase in prolactin levels is slow during the first trimester.

In the second trimester of pregnancy, the effects of progesterone cause the lobular formation to exceed the ductal sprouting. During this time, prolactin levels continue to rise and by the third trimester, blood levels of prolactin are three to five times higher than normal.

At this point the alveoli contain colostrum, but no fat. The breast continues to enlarge, but this is not due to epithelial proliferation but rather the filling of the alveoli with colostrum, as well as the hypertrophy of myoepithelial cells.

In the third trimester of pregnancy, the stroma surrounding the lobules diminishes to make room for the hypertrophied lobules. As pregnancy continues, colostrum composed of desquamated epithelial cells and fluid accumulates. This is released in the immediate postpartum period.

Lactation

During pregnancy, prolactin is being produced, starting during the eighth week of pregnancy and increasing until birth. During that time, the high levels of estrogen and progesterone block the prolactin receptors and inhibit milk production. After birth, there is a decline in the serum levels of estrogen and progesterone over several days. This removes the inhibition of milk production and lactogenesis begins.

Prolactin is one of two hormones responsible for milk production, with the other being oxytocin. Prolactin levels were increasing until birth, and after delivery begin to decline. If the mother is not nursing, the prolactin levels will drop slowly (>14 days). In the nursing mother, prolactin will also drop, but much more slowly, dependent on the time that the infant nurses. Prolactin drives the synthesis and secretion of milk into the alveolar spaces. When the myoepithelial cells contract, the milk passes through the ductal system and out of the breast.

Oxytocin is the second hormone responsible for milk production and delivery. When an infant suckles at the mother's breast, this causes the increase in both prolactin, to stimulate more production, and oxytocin, to increase milk delivery.

During the first few days after delivery, the body does not produce milk but rather a liquid substance called *colostrum*. This is high in immunoglobulins, which help protect the infant against infections at a time when the infant's own immune system has not fully developed. Colostrum may help decrease the infant's chances of developing asthma and other allergies.

When breast-feeding stops, it may take several months for milk production to completely stop. The breasts usually return to their previous size, although they may be smaller after breast-feeding is completed.

Suggested Readings

1. Abramson RG, Mavi A, Cermik T, et al. Age-related structural and functional changes in the breast: Multimodality correlation with digital mammography, computed tomography, magnetic resonance imaging and positron emission tomography. Semin Nucl Med 2007;37(3):146–153.
2. Anderson E. The role of oestrogen and progesterone receptors in human mammary development and tumorigenesis. Breast Cancer Res 2002;4(5):197–201.
3. Aupperlee M, Kariagina A, Osuch J, Haslam SZ. Progestins and breast cancer. Breast Dis 2005-2006;24:37–57.
4. Kass R, Mancino AT, Rosenbloom A, et al. Breast physiology: Normal and abnormal development and function. In Bland KI, Copeland EM, eds. The Breast: Comprehensive Management of Benign and Malignant Disorders. St. Louis: Elsevier, 2004.
5. Romrell LJ, Bland KI. Anatomy of the breast, axilla, chest wall and related metastatic sites. In Bland KI, Copeland EM, eds. The Breast: Comprehensive Management of Benign and Malignant Disorders. St. Louis: Elsevier, 2004.
6. Russo J, Russo IH. Development of the human breast. Maturitas 2004;49(1):2–15.
7. Osborne MP. Breast anatomy and development. In Harris JR, Lippman ME, Morrow M, Osborne CK, eds. Diseases of the breast, 3rd ed. Philadelphia: Lippincott Williams & Wilkins, 2004.

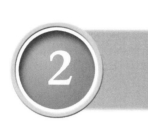
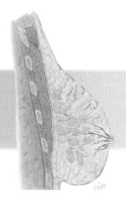

Principles of Breast Cancer Screening

Key Points

- Describe how mammography is performed for screening and additional techniques used for diagnostic mammography.
- Know the differences between film and digital mammography.
- Be familiar with the BI-RADS system and the abnormalities on mammogram that warrant close observation versus biopsy.
- Describe how ultrasound is performed and its indications.
- Know the strengths and limitations of breast MRI in both screening and diagnosis.
- Understand the principles of cancer screening.

Breast imaging has changed the management of breast disease dramatically over the past few decades. Not only has screening changed the face of breast cancer, but improvements in technology and newer modalities have altered the approach to the diagnosis of breast abnormalities. Understanding the indications, benefits and limitations of the various modalities used in the evaluation of the breast is critical to the breast surgeon.

Modalities of Breast Imaging

Mammography

Technique

Mammography is by far the most important imaging modality used today for the evaluation of breast disease. Mammography is used both for screening the asymptomatic woman and helping diagnose women who present with a complaint regarding the breasts. When a screening mammography is performed, two standard views are used; the mediolateral oblique (MLO) view and the craniocaudal (CC) view (Fig. 2–1). The MLO view compresses the breast along a plane of approximately 45 degrees extending from the upper inner quadrant to the lower outer quadrant, with the x-ray tube rotated parallel to the pectoralis muscle fibers. The natural mobility of the breast is used to get as much breast tissue as possible included, and when done properly in the MLO view, shows both axillary tail and abdominal wall. The CC view positions the breast directly on top of the x-ray cassette holder, with the x-ray tube positioned for superior to inferior imaging.

For both the MLO and CC views, maximum compression of the breast is necessary to decrease the thickness of the breast, and to make the breast more uniform in appearance, spreading out overlapping structures. If there is an abnormality detected on a screening mammogram, or if a diagnostic mammogram is being performed, additional views beyond the MLO and CC views are often necessary (Table 2–1). These are done under the direct supervision of the radiologist, who reviews the results of the procedure with the patient at the time of the examination.

Digital Mammography

Standard mammography uses film for the acquisition of the image, display for the radiologist, and storage. In contrast to what some people believe, both traditional and digital mammography use x-rays to obtain the image (Fig. 2–2). The difference is that with digital mammography the image is stored on a computer rather than film. This does have several advantages, however. On the computer screen, the image can be manipulated. Postexposure processing may be performed to adjust

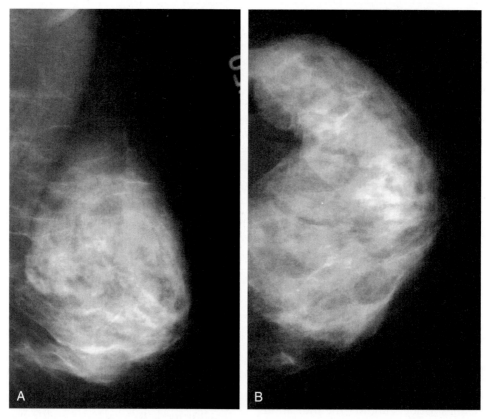

Figure 2–1. The MLO view **(A)** compresses the breast along a plane of approximately 45 degrees extending from the upper inner quadrant to the lower outer quadrant, with the x-ray tube rotated parallel to the pectoralis muscle fibers. When done properly, the MLO view shows both axillary tail and abdominal wall. The CC view **(B)** positions the breast directly on top of the x-ray cassette holder, with the x-ray tube positioned for superior to inferior imaging. The CC and MLO views of the right breast are negative for malignancy. (Image courtesy of Dr. Alexis Nees, Department of Radiology, University of Michigan.)

TABLE 2–1 • *Additional Views Obtained During Diagnostic Mammography*

Magnification views	Magnified views are taken of a specific area, with increased resolution to better look at the lesion.
Spot compression views	A small compression paddle is used to spread out the tissue, bringing the area of concern closer to the film.
Exaggerated CC views	Typically the CC view starts at the medial aspect and includes as much of the lateral breast as possible. However, in some women, additional views are obtained to include the entire lateral half of the breast.
Rolled views	The breast tissue is reoriented about the axis of the nipple to determine whether an abnormality is real or simply overlapping tissue.
Tangential views	For palpable lesions, a metallic BB is placed on the skin and then the area is rolled, placing it tangential to the x-ray beam.

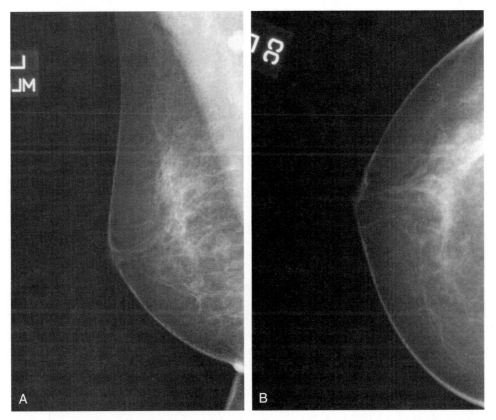

Figure 2–2. Digital mammographic MLO and CC views are negative for malignancy. (Images courtesy of Dr. Alexis Nees, Department of Radiology, University of Michigan).

contrast, brightness, and magnification without the need to obtain additional images. There is greater contrast resolution than with film, and less "noise," which may enhance sensitivity and specificity. It also allows for the rapid and easy transmission of images so that second reads can be easily obtained.

Digital mammography is not without its drawbacks as well. Primarily, the cost is significant; in addition to the new machines, monitors and digital workstations are needed for the radiologists. As the transition is made from film to digital imaging, problems may arise when trying to compare a digital image to a previous mammogram on film. Plus, the spatial resolution is less than that of film mammography, which can limit the evaluation of microcalcifications or the margins of masses.

Digital mammography may provide better screening in women with dense breasts, particularly younger women. The multicenter Digital Mammographic Imaging Screening Trial showed improved performance of digital mammography in women who had dense breasts, with 70% sensitivity compared with 55% sensitivity for film-screen mammography. In addition to the previously mentioned benefits of digital mammography, computer systems have been designed to recognize mammographic patterns and deviations from normal patterns, which may help radiologists identify suspicious areas. This technology is rather new, but could possibly decrease the time it takes to read a mammogram, as well as improve accuracy.

Indications and Uses

Screening

The benefits of mammographic screening are well documented. Although it was clear from the outset that x-ray mammography could identify cancers at a smaller size than physical examination, it was not clear whether this would have an impact on survival. Ultimately this led to eight randomized trials that demonstrated that mammographic screening can decrease breast cancer mortality in women age 50 and older (Table 2–2). A meta-analysis estimated this reduction to be approximately 34% by 7 years. The overall decreases in breast cancer–specific mortality seen over the past decade also attest to the impact of screening. Screening is discussed in further detail later in the chapter.

For the benefits of screening to be optimized, the process needs to be cost and time efficient. The most commonly applied approach is to separate screening from diagnosis. Thus women come to screening centers where two views are obtained of each breast, the medial lateral oblique (MLO) and the craniocaudal (CC) views. The patient leaves and the images are read at a later time, allowing for efficiency and for "double reading," meaning two radiologists review the films, which increases the number of cancers detected. This may be facilitated by the use of digital images. The main disadvantage is that women leave, only to be called back if there is an abnormality requiring additional diagnostic images. Approximately 5% to 10% of women are called back. This can cause undue concern for women, even though most of the women called back will be found to have nothing (e.g., the benign overlap of tissue) or benign findings requiring nothing or short-interval follow-up. Simply receiving a telephone call that there was an abnormality on the mammogram can lead to increased stress in that time period between the telephone call and when the additional imaging is done. This has prompted calls for immediate reading, but this is not only cost-ineffective but also pressures the radiologists to read quickly, which leads to increased errors.

TABLE 2–2 • *Randomized Trials of Breast Cancer Screening*

Study	Years	Mammogram	Frequency	Breast Examination	Relative Risk (CI)	
HIP Study	1963-69	2 Views	q 1 year 4 rounds	Yes	40-49 50-64	0.77 (.53,1.11) 0.80 (.59,1.08)
Edinburgh	1979-88	1 or 2 Views	q 2 years 4 rounds	Yes	45-49 50-64	0.83 (.54,1.27) 0.85 (.62,1.15)
Kopparberg	1977-85	1 View	q 2 years 4 rounds	No	40-49 50-74	0.76 (.42,1.40) 0.52 (.39,.70)
Ostergotland	1977-85	1 View	q 2 years 4 rounds	No	40-49 50-74	1.06 (.65,1.76) 0.81 (.64,1.03)
Malmo	1976-90	1 or 2 Views	q 1.5 to 2 years × 5 rounds	No	45-49 50-69	0.64 (.45,.89) 0.86 (.64,1.16)
Stockholm	1981-85	1 View	q 2 year × 2 rounds	No	40-49 50-64	1.01 (.51, 2.02) 0.65 (.4, 1.08)
Gothenburg	1982-88	2 Views	q 1.5 year × 5 rounds	No	39-49 50-59	0.56 (.32, .98) 0.91 (.61,1.36)
CNBSS	1980-87	2 Views	q 1 year × 4 to 5 years	Yes	40-49 50-59	1.07 (.75,1.52) 1.02 (.78,1.33)

Diagnostic Mammography

Diagnostic mammography is defined as the evaluation of individuals with an abnormality of the breast, whether that is a clinical complaint (e.g., a mass, skin changes, nipple inversion or discharge, or breast pain) or an irregularity detected on a screening mammogram. In some cases, the goal of the diagnostic mammogram is to characterize a specific area, such as a palpable mass. In other cases, it is to "screen" the breasts for an occult unsuspected cancer that may or may not be related to the complaint, such as with breast pain.

When a diagnostic mammogram is performed on the basis of a callback from a screening mammogram, the goal is to characterize the suspect lesion as normal tissue, a benign finding, or a possible breast cancer. To do this, the radiologist obtains additional views, using special techniques to better visualize the area of concern (see Table 2–1). With these additional views, the goal of the radiologist is to then classify the findings into one of five categories known as *BI-RADS*; the Breast Imaging Reporting and Data System (Table 2–3). On mammography, some abnormalities that appear benign may be malignant and vice versa. It is very rare that the radiologist can make a definitive diagnosis, only an estimation of the likelihood of a specific lesion representing a cancer. The BI-RADS system helps classify that risk, as well as provide some national uniformity to mammography.

Categories 1 and 2 represent a normal mammogram without findings suspicious for malignancy. Whereas category 1 refers to a perfectly normal mammogram, category 2 refers to findings that are clearly benign. Examples include an involuting, calcified fibroadenoma, an intramammary lymph node, stable, benign-appearing calcifications, cysts, lipomas, or hamartomas. Patients with a category 1 or 2 mammogram do not need any specific intervention or follow-up. Category 3 represents those findings that are probably benign. The risk of malignancy for a category 3 lesion should be less than 2%; however, short-term follow-up is needed to assure stability. The mammogram should be repeated 6 months after the initial evaluation and possibly every 6 months for up to 2 years. Biopsy should rarely be needed for a category 3 finding unless stability cannot be assured. If the lesion remains stable for 2 years, then it can be reclassified as benign.

Categories 4 and 5 include abnormalities for which cancer cannot be ruled out. Category 5 includes those abnormalities with classic hallmarks of cancer. The risk of cancer should be above 75%, and biopsy is absolutely indicated. Category 4 therefore includes those lesions in between probably benign and probably malignant. These are the lesions that do not have the characteristic findings of cancer but have a good chance of representing malignancy. Biopsy should be considered for any category 4 finding; however, this category represents a broad range of risk (3% to 74%). Thus the clinician needs to work with the radiologist to assess a reasonable risk assessment and then discuss with the patient the relative risks and benefits of short-term observation versus tissue biopsy. It is important to keep in mind that a category 4 mammogram will have a reading of "Suspicious abnormality—biopsy should be considered," so it should be well documented as to why a patient opted not to have a biopsy if she chooses observation.

Even though mammography cannot make a definitive diagnosis, there are aspects that are highly suggestive of either benign or malignant lesions. These findings may help assign relative risk and help the patient and the physician determine whether the risk of a biopsy outweighs the risk of missing a cancer; very few of these descriptive findings can be used to absolutely designate a lesion as benign.

A *mass* is any space-occupying lesion that can be detected in two different projections. Lesions seen in only one projection are referred to as *densities*. Masses are characterized by their shape, density, and margin (Fig. 2–3). Masses that are irregular or lobular are more likely to

TABLE 2–3 • Breast Imaging Reporting and Data System (BI-RADS)

Category 0	*Incomplete assessment.* Additional imaging is needed.
Category 1	*Negative.* The breasts are normal in appearance.
Category 2	*Benign finding.* A finding is present that is characteristic of a benign lesion.
Category 3	*Probably benign finding.* A finding is present that has a high probability of being benign.
Category 4	*Suspicious abnormality.* A finding is present that has a possibility of being cancer.
Category 5	*Highly suggestive.* A lesion is present that has the typical morphology of a cancer.

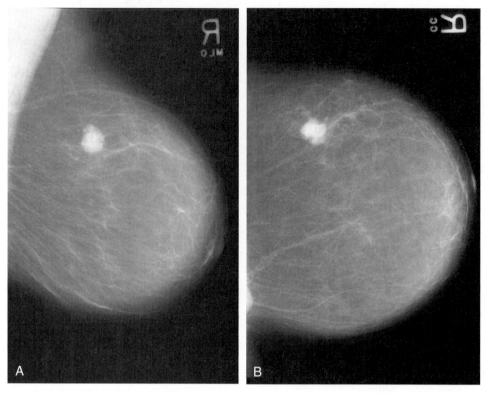

Figure 2–3. MLO and CC views of the right breast demonstrate a spiculated mass in the upper outer quadrant. Pathology demonstrated invasive ductal carcinoma. (Images courtesy of Dr. Alexis Nees, Department of Radiology, University of Michigan.)

be malignant than round or oval masses. Although mammography can rarely distinguish benign from malignant, there are some lesions that can be called benign based on their density. Lesions that are fat dense (these appear black on a mammogram) are benign, representing either lipomas or areas of fat necrosis with oil cyst formation. Tissue biopsy is not necessary. Benign hamartomas may also have a pathognomonic appearance and may be characterized as BI-RADS category 2 (Fig. 2–4). Finally, the margins surrounding a mass are an important feature in analyzing a mammographic mass. Benign lesions tend to have well-defined circumscribed margins. Cancers on the other hand more often have indistinct or microlobulated margins. Masses with spiculated margins, forming a stellate pattern of radiating lines, are almost always malignant (Fig. 2–5).

Because calcium absorbs x-rays, *calcifications* are easily detected by mammography, even calcifications as small as 0.2 to 0.3 mm. Calcifications often form in response to cell turnover, which may be related to cancer but can also be related to benign changes in the breast.

The fact that they can be seen so readily on mammogram is why mammography is particularly useful in detecting early stage cancer, particularly ductal carcinoma in situ (DCIS). However, there are many different types of calcifications, and their morphologies and distribution can provide clues to their etiology. Some types of calcifications are clearly benign, such as the popcorn-like macrocalcifications seen in an involuting fibroadenoma. As a general rule, larger, round or oval-shaped calcifications uniform in size have a higher probability of being associated with a benign process and smaller, irregular, polymorphic, branching calcifications that are heterogeneous in size and morphology are more often associated with a malignant process (Figs. 2–6 and 2–7).

Calcifications are analyzed according to their size, shape, number, location, and distribution (Table 2–4). Size is an important characteristic because macrocalcifications are typically associated with a benign process and microcalcifications are associated with malignancy; however, there is no strict measurement cutoff between micro and macro. Most radiologists classify calcifications of 0.5 mm or

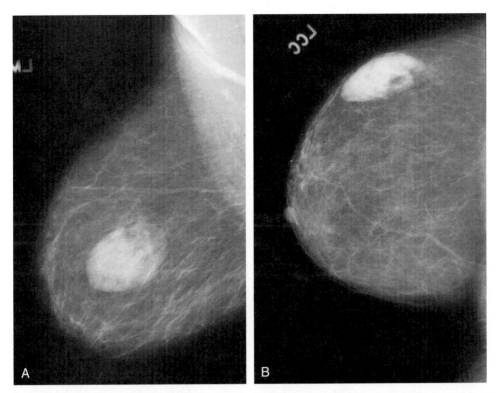

Figure 2–4. Hamartomas have a very characteristic appearance on mammography, possessing a combination of fatty and soft tissue densities surrounded by a fibrous capsule. **A,** The MLO view shows the classic "breast within a breast" appearance of hamartoma. **B,** The CC view. (Images courtesy of Dr. Alexis Nees, Department of Radiology, University of Michigan.)

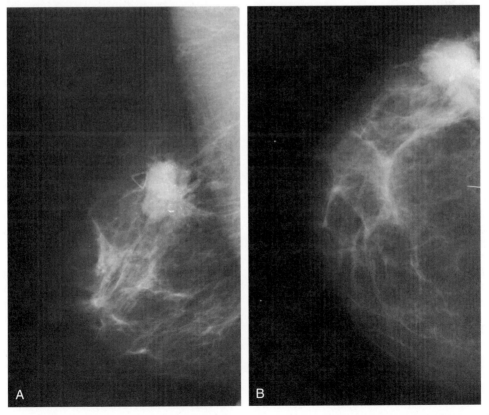

Figure 2–5. MLO and CC of the left breast demonstrate an irregular mass with spiculated margins and pleomorphic calcifications. Pathology demonstrated invasive ductal carcinoma. (Images courtesy of Dr. Alexis Nees, Department of Radiology, University of Michigan.)

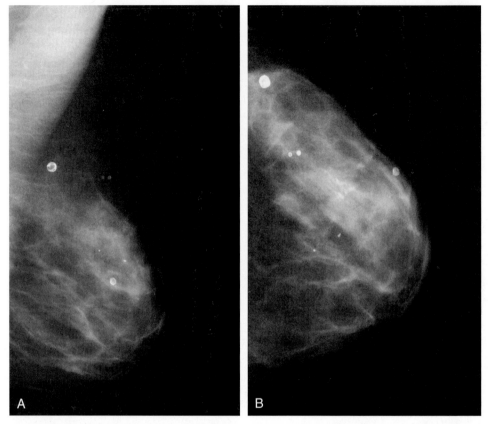

Figure 2–6. MLO and CC views of the right breast demonstrate benign calcifications of posttraumatic oil cysts. (Images courtesy of Dr. Alexis Nees, Department of Radiology, University of Michigan.)

less as having a high probability of association with cancer; calcifications of 2.0 mm or larger are typical of a benign process. The number of calcifications can also be used as a rough indicator of malignancy. Rarely will four or fewer calcifications lead to the detection of breast cancer, even when two or three calcifications with a worrisome morphology warrant a biopsy. Calcifications that are irregular in shape and size (resembling small fragments of broken glass) are often associated with malignancy.

Calcifications in the skin are rarely due to cancer, although they may appear to be parenchymal and require incremental imaging to prove they are in the skin. Otherwise the location of the calcifications provides little direction. The distribution of the calcifications is more important. Calcifications in arteries appear as parallel lines. Calcifications containing lucent centers ("eggshell" or "rim" calcifications) are associated with calcified fat necrosis or cysts and are benign. Calcifications that are fine linear or fine linear branching in appearance (resembling the casting pattern of a duct) are particularly worrisome for DCIS or invasive cancer.

Architectural distortion can be either obvious or quite subtle on mammography (Fig. 2–8). This refers to an unusual pattern in the breast parenchyma. This may include spiculations or retraction. In some cases, this may be associated with postsurgical changes or infection. Otherwise, however, architectural distortion should prompt a biopsy because there is strong association with malignancy. One benign entity that can cause architectural distortion is *radial scar* (see Chapter 3) but a biopsy is necessary to establish the diagnosis. Other worrisome findings on mammography include evidence of skin or nipple retraction and focal skin thickening.

Guidance of Interventional Procedures

One of the most significant advances in the management of breast disease has been the advent of stereotactic-guided breast biopsy. This allows for the percutaneous biopsy of an

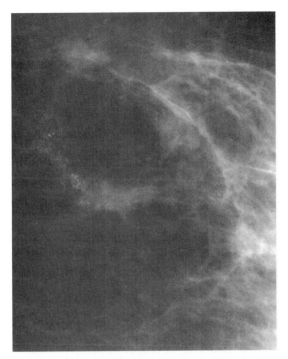

Figure 2–7. Magnification CC view demonstrates segmentally distributed, pleomorphic calcifications. Pathology demonstrated DCIS and invasive ductal carcinoma. (Image courtesy of Dr. Alexis Nees, Department of Radiology, University of Michigan.)

abnormality detected on mammography, eliminating the need for wire-localized biopsy for many women.

Stereotactic biopsy uses radiographic imaging to target the abnormality. The most common approach is the use of a dedicated stereotactic table, in which a patient is positioned prone with the breast placed through an aperture on the table. The breast is then compressed and imaged with mammographic equipment located beneath the table (Fig. 2–9). Stereotactic biopsy can also be done upright with equipment added onto existing mammographic equipment; however, there is more patient movement and may be increased vasovagal reactions.

Initial scout images are obtained and the radiologist uses these to determine the lesion position in the x- and y-axes and the shortest skin to lesion distance. Stereotactic images are then obtained 15 degrees from midline in both the positive and negative directions. By calculating the shift of the lesion on these images from the midline location, the radiologist can determine the depth of the lesion. Once all the coordinates have been determined, the skin is prepped and anesthetized. After a small incision in the skin is made with a number 11

blade, a biopsy needle (either spring-loaded or vacuum-assisted) is introduced into the breast and guided to the lesion using the stereotactic images. Once confirmed, the needle is fired. Post-fire images are obtained to confirm that the needle is positioned within the lesion. Specimen radiographs can also be obtained to ensure that calcifications are in the specimen. Typically, several biopsies of the area are obtained. When finished, a marker clip is inserted at the site of the biopsy. After needle removal, pressure is held to achieve hemostasis, and a sterile dressing is applied. The most common complication is hematoma, which occurs in less than 0.5% of cases.

It is important that the radiologist and the surgeon follow up on the results of the biopsy and determine whether the pathology is *concordant*, meaning the histologic diagnosis is reasonable given the appearance on mammography. A *discordant* finding requires a surgical biopsy. The physicians must also appreciate the limitations of percutaneous biopsy. Patients with atypia (atypical ductal hyperplasia [ADH], atypical lobular hyperplasia [ALH], and lobular carcinoma in situ [LCIS]) diagnosed on needle biopsy also require a surgical biopsy because there may be associated DCIS or invasive carcinoma missed by the needle (see Chapter 8).

Ultrasound

Ultrasound now plays a significant role in the diagnosis and treatment of breast cancer and many breast surgeons perform ultrasound in their office. Even though it cannot reliably detect microcalcifications and therefore plays a minor role in breast cancer screening, it can identify and characterize masses in the breast, as well as evaluate the axillary lymph nodes.

Technique

The entire breast can be imaged with ultrasound, but the most common use of ultrasound of the breast is to evaluate a mass or lesion that has been detected on physical examination or on mammography. Although it has primarily been used to differentiate solid from cystic lesions, several criteria can be used to help characterize solid lesions as more likely benign or malignant. Ultrasound is performed with high-resolution linear array transducers with a frequency of at least 7.5 MHz. Scans are performed around the lesion in the longitudinal, transverse, and radial orientations. Several techniques can also be used to better characterize the mass. The transducer can be

TABLE 2–4 • Calcifications on Mammography

Benign Calcifications

Skin calcifications	Not in the parenchyma but may appear as such. Tangential views should help differentiate. Typically have a lucent center that can be seen on magnification views.
Vascular calcifications	Vascular calcifications can be seen as parallel tracks that run along a blood vessel.
Coarse or popcorn-like calcifications	Typically found in involuting fibroadenomas.
Rod-shaped calcifications	Large rodlike calcifications are typical of secretory disease but not of breast cancer. They are usually >1 mm, are occasionally branching, and may have lucent centers. They form in debris that collects in the duct lumen or cause an inflammatory reaction around a duct.
Round calcifications	Smooth round calcifications are associated with a benign process. Variable in size. When <1 mm they are often found in the acini of lobules. When <0.5 mm the term *punctuate* is used.
Spherical or lucent-centered calcifications	Spherical or lucent-centered calcifications can range from <1 mm to >1 cm. They may be found as debris collected in a duct, in areas of fat necrosis, and occasionally in fibroadenomas.
Rim or eggshell calcifications	These are thin calcifications that surround all or part of the margin of a mass. They are typically found in the wall of cysts. Breast cancer rarely produces this type of calcifications.
Milk or calcium calcifications	This form of calcium precipitates and settles in the bottom of cysts. Their morphologies change between the CC and MLO views.
Dystrophic calcifications	These calcifications are irregular in shape but they are usually large, that is, >0.5 mm in size. They often form in the irradiated breast or after trauma to the breast.

Concerning for Malignancy

Indistinct or amorphous microcalcifications	Round or flake-shaped calcifications that are sufficiently small or hazy such that their morphology cannot be reliably ascertained.
Pleomorphic or heterogeneous calcifications	A cluster of heterogeneous or pleomorphic calcifications, irregular in shape and size, generally <0.5 mm. These raise suspicion of a malignant process.
Fine linear or branching calcifications	Thin, irregular calcifications that appear linear from a distance. Closer examination reveals that they are distinct and <1 mm in width. They result from irregular calcifications of necrotic tumor in the lumen of a duct involved by breast cancer.

used to compress the breast during evaluation to clear or confirm the presence of artifacts. Color Doppler imaging can be used to assess its vascularity. When performing breast ultrasound, it is important to carefully document the position of any findings, including the depth from the skin, and label all images as to their location and the orientation of the transducer.

When evaluating a mass by ultrasonography, several features of the mass must be noted (Table 2–5). The margins of the mass are important because ductal carcinomas may have markedly irregular or spiculated margins. Fibroadenomas and other benign lesions often have smoother margins. However, there are several types of circumscribed carcinomas, such as medullary, mucinous (colloid), or papillary carcinomas, which can have smooth margins. The shape of the mass is also important. A mass that is taller (anterior-posterior) than it is wide is concerning for malignancy. *Echogenicity* represents the ability of the tissue to generate echoes on ultrasound that are detected by the transducer and appear white on the ultrasound image. Fluid does not produce echoes, which is why cysts appear black on ultrasound. Benign lesions tend to have a more homogeneous, hypoechoic appearance (less echo, appearing darker than the surrounding tissue) (Fig. 2–10). The more heterogeneous the echo texture of the mass, the more suspicious for malignancy. Dense fibrosis within some ductal carcinomas may cause massive acoustic shadowing (Fig. 2–11). An echogenic rim around a mass is also concerning for malignancy in that this may be caused by a desmoplastic reaction around the tumor.

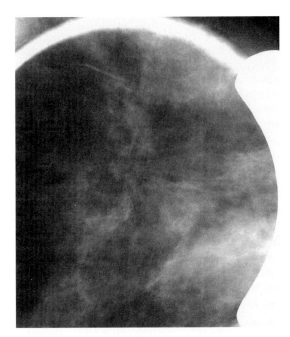

Figure 2–8. Spot compression magnification view demonstrates architectural distortion. Pathology demonstrated a radial sclerosing lesion. (Image courtesy of Dr. Alexis Nees, Department of Radiology, University of Michigan.)

TABLE 2–5 • *Features Suspicious for Malignancy on Ultrasound*		
	Likely Benign	**Likely Malignant**
Margins	Smooth	Irregular
Echogenicity	Homogenous	Heterogeneous
Shape	Ellipsoid (transverse greater than anteroposterior)	Irregular
Echogenic capsule	None or thin	Present

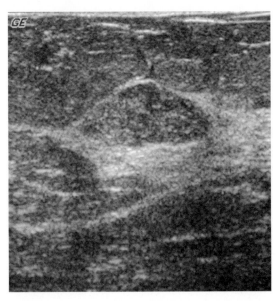

Figure 2–10. Radial US image of circumscribed oval hypoechoic mass. This is a pathologically proven fibroadenoma. (Image courtesy of Dr. Alexis Nees, Department of Radiology, University of Michigan.)

The absence of a mass on ultrasound does not preclude cancer because lobular carcinomas may be very difficult to detect on ultrasound, just as they are on mammography. Although they may present as a well-defined mass, more often they may appear as a vague area of shadowing. Color Doppler imaging may reveal some suspicious vascularity at the periphery of the lesion.

Indications and Uses

Diagnostic Evaluation of a Breast Mass

When a patient presents with a palpable mass or when an abnormality is detected on mammography, ultrasound can be particularly useful in helping to characterize it further. It is most accurate at diagnosing simple cysts, which

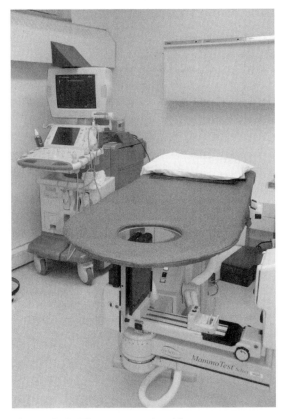

Figure 2–9. The stereotactic table.

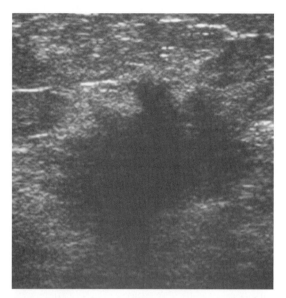

Figure 2–11. Ultrasound demonstrates an irregular hypoechoic mass with spiculated margins. Pathology demonstrated invasive ductal carcinoma. (Image courtesy of Dr. Alexis Nees, Department of Radiology, University of Michigan.)

appear as round or oval masses with smooth walls and no internal echoes (Fig. 2–12). Complicated cysts tend to have some internal echoes, wall thickening, or other abnormalities. Complex cysts (or complex masses) contain mixed cystic and solid components. Whereas simple cysts are never cancer and do not require any intervention, complicated and complex cysts cannot be written off as easily. For complicated cysts, often the internal echoes are due to proteinaceous

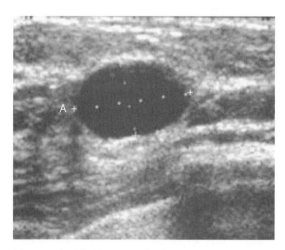

Figure 2–12. Ultrasound demonstrates circumscribed oval anechoic lesion with posterior acoustic enhancement. Findings are consistent with simple cyst. (Image courtesy of Dr. Alexis Nees, Department of Radiology, University of Michigan.)

debris, hemorrhage, or calcium deposits. Depending on their appearance and the clinical history, diagnosis by fine needle aspiration (FNA) biopsy may be necessary. While complicated cysts have a cancer risk of less than 1%, complex cysts have a high rate of cancer, ranging from 20% to 40%. Core needle biopsy or even wire-localized biopsy is recommended.

Beyond solid versus cystic, the breast surgeon must be aware of the limitations of ultrasound in differentiating between benign and malignant masses. On ultrasound, benign characteristics include smooth lesions with few or no lobulations, homogenous echogenicity, a parallel orientation with the width greater than the height, and mild posterior acoustic enhancement. On the other hand, malignant lesions have an irregular shape with heterogeneous echogenicity, strong posterior shadowing, and an echogenic rim. They may be spiculated and may be taller than wide. When combined with the clinical information, ultrasound can be helpful, but one must remember that some cancers have all the classic characteristics of a benign lesion, and vice versa.

Local and Regional Staging

Upon the diagnosis of breast cancer, ultrasound is becoming increasingly important in the clinical staging of the disease. Ultrasound of the primary mass may allow for a more accurate measurement of the tumor size, as well as detect additional foci of disease. This can directly impact the decision to perform breast conservation. More important, ultrasound of the axilla can demonstrate abnormal lymph nodes suspicious for metastases (see Chapter 13). This also allows for the ultrasound-guided FNA of these lymph nodes, which can allow patients with documented axillary disease to bypass sentinel lymph node biopsy and proceed directly to axillary lymph node dissection (Fig. 2–13).

Guidance of Interventional Procedures

Ultrasound is often used to help guide interventions such as FNA biopsies or core needle biopsies (see Chapter 3). If a lesion is visible on both mammogram and ultrasound, ultrasound-guided biopsy offers several advantages. It is faster and requires no radiation or breast compression. It is usually much more comfortable for the patient.

The patient is positioned supine, or in some cases depending on the position of the lesion, obliquely on a table, with the arm raised above

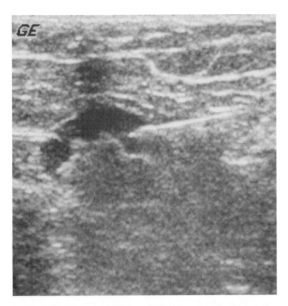

Figure 2–13. Image demonstrates a spinal needle with tip in thickened cortex of abnormal axillary lymph node in a woman newly diagnosed with breast cancer. Cytology demonstrated metastatic disease. (Image courtesy of Dr. Alexis Nees, Department of Radiology, University of Michigan.)

the head. Once the lesion is identified with the ultrasound, the skin is marked and then prepped. After anesthetizing the skin, a number 11 scalpel is used to make a small incision and the biopsy needle introduced. One hand holds the transducer (and remains fixed) while the other hand advances the needle. The needle is easily visualized on ultrasound, particularly when the transducer is kept parallel to the needle. As with stereotactic biopsy, either a spring-loaded or vacuum-assisted needle can be used. Once the needle is in position, it is fired and a post-fire image is obtained. Several specimens are obtained and a metal clip can be placed at the site. Afterward direct pressure is applied, followed by a sterile dressing once hemostasis has been assured.

Magnetic Resonance Imaging

Technique

Advances in surface coil technology and imaging sequences have allowed magnetic resonance imaging (MRI) to emerge as a method for imaging the breasts. The use of contrast attempts to overcome one of the major limitations of other breast imaging modalities (mammography, ultrasound), specifically the differentiation of benign and malignant lesion. Contrast-enhanced breast MRI (CE-MRI) takes advantage

of the production of angiogenic substances by tumors that result in the development of new vessels to supply the tumor. These new vessels are abnormal, with increased capillary permeability and arterial to venous shunting. This neovascularity results in rapid uptake of contrast agent to the tumor relative to the normal tissue. CE-MRI uses magnetic and radiofrequency fields to visualize the uptake of an MRI-specific contrast agent (gadolinium-DTPA). Breast CE-MRI involves evaluation of the breasts before and after the administration of the intravenous gadolinium-DTPA. Images of the breasts are obtained immediately after the administration of the contrast bolus and are repeated three to five times over several minutes. This results in multiple images of each slice of breast tissue, demonstrating the change in contrast enhancement over time. Suspicious lesions are then evaluated based on both their morphology and the kinetics of contrast enhancement (Fig. 2–14).

Without the contrast agent, MRI is not terribly useful. However, the time course of the contrast helps differentiate benign from malignant lesions. Cancers show a sharp increase in signal intensity due to rapid contrast enhancement, followed by a plateau, and early washout. Benign lesions show a slower, more gradual rise in enhancement. CE-MRI appears to be the most sensitive modality to detect invasive breast cancer, ranging from 88% to 100%. The sensitivity is not dependent upon

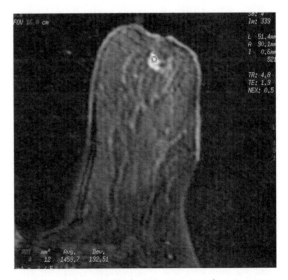

Figure 2–14. Sagittal MR image demonstrates enhancing retroareolar mass with ill-defined margins and area of central hypoenhancement. Pathology demonstrated invasive ductal carcinoma. (Image courtesy of Dr. Alexis Nees, Department of Radiology, University of Michigan.)

the density of the breast, unlike mammography. Also unlike mammography, MRI does not use ionizing radiation. Thus MRI should be the optimal examination for the breast. However, CE-MRI has several drawbacks.

Although it is extremely sensitive (approaching 100% for invasive cancer), the foremost drawback is the specificity. The specificity of MRI ranges from 37% to 96% depending on the indication, and this variable specificity greatly limits its use. Particularly in young women, MRI has difficulty discriminating between cancers and benign lesions such as fibroadenomas, adenosis, or even hormone-induced enhancement of normal parenchyma. As of yet, there is a lack of standardized protocol interpretation guidelines, so there can be great variations in interpretation between radiologists and between institutions. This makes it challenging for a radiologist to offer a second opinion on an MRI from an outside institution.

Another challenge for incorporating MRI into clinical use is the ability to obtain histopathologic proof of suspicious lesions. Abnormalities seen on mammography or ultrasonography can easily be targeted for an image-guided biopsy. However, abnormalities seen only on MRI may present a challenge. If a targeted second-look ultrasound can identify a lesion in the area, this may be an option for biopsy. However, if the lesion is not visualized on mammogram or ultrasound, the only option is an MRI-guided biopsy. As of now, these are only available at a handful of institutions and they are limited in their ability to biopsy lesions less than 1 cm in diameter. Some institutions can do MRI-guided wire localization, but this may lead to an excessive use of excisional biopsies for benign lesions. Hospitals and physicians that use MRI but do not have the capability to biopsy MRI-only visible lesions can put their patients in a difficult position, knowing there is a suspicious lesion but being unable to identify it.

MRI has several additional drawbacks. Although it has a high sensitivity for invasive cancer, the sensitivity for DCIS is inferior to that of mammography, possibly as low as 50%. The high cost of MRI is a notable problem. Hormone-induced enhancement can be a problem in premenopausal women, so it is best to perform the examination during the second week of the cycle. Patients with pacemakers or aneurysm clips cannot undergo MRI, and a reasonable percentage of patients are bothered by claustrophobia and have difficulty with the examination.

Indications and Uses

Imaging of Silicone Breast Implants

One of the first accepted uses of breast MRI was the imaging of silicone breast implants when a rupture was suspected. Implants may be placed either beneath the gland or beneath the pectoralis major muscle. When the implant ruptures, the silicone may still be contained by the fibrous capsule surrounding the implant. This is known as an intracapsular rupture. An extracapsular rupture occurs when the silicone escapes beyond the fibrous capsule. The "linguine sign," the appearance of curvilinear lines representing the collapsed elastomer shell, is a highly reliable sign of intracapsular rupture. When the rupture is extracapsular, the high-signal silicone can be seen outside of the fibrous capsule.

The Occult Primary Breast Cancer

Occasionally, breast cancer patients present with axillary metastasis without clinical or radiographic evidence of the primary tumor. In most cases in which the primary tumor cannot be found, modified radical mastectomy is recommended. MRI is being used increasingly to identify a primary tumor when mammography and whole-breast ultrasound is negative. Several small studies have demonstrated that with the use of contrast-enhanced breast MRI, more than 70% of primary tumors can be identified. If a primary tumor is identified, the patient can undergo breast conservation therapy. If the MRI is negative, treatment options include a modified radical mastectomy or an axillary lymph node dissection followed by whole breast irradiation.

The low specificity of MRI must be considered when a lesion is discovered, because false-positive results can occur. Repeat mammograms and ultrasounds should be obtained, directed at the area suggested by the MRI. If a lesion is seen, than a stereotactic or ultrasound-guided biopsy should be performed. If ultrasound fails to identify a lesion, MRI-directed biopsy can be performed at facilities with the appropriate equipment.

Assessing Candidacy for Breast Conservation

Although breast conservation has radically changed the surgical treatment of breast cancer, allowing many women to avoid mastectomy, it often requires more than one operation to achieve negative margins and some women who initially pursue lumpectomy are found to have more extensive disease requiring mastectomy. MRI has emerged as a possibly improved method of staging the local extent of the tumor and identifying women who might not be suitable candidates for breast conservation due to either the extent of the primary or multicentric disease.

Indeed, MRI has been shown to detect both additional foci of disease within the ipsilateral breast and undiagnosed contralateral cancers. The majority of the data are from single institutions, showing the increased detection of unrecognized foci of disease from between 10% and 30%. The impact on surgical therapy is significant. Several authors have described MRI prompting wider excisions in 3% to 13% of women and mastectomies in 7% to 25% of women otherwise planning on lumpectomy. Based on these studies, many surgeons and radiologists have initiated the routine use of MRI in the preoperative staging of breast cancer.

These data, however, must be interpreted carefully. In series of patients treated by breast conservation without preoperative MRI, the conversion to mastectomy and the local recurrence rates are not nearly as high as the series of MRI would suggest they should be. Even lobular carcinomas, whose size is notoriously underestimated by mammography and ultrasound, do not seem to fail breast conservation therapy (BCT) or locally recur to the degree that the MRI studies might imply.

Taken together, this suggests that MRI is detecting multifocal or multicentric foci of disease that might not have led to local recurrence after lumpectomy, radiation, and systemic therapy. Many studies using serial subgross sectioning to evaluate the breasts of women with known cancers have shown additional foci of disease in 20% to 60% of patients. These data were often used to argue against breast conservation, but 30 years of experience have clearly demonstrated that local recurrence rates are acceptably low after lumpectomy, whole breast irradiation, and when indicated systemic therapy. There is no evidence that the use of MRI for patient selection improves local control. There is also no evidence that it decreases the reexcision rate. It thus seems possible that the use of MRI in this setting may be leading to women undergoing more extensive surgery than necessary.

When staging a woman with breast cancer (see Chapter 10), the use of MRI should not be performed routinely, even in women with lobular carcinoma. A balanced discussion must be held with the woman about the potential benefits and risks of undergoing an MRI before surgery, how this information might alter the surgery, and whether this is worthwhile. It is also important that MRI only be done at institutions that also have the capability to perform MRI-guided biopsy of any newly identified lesions. If that capability is not present and the MRI-detected lesion cannot be found on a directed mammogram or ultrasound, the woman may be facing an awkward decision of undergoing mastectomy for what might be a benign lesion versus ignoring a possible second cancer in pursuit of breast conservation.

Screening

Mammography remains the standard of care for breast cancer screening. However, there has been great hope that MRI, with its increased sensitivity even in the face of dense breast tissue, could help increase early detection, especially among younger women. The detection of cancer with MRI is dependent upon the increased vascularity of cancer. This results in enhancement of the lesion after the injection of contrast material. As opposed to mammographic detection, MRI detection is not limited by the density of the breast. However, because benign lesions may also enhance with contrast material, enhancement alone is not diagnostic. Thus distinguishing between benign and malignant lesions requires evaluation of the kinetics of the enhancement as well as the morphology of the lesion.

Initial trials of MRI screening focused on women with a high risk of developing breast cancers. In women with known BRCA1/2 mutations, MRI screening was shown to decrease the stage (tumor size, nodal status) at which cancer is detected. Eventually, several single and multi-institutional trials demonstrated the superiority of MRI screening as compared to mammography and ultrasound. This led to five prospective randomized trials comparing the use of mammography and MRI in high-risk women. All but one demonstrated an increased sensitivity of MRI for the detection of cancer.

Based on these results, screening with MRI is recommended for women at particularly high risk of developing breast cancer (Table 2–6). However, there are still several issues that need to be addressed. First, no studies have been done on other groups of high-risk women,

TABLE 2-6 • *American Cancer Society Guidelines for Screening with MRI*
Recommended Annually Based on Evidence
BRCA Mutation Carriers
Untested first-degree relative of BRCA carrier
Lifetime risk >20% to 25% defined by BRCAPRO or other family history model
Recommended Based on Expert Consensus Opinion
Radiation to chest from age 10 to 30
Li-Fraumeni syndrome and first-degree relatives
Cowden syndrome (and variants) and first-degree relatives
Insufficient Evidence to Recommend For or Against
Lifetime risk 15% to 20%
LCIS
ALH or ADH
Dense breasts on mammography
Personal history of intraductal or invasive breast cancer
Recommend Against Based on Expert Consensus
Lifetime risk <15%

such as those with LCIS, ALH, or ADH (see Chapter 8). Retrospective studies in this population have shown minimal benefit but a high number of biopsies secondary to MRI's decreased specificity. In the five randomized trials in high-risk women, the specificity was lower than that of mammography, and MRI will lead to an increased number of follow-up studies and biopsies. This will further increase the costs of screening with MRI, which is already significantly higher than that of mammography alone.

It is important to note that MRI is an adjunct to mammography, not a replacement. As many cancers detected by MRI and missed on mammography are found on mammography and missed on MRI. MRI is also not used to determine whether a suspicious lesion on mammography should be biopsied. It is also worth noting that the data to date suggest the usefulness of MRI screening is in high-risk individuals. When screening is applied to a low or intermediate risk population, the utility drops because this population has fewer cancers. The positive predictive value (PPV) is the percentage of abnormal lesions that turn out to be cancer. This is extremely variable

with MRI depending on the method of imaging, how an abnormal lesion is defined, and the incidence of cancer within the population being screened. Therefore it is difficult to assess whether MRI is cost-effective outside of the highest risk populations, and at this time cannot be recommended.

Response to Neoadjuvant Therapy

Neoadjuvant chemotherapy as a method of downstaging primary tumors and evaluating response to chemotherapy is becoming increasingly popular (see Chapter 18). Throughout the course of chemotherapy, the response is monitored by physical examination, mammography, and ultrasound, and after treatment these modalities are used to determine whether BCT is appropriate. Several investigators have examined the use of MRI in this regard. However, the data from these studies have been variable and MRI can neither accurately predict complete response (women with no residual disease on MRI still have pathologic disease) nor incomplete response (women with a residual lesion have no disease on pathology). MRI can be very helpful in the determination of eligibility for BCT after neoadjuvant chemotherapy, but it cannot be used to identify women who may not require surgery at all.

Follow-up of Breast Cancer Patients

The increased sensitivity of MRI has also raised the question of whether it might be appropriate for the surveillance of patients after breast conservation surgery. However, it is unclear whether the earlier identification of local recurrence impacts outcome or would change treatment. There are also few data on the ability of MRI to detect recurrences any earlier than mammography in breasts that have undergone surgery and radiation. Therefore, at this time, MRI should not be used as a surveillance tool.

Positron Emission Tomography

Technique

The above described modalities are anatomic in nature. Positron emission tomography (PET) scanning demonstrates physiologic changes, based on the uptake of neutron-deficient radionuclides (positron emitters) tagged to a metabolic tracer. ^{18}F-FDG (fluorodeoxyglucose labeled with fluorine-18) is the most commonly used agent and is transported across

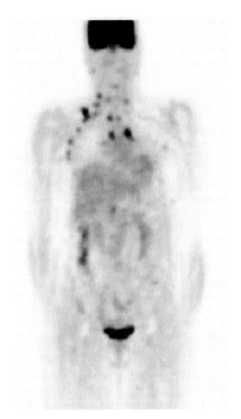

Figure 2-15. PET scan showing metastatic disease in a patient with a history of breast cancer. The PET scan shows multiple metabolic foci involving the suprahilar, supraclavicular, and axillary regions on the right. Small nodes are also seen along paratracheal region bilaterally, extending into the supraclavicular on the left. Metabolic foci are also seen along the periaortic nodes bilaterally.

the cell membrane through glucose pathways. As most tumors have a high aerobic glycolytic rate than normal tissue, there is increased uptake of the FDG. The emitter decays, releasing a positron, which then interacts with an electron, ultimately releasing two photons in opposite directions. The PET scanner detects these photons with detectors placed 180 degrees apart (Fig. 2–15).

Indications and Uses

At this time, the use of PET scanning offers little assistance in the identification of a primary tumor. Although early, small studies suggested that PET might be very accurate, subsequent larger studies failed to confirm these findings. This is primarily because the sensitivity of PET drops significantly as the tumor gets smaller, with a sensitivity of less than 25% for

tumors less than 1 cm. PET scan adds very little to present imaging studies of the breast, such as mammography or ultrasound. It also has not been demonstrated to be very helpful in those situations in which mammography is limited, such as the identification of multifocal disease that might preclude breast conserving surgery or in identifying lobular carcinomas. However, a promising technology is that of PET-mammography (PEM), which may prove to be a useful adjunct in the identification and staging of primary breast cancers. At this time, PET-mammography is experimental.

PET scanning has also been examined as a method of detecting metastases in the axillary lymph nodes. If accurate, this might preclude the need to perform sentinel lymph node biopsy in clinically node-negative patients. However, when compared with sentinel lymph node biopsy, the sensitivity of PET was quite low and often missed small volume disease. One promising area for PET might be the identification of disease in the internal mammary lymph nodes, although more studies are necessary.

Perhaps the best use of PET scans in breast cancer is for the detection of distant disease. One significant advantage is that, as compared to a CT of the chest, abdomen, and pelvis and a bone scan, PET allows for a one-step procedure with a minimal radiation exposure. When compared with CT or MRI, PET does appear to be equally sensitive and specific in identifying distant disease. Although PET is not typically used as the first modality for identifying metastases, it is often used when a CT scan shows a borderline suspicious lesion, especially when biopsy of this lesion would be difficult. It can also be used to differentiate scar tissue or radiation-induced fibrosis from recurrent tumor. This is particularly true in patients with brachial plexopathy.

Principles of Breast Cancer Screening

The decision to recommend screening an asymptomatic population for cancer must be based on several well-established criteria (Boxes 2–1 and 2–2). First, the disease needs to be prevalent and serious enough to justify the cost and effort of screening. Screening large populations for a rare disease would not be appropriate from a cost-analysis standpoint. Of course, this partly depends upon the cost of

BOX 2–1 TERMS RELEVANT TO SCREENING EXAMINATIONS

- Incidence: The number of new cases diagnosed during a fixed time period divided by the total population at risk.
- Prevalence: The number of people living with the disease during a fixed time period divided by the total population at risk.
- Sojourn time: The time between when a cancer is detectable on a screening test and when it would be clinically detectable.
- Interval cancers: Cancers that are diagnosed between scheduled screening examinations.
- Lead time bias: The appearance that screening impacted survival when in fact it did not because survival is measured from the time of diagnosis and not from the time screening is initiated.
- Length time bias: The appearance that screening impacted survival when in fact it did not because screening tended to detect a higher percentage of slower-growing, more biologically favorable cancers.
- Selection bias: The appearance that screening impacted survival when in fact it did not because the women who opted to undergo screening have a different probability of developing cancer (or dying from it) than those who refused to undergo screening.

BOX 2–2 PRINCIPLES OF APPROPRIATE CANCER SCREENING

- The disease needs to be prevalent and serious enough to justify the cost and effort of screening.
- The screening test must have acceptable levels of both sensitivity and specificity.
- The disease has to have an asymptomatic phase where it is detectable (*sojourn time*)
- Intervention offers a better outcome than if treatment is initiated when the disease is symptomatic.

the examination. The screening test must have acceptable levels of both sensitivity and specificity (Fig. 2–16). If a test accurately detects the disease, but also prompts needless workups because it also picks up many false-positive results, then it is not a suitable screening examination. Finally, the disease has to have an asymptomatic phase when it is detectable (sojourn time) *and* intervention must offer a better outcome than if treatment is initiated when the disease is symptomatic. Assume that the average tumor size found by a screening test is 1 cm. If you wait for symptoms, or for the tumor to be detectable by physical examination, the average size is 3 cm. If there is a 25% improvement in survival between treating a 1-cm tumor and a 3-cm tumor, then screening would be worthwhile. However, if the improvement in survival is only 1% to 2%, then this does not justify the cost and effort involved in screening the population.

So does breast cancer meet these criteria? There is no doubt that the disease is prevalent. Breast cancer is the most common cancer in women in the United States and the second most common cause of cancer death among women. Approximately 1 in 8 women will be diagnosed with breast cancer and 1 in 33 will die of their disease. The sensitivity and specificity of mammography is reasonable, although this is dependent upon how aggressive we are in recommending biopsies. If the bar is set low, so that any mildly suspicious lesion is recommended for a biopsy, then very few cancers will be missed but many additional biopsies will be performed. On the other hand, if the bar is set high, so that only the most suspicious lesions are referred for biopsy, then fewer unnecessary procedures will be performed but more cancers will go undiagnosed for another 6 months to 1 year.

What about the sojourn time and the impact of initiating treatment at an earlier time point? There is little doubt that the earlier you treat breast cancer, the better the survival. Consistently, across all age groups, there exists an inverse relationship between the size of the tumor and long-term survival. The sojourn time, the time between when a tumor is detected by screening and when it would be detected by symptoms, will vary greatly among individuals. For example, younger women will have a smaller sojourn time because mammography is less sensitive. It has been estimated that for women between 60 and 69 years of age, the sojourn time for mammographic screening of breast cancer is 4.2 years (Box 2–3). This means that screening will find the cancer 4 years earlier than if we wait for the patient (or their doctor) to detect it on examination. The sojourn time will also be quite variable depending upon the body habitus of the patient and the histology.

True disease status

		Patient has disease	Patient does not have disease
Test result	Positive	A True positive	B False positive
	Negative	C False negative	D True negative

True-positive rate (sensitivity)	$\dfrac{\text{People with positive test and disease}}{\text{All people with disease}}$	$\dfrac{A}{A+C}$
False-negative rate	$\dfrac{\text{People with negative test and disease}}{\text{All people with disease}}$	$\dfrac{C}{A+C}$
True-negative rate (specificity)	$\dfrac{\text{People with negative test and no disease}}{\text{All people without disease}}$	$\dfrac{D}{B+D}$
False-positive rate	$\dfrac{\text{People with positive test and no disease}}{\text{All people without disease}}$	$\dfrac{B}{B+D}$
Positive predictive value	$\dfrac{\text{People with positive test and disease}}{\text{All people with positive test}}$	$\dfrac{A}{A+B}$
Negative predictive value	$\dfrac{\text{People with negative test and no disease}}{\text{All people with negative test}}$	$\dfrac{D}{C+D}$
Accuracy	$\dfrac{\text{All true test}}{\text{All tests}}$	$\dfrac{A+D}{A+B+C+D}$

Figure 2–16. Measures of the accuracy of diagnostic and screening tests.

BOX 2–3

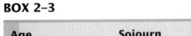

Age	Sojourn Time
40 to 49	2.4 years
50 to 59	3.7 years
60 to 69	4.2 years

Tabar L. The swedish two-county trial twenty years later: Updated mortality results and new insights from long-term follow-up. Radiol Clin North Am 2000; 38(4): 625–651.

It is important to remember that the impact of screening on a population will be variable over time as screening tests and treatments improve. If screening tests become better at detecting cancers at earlier time points, the sojourn time will increase. On the other hand, if treatments improve to the point that the survival of a 3-cm tumor is not much worse than that of a 1-cm tumor, then the impact of screening will decrease. For this reason, the impact of screening needs to be constantly reassessed.

Based on what we know about breast cancer and the criteria for an ideal screening test, breast cancer seems to be an ideal cancer for screening. However, the only way to know this for sure is the performance of randomized controlled trials (RCTs). Retrospective studies of screening tests are often misinterpreted because of several biases (Box 2–1). Lead time bias refers to the calculation of survival from the point of diagnosis to the time of death. This can easily give the appearance that subjects live longer when the disease is diagnosed early, but survival should be measured from the beginning of screening, not from the diagnosis of cancer (Fig. 2–17). Otherwise the only thing that has been lengthened is the time the patient knows he or she has the cancer, while death occurs at the same point in the natural history of the disease. Another type of bias is

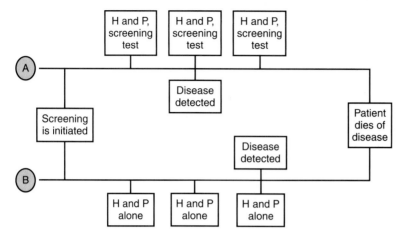

Figure 2–17. Lead time bias occurs when the survival is measured from the point where disease is detected to when the patient dies. This gives the appearance that screening lengthened the survival. However, if survival is measured from the point that screening was started to the moment the patient dies, one sees that screening had no impact on survival.

length time bias. This refers to the tendency of screening to detect the slower growing and less aggressive tumors. In this case, the screening test may only identify those tumors with a better prognosis, those that do just as well if therapy is initiated in another year or 2. Thus it appears that screening is improving survival (because the patients with cancer in the screening group do better), but in reality the survival is the same as if screening had not been performed. Finally, these studies often suffer from a selection bias, because patients who are more health-conscious or those with fewer comorbidities, undergo the screening. Again, this leads to the false assumption that the group undergoing the screening lived longer because of the screening, when in reality they lived longer because they were healthier.

In a population-based RCT, these biases are eliminated because the analysis is based on mortality differences between the two groups from the beginning of the screening period, and because the randomization should equally distribute any confounding factors. However, even RCTs can suffer from bias or misinterpretation.

Screening for Breast Cancer

There are several methods by which patients and physicians screen for breast cancer (Box 2–4). Besides mammography, women are encouraged to perform self-breast examinations on a monthly basis and to undergo a clinical examination by a physician at least once a year. Given the improved survival associated with finding breast cancer at an earlier stage, particularly when it is noninvasive, there is a strong motivation to develop new, more sensitive screening examinations.

The evidence for mammographic screening is strong, although it has come under fire recently. There have been several RCTs examining the benefits of breast cancer screening. These trials demonstrated a benefit in women ages 50 years and older, with an approximate 34% reduction in the risk of dying from breast cancer at 7 years. A follow-up analysis of four randomized trials in Sweden, with a median follow-up of 15.8 years, demonstrated a 21% reduction in the risk of breast cancer mortality.

The benefit of mammography came into question when a Cochrane review questioned whether five of the eight studies were appropriately designed and concluded that the effectiveness of screening mammography, based on the remaining three studies, was not evident. However, many reviewers subsequently questioned the Cochrane review itself, and most experts believe that the evidence that mammography decreases breast cancer mortality is solid.

This is not to say that there are not still questions regarding the use of mammography,

BOX 2–4 BREAST CANCER
SCREENING RECOMMENDATIONS

American College of Surgeons:
  Begin self-examinations and every
    3 years clinical breast examination
    at age 20.
  Begin annual mammograms and yearly
    clinical breast examination at age 40.
American College of Radiology
  Begin annual mammograms and yearly
    clinical breast examination at age 40.
National Cancer Institute
  Begin every 1- to 2-year mammograms at
    age 40.

specifically when mammographic screening should begin and when it should end. Even though there is a clear benefit for women older than 50, the benefits are less clear for women in their 40s. Initially, a 1993 meta-analysis showed no benefit to women in their 40s after 7 years of follow-up. However, subsequent meta-analyses, which included more recent results and longer follow-up, demonstrated an approximate 15% reduction in breast cancer mortality among women in their 40s.

Even though the evidence suggests there is a benefit to women in their 40s, the cost effectiveness of screening this age group remains in question. Similar to the number needed to treat (NNT) as a way of evaluating the clinical benefit of therapeutic interventions, the number needed to screen (NNS) can help put into perspective the benefit of screening examinations. When one looks at mammography, between 1500 and 2500 women in their 40s need to be screened regularly for 10 years to prevent 1 breast cancer death. In addition, of all these women undergoing screening, mammography will reveal abnormalities resulting in call-backs, short-term follow-up, and biopsies. When one takes this into account, the cost of screening mammography for women in their 40s can be almost 5 times that of older women.

These questions apply to the general population, but most physicians recommend that mammographic screening should be started at a younger age in women with a strong family history of breast cancer. In women with a first-degree relative with breast cancer, particularly if that cancer was premenopausal, screening should begin 5 to 10 years earlier than the age of the family member. However, for many women, this will mean screening begins in their 20s and 30s, when the sensitivity of mammography is relatively low. This fact, along with the lack of data regarding the impact on mortality of screening high-risk patients earlier, makes it difficult to know the true benefit of these recommendations.

Another question is when to discontinue screening. The randomized trials included almost no women over the age of 70. Case control studies of mammographic screening in older women have failed to demonstrate an impact on mortality in women older than 75. This is secondary to both the lower incidence of DCIS in this population and the reduced life expectancy among this population. Thus the cost effectiveness and efficacy of continuing screening past age 70 is unclear. The decision to continue screening should be decided on an individual basis, based on the woman's health and life expectancy, breast cancer risk, and other factors.

When screening is performed separate from diagnostic procedures, approximately 5% to 10% of women will be called back for additional images because of a concern on the screening mammograms. Approximately 40% of these women will have nothing that requires further intervention; there may be overlapping tissue that disappeared on subsequent images or the finding is clearly benign, such as a cyst or benign calcifications. Of the remaining women, they will have abnormalities that require either short-interval follow-up images (less suspicious lesions) or biopsy (more suspicious lesions). Where to set that threshold remains a question. Setting that threshold low, meaning biopsy is recommended for a large percentage of atypical lesions, results in very few missed cancers but a large number of benign biopsies. Setting that threshold high will minimize the number of biopsies but delay the diagnosis of several cancers for several months. The impact this has on survival is unclear. Most breast imagers strive for a 20% to 25% cancer detection rate, meaning one fifth to one fourth of patients referred for biopsy have cancer.

While mammography remains the standard of care for breast cancer screening, MRI has emerged as a useful adjunct in appropriate patients. In very high-risk women, such as those with documented BRCA mutations, MRI screening has been shown to increase the detection of cancer and decrease the stage (tumor size, nodal status) at which cancer is detected. Yearly screening with MRI in addition to clinical examination and mammography is recommended for women at particularly high risk of developing breast cancer. It is not, however, recommended for women at lower risks of developing breast cancer.

Suggested Reading

1. Bevers TB, Anderson BO, Bonaccio E, et al. National Comprehensive Cancer Network. Breast cancer screening and diagnosis. J NCCN 2006;4(5): 480–508.
2. Bartella L, Smith CS, Dershaw DD, et al. Imaging breast cancer. Radiol Clin North Am 2007;45(1): 45–67.
3. Dershaw DD. Film or digital mammographic screening? N Engl J Med 2005;353:1846–1847.
4. Humphrey L, Helfand M, Chan B, et al. Breast cancer screening: A summary of the evidence. In U.S. Preventive Services Task Force, 2002, Vol 2003.

5. Kriege M, Brekelmans CT, Boetes C, et al. Efficacy of MRI and mammography for breast-cancer screening in women with a familial or genetic predisposition. N Engl J Med 2004;351:427–437.

6. Lacquemant MA, Mitchell D, Hollingsworth AB. Positive predictive value of the Breast Imaging Reporting and Data System. J Am Coll Surg 1999;189:34–40.

7. Liberman L. Breast cancer screening with MRI—what are the data for patients at high risk? N Engl J Med 2004;351:497–500.

8. Olsen O, Gotzsche PC. Cochrane review on screening for breast cancer with mammography. Lancet 2001;358:1340–1342.

9. Orel SG, Kay N, Reynolds C, Sullivan DC. BI-RADS categorization as a predictor of malignancy. Radiology 1999;211:845–850.

10. Pisano ED, Gatsonis C, Hendrick E, et al. Diagnostic performance of digital versus film mammography for breast cancer screening. N Engl J Med 2005; 353:1773–1783.

11. Shen Y, Zelen M. Screening sensitivity and sojourn time from breast cancer early detection clinical trials: Mammograms and physical examinations. JCO 2001;19:3490–3499.

12. Thomas DB, Gao DL, Ray RM, et al. Randomized trial of breast self-examination in Shanghai: Final results. J NCI 2002;94:1445–1457.

13. Thompson M, Klimberg VS. Use of ultrasound in breast surgery. Surg Clin N Am 2007;87(2): 469–484.

14. Warner E, Plewes DB, Shumak RS, et al. Comparison of breast magnetic resonance imaging, mammography, and ultrasound for surveillance of women at high risk for hereditary breast cancer. J Clin Oncol 2001;19:3524–3531.

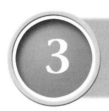

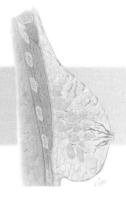

The Breast Mass, Breast Biopsies, and Benign Lesions of the Breast

EVALUATION
History
Physical Examination
Directed Breast Imaging
Breast Biopsies of Palpable
  Lesions
Breast Biopsies of Nonpalpable
  Lesions

MANAGEMENT OF BENIGN
BREAST MASSES
Fibroadenoma

Cysts
Lipoma
Hamartoma
Trauma/Hematoma/Fat
  Necrosis
Diabetic Mastopathy
Sclerosing Adenosis and Radial
  Scar
Papilloma and Papillomatosis

The Breast Mass, Breast Biopsies, and Benign Lesions of the Breast: Key Points

Describe a complete history and physical for the woman with a breast complaint.

Know when imaging is indicated and what imaging tests are most helpful.

Describe the technique for performing a fine needle aspiration biopsy and core needle biopsy, and know the relative pros and cons of each technique.

Explain the principles of the surgical breast biopsy.

Recognize the classic features of cysts and fibroadenomas and describe the management options.

Understand when and why excisional biopsy of benign lesions such as radial scars or papillomas is necessary.

One of the most common problems in primary care and specifically for the breast surgeon is the evaluation of a newly discovered breast mass. Complaints of a breast lump are extremely common. In one study, 16% of women between the ages of 40 and 70 saw a physician for a breast problem, and 40% of these were breast lumps. The overwhelming majority of these will be benign, even in referral practices, the most common causes being a cyst or fibroadenoma.

When evaluating a patient who presents with a breast mass, the clinician needs to carefully balance the risk of missing a cancer with performing too many biopsies. In addition to the time and expense, breast biopsies are not without morbidities. These may include bruising or hematoma, infection, or a misdiagnosis. More than 500,000 breast biopsies are performed in the United States each year; 75% to 80% are benign. The reason for this high use of biopsies in the United States is not surprising when one realizes that the failure to diagnose breast cancer has led malpractice claim lists in the United States for several years.

Evaluation

History

The first question to ask a patient presenting with a breast mass (or derive from the chart) is her age. Breast masses are different entities in women younger than 30, between 31 and 50, or older than 50 years old. As the incidence of breast cancer increases with age, so too will the aggressiveness of the evaluation. On a statistical basis, 9 of 10 new masses in premenopausal women are benign.

A careful history of the lump should include the precise location of the mass and how it was first noted (Box 3–1). Was this felt by the patient and if so was it incidental or during a monthly self-breast examination? If it was felt by a doctor on a routine physical, did the patient know about it and can she now locate it? The physician should inquire about how often the patient does self breast examinations. If she does not do self-examinations, the mass may have been present for longer. How long has it been present and has it changed in any way since she first noted it? This includes not only getting larger since first noticing it, but does it get larger or smaller at particular times in the menstrual cycle. Are

BOX 3–1 ESSENTIAL COMPONENTS OF THE HISTORY IN THE EVALUATION OF THE BREAST MASS

- Patient age
- Method of detection (self-examination, incidental, physician's examination)
  - Does the patient do monthly self-examinations?
- Length of time it has been present
- Any change in size (particularly with menstrual cycle)
- Associated symptoms (pain, skin changes, nipple discharge)
- History of other breast masses or fibrocystic disease
- History of previous breast biopsies and pathology
- Menstrual history (age of menarche, age at first pregnancy, number of pregnancies, age at menopause)
- Personal history of cancer and how was it treated
  - Hodgkin's disease and chest wall radiation
- Use of hormone replacement therapy
  - How long, what kind (estrogen only or estrogen and progestin)?
- Family history of all cancers, mother's and father's side
  - Age of onset, bilateral disease?

there any associated symptoms such as nipple discharge (and if so, the nature of that discharge) or breast pain? Has she ever had any breast masses or symptoms before, and if so, how were they managed?

The physician should then gather information to assess the risk of breast cancer in this patient. Has she had breast cancer in the past? How many previous biopsies has the patient had, and does she know the pathology? This is particularly important if a previous biopsy demonstrated atypical hyperplasia or lobular carcinoma in situ (LCIS) (Chapter 8). Sometimes it is useful to obtain the histologic slides. The age of menarche, number of pregnancies, age at first pregnancy, age of menopause, and use of hormonal replacement therapy should be documented. If hormone replacement is used, what type (estrogen only or estrogen plus progestin)? If the patient has had a hysterectomy, what was the reason for the operation and were the ovaries removed? A social history, including both alcohol and tobacco use, is also important. A full family history should be obtained. This should not be limited to breast cancer, nor to the maternal side of the family. Rather it should include all cancers and document the age of the family members who had cancer. If a family member did have breast cancer, was it bilateral?

Physical Examination

The breast examination includes inspection of the breast and palpation of both the breast and the regional lymph nodes (axillary, supraclavicular, and cervical) (Box 3–2). Although there are several approaches to the examination, the breast surgeon should develop his or her own systematic approach. Always keep in mind that this is an awkward examination for most women, and every attempt should be made to keep the patient comfortable and relaxed, maintain her privacy, and perform the examination in a professional manner.

The examination should begin with the patient in the sitting position. For premenopausal women, you should document where the woman is her menstrual cycle. The optimum examination is 1 week after the onset of the last period. At this time point, swelling and tenderness of the breasts are at a minimum.

With the patient in the seated position, ask her to point out the problem area. Some women will tell you the abnormality is best felt while sitting up; others need to lie back or on their side. With the woman sitting straight, note whether the breasts are symmetric. It is normal for one breast to be larger than the other. Are the nipples both everted (or both inverted) and do they point in the same direction? Is the color of the skin and venous pattern the same on both sides? Is there any dimpling, retraction, or redness? Are there any previous scars? Is a distortion obvious? The woman should then raise her hands above her head and touch them together. She should also put them on her hips and press inward (Fig. 3–1). Both of these maneuvers will exaggerate any retraction of the skin or deviation of the breast.

With the patient still sitting up, the next step is palpation of the axillary nodes. This should begin with the cervical lymph nodes along the anterior border of the sternocleidomastoid muscle. As you palpate downward, you should examine the supraclavicular fossa. There may be some infraclavicular nodes within the deltopectoral groove. To examine

BOX 3–2 KEY COMPONENTS OF THE BREAST EXAMINATION

- Patient sitting up, facing the examiner, arms to the side
  - Inspection for symmetry, contour, scars, skin lesions, erythema, nipple inversion
  - Palpation of the cervical and supraclavicular basins
  - Palpation of the mass in the upright position
- Patient sitting up, arms above head, touching
  - Inspection for dimpling, retraction, protruding mass
- Patient sitting up, arms on hips, pressing inward
  - Inspection for dimpling, retraction, protruding mass
- Patient sitting up, physician supporting weight of the arm
  - Palpation of bilateral axilla
- Patient in the supine position, arm raised over the head
  - Inspection for contour, scars, skin lesions, protruding masses, dimpling, or retraction
  - Examination of the nipple including gentle attempt to express discharge
  - Palpation of the mass in the supine position. Note size, consistency, borders, fixation, and location (including clock position and distance from areola)
  - Palpation of the entire breast parenchyma including inframammary fold, axillary tail
  - Note locations of any additional masses including size and location
- Examine the opposite breast in same way, noting symmetry between any areas of concern

the axillary nodes, you should face the patient or stand slightly to her side. You should use the nonpalpating hand to either steady the patient's shoulder, or support her arm, asking her to let it go loose. This will relax the pectoralis major and axillary fascia, allowing for a better examination of the axilla (Fig. 3–2).

Begin high in the axilla with your examination. In this way, the axillary nodes are trapped lower rather than initially pushed upward.

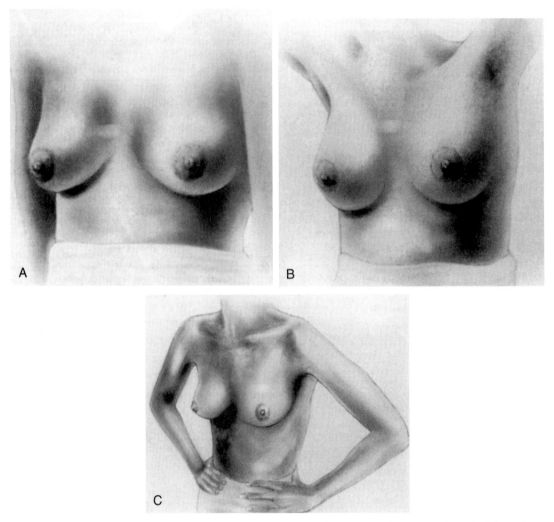

Figure 3–1. Inspection of the breast in the upright position with the patient's arms to the side **(A)**, in the air **(B)**, and hands on hips **(C)**. (From Bland KI, Copeland EM III. The breast, 3rd ed. Philadelphia: WB Saunders, 2004.)

Gently palpate back and forth to feel whether any nodes are apparent. Several passes should be made from top to bottom, both anteriorly and posteriorly in the axilla. If any lymph nodes are detected, their size, consistency, and fixation should be noted. Several points should be highlighted. In thin women, it is not unusual to palpate axillary nodes. These should be soft, mobile, and less than 1 cm in size. It is also not unusual to run your fingers over the lateral edge of the pectoralis minor muscle, or tonguelike extensions of breast tissue within the axilla. These should not be mistaken for lymph nodes.

Once the right and left axillary examinations are completed, the patient should be placed in the supine position. The patient's arm is brought over her head and her hand placed behind her back. Some patients will have difficulty with this maneuver because of shoulder problems. The breast often falls laterally. This can be corrected for by placing a small pillow under the back, or more commonly by displacing the breast medially with the opposite hand during palpation. Some surgeons prefer to stand on the same side of the breast being examined; some prefer the opposite side. The examiner should map out an approach to the breast so that the entire area is examined; some use concentric circles or spirals, some use a pattern like the spokes of a wheel, others use up-and-down columns (Fig. 3–3). The best method for palpating the breast is a rotating or kneading motion with

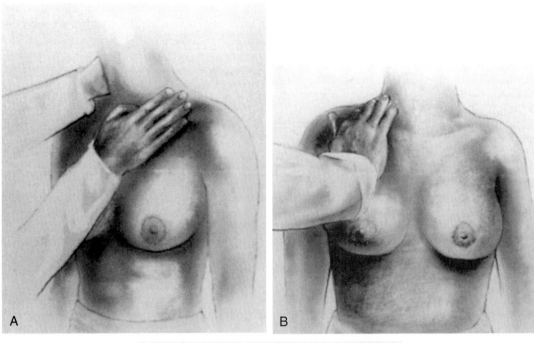

Figure 3–2. Examination of the cervical **(A)**, supraclavicular **(B)**, and axillary nodes **(C)**. (From Bland KI, Cope-land EM III. The breast, 3rd ed. Philadelphia: WB Saunders, 2004.)

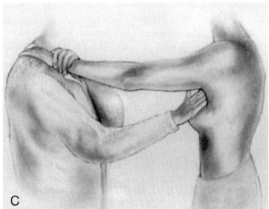

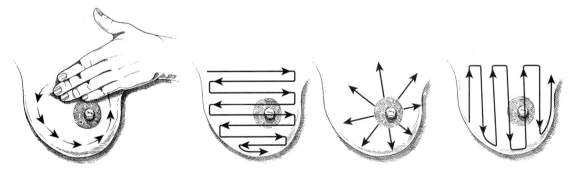

Figure 3–3. Methods of clinical breast examination. To ensure that the entire breast is examined, physicians use a number of patterns, including concentric circles, back and forth, spikes of a wheel, or up and down. (From Roses D. Breast Cancer. Philadelphia: Elsevier, 2005.)

the fingers that causes the breast tissue to move back and forth beneath the skin. The surgeon should note the overall consistency of the breast tissue (e.g., soft, firm, dense.). In general, younger women have denser fibroglandular tissue, but one should not be surprised to find dense parenchyma in women in their 60s.

The distribution of the fibroglandular tissue is not always even throughout the breast, and this often causes confusion during the breast examination. Often the tissue is concentrated in the upper outer quadrant, causing some inexperienced clinicians to think they have discovered a large breast mass when in reality they are just feeling the normal parenchyma. Breast tissue may extend up into the axilla, and should not be confused for an axillary mass or lymph node. Always compare these asymmetries to the contralateral breast. There may also be a vacancy of tissue beneath the areola, with the normal tissue being configured as a "doughnut." This often leaves a ridge of normal parenchyma, which can be confused for a mass. The same can be said for defects under scars from sites of previous excisions. Other areas that are sometimes confused for masses include the ribs and a firm inframammary ridge.

The nipple should be inspected for retraction, overlying skin changes, or discharge. It is not always abnormal for the nipple to be inverted. If this is the case, determine whether it can be everted. There may be some cutaneous debris that is not necessarily a nipple discharge. Beginning at the border of the areola and sliding toward the tip, the nipple should be *gently* squeezed to determine if there is a discharge, as well as to feel any mass underneath the nipple-areolar complex.

During the breast examination, the examiner might identify a mass or nodule, or several. Breast tissue in normal women is often "lumpy." The key is to identify masses that are different from the remainder of the examination. If a mass is noted, the examiner should take note of whether the mass has a complete periphery that is distinct from the surrounding tissue. Is the mass mobile? If not, why not? Is it fixed to the skin or to the underlying muscle? Is there tenderness associated with it? What is the consistency; is it soft or hard? What are the borders like; smooth or irregular?

For each mass found, the examiner should accurately document the location and size. In this manner, if it is to be managed by observation, the surgeon knows exactly what to expect when the patient returns 4 to 6 months later for a repeat examination. The location should be documented as not only the position on a clock, but also the number of centimeters from the areolar border.

Directed Breast Imaging

The next step in the evaluation of the patient with a breast mass is that of diagnostic breast imaging. Mammography is indicated in any patient age 35 years or older with a breast mass. This is not only important for characterizing the mass in question, but also looking for clinically occult lesions or other findings that may guide surgical therapy in case this mass proves to be cancer. For women younger than age 35, mammography should be obtained more selectively. This should be based on the level of suspicion associated with the mass and the density of the breast. The breast tissue in younger women is often too dense to allow for accurate imaging and interpretation.

The results of the mammogram must be interpreted carefully. When evaluating a breast mass, the mammogram results are only one piece of information, and the decision to biopsy should not be based on these films alone. If the mass is clinically suspicious, either because of the patient's history or the physical examination, then biopsy is indicated whether or not the mammogram shows anything. Cancers may be mammographically occult. This is especially true in younger women or with invasive lobular carcinoma. The lump may be visible but indeterminate. Even though the mammogram adds little to the diagnosis or the decision to biopsy, it is still necessary to screen the remainder of the breast and the contralateral side.

On the other hand, the mammogram may demonstrate a classic benign appearance for a mass that otherwise feels suspicious, such as fat necrosis, a benign calcifying fibroadenoma, or a hamartoma. In other cases, a lump that otherwise does not feel suspicious on examination, may have very worrisome findings on mammography, prompting a biopsy. Although both of these scenarios are less common, they do support the strong role of diagnostic mammography in evaluating breast masses.

Ultrasound can be a useful tool to determine whether a breast mass is a solid mass, a simple cyst, or a complex cyst. It is particularly useful in the evaluation of a breast mass in a woman younger than age 35 years. It may also be used in conjunction with mammography in women older than 35. Increasingly, breast surgeons are becoming certified in breast ultrasound so they can easily perform ultrasonography in the office. This allows for not only a rapid assessment of breast masses but also for image guidance for aspiration or core needle biopsy.

The benefits of magnetic resonance imaging (MRI) in the diagnosis and staging of breast cancer have been touted recently. MRI has emerged as an imaging modality for the breast with a wide array of purported uses (see Chapter 2). In the clinical assessment of a benign mass, however, there is limited data to suggest that a suspicious lesion found on clinical examination or mammography but seen as benign on MRI is unlikely enough to represent cancer that a biopsy can be avoided. MRI, with its high sensitivity and lower specificity, may also lead to the detection of other lesions that require biopsy. Not all institutions that perform breast MRI have the ability to perform MRI-guided biopsies. Even though MRI may have benefits in defining the extent of a known breast cancer, or screening the remainder of the breast and contralateral breast in patients with breast cancer, its use in the evaluation of a palpable breast mass is limited. MRI is indicated in the evaluation of a breast mass in a woman with silicone breast implants, as well as in women with documented axillary metastases but no primary lesion identified on breast imaging studies (the "occult breast cancer").

Triple Diagnosis

One of the greatest fears among breast surgeons is that of misdiagnosing a breast cancer presenting as a palpable mass, leading to a delay in diagnosis. Unfortunately, this fear (both on the part of the patient and the doctor) has probably led to a large number of unnecessary excisional breast biopsies.

When can a breast mass be safely observed? The term "triple diagnosis" refers to the combination of physical examination, mammography, and fine-needle aspiration biopsy (FNAB) for diagnosing palpable breast masses (Table 3–1). If all three tests are suggestive of benign disease, the likelihood of missing a cancer is extremely low (0% to 0.6%). This approach is clearly more cost-effective than subjecting these women to an excisional biopsy.

If all three tests suggest benign disease, the patient should return in 4 to 6 months for a repeat clinical examination to assure stability or regression. The patient should then be seen again at 1 year. If either the mammogram or the FNAB is suggestive of malignancy, then a more definitive tissue biopsy is strongly indicated. If the physical examination is concerning, but the mammogram and FNAB are both benign, then a detailed discussion should be held with the patient regarding the risks and benefits of biopsy versus observation.

Breast Biopsies of Palpable Lesions

In some cases, the history, physical examination and directed breast imaging will suggest that observation without a biopsy may be a reasonable approach. In these cases, the patient should return for a follow-up clinical appointment in 4 to 6 months to assure stability. The patient should also be instructed to perform monthly self-examinations and return earlier if she notices any change in symptoms or size. In these situations, it is not prudent to simply reassure the patient this is likely benign and give her an

TABLE 3–1 • *Percent Probability of a Cancer after Triple Diagnosis (Physical Examination, Mammogram, Fine-Needle Aspiration)*

Benign Physical Examination			
Mammogram Findings	FNA Benign	FNA Suspicious	FNA Positive
Benign	0.6%	16.0%	100%
Suspicious	4.1%	32.4%	100%
Positive	5.7%	55.7%	100%
Suspicious Physical Examination			
Mammogram Findings	FNA Benign	FNA Suspicious	FNA Positive
Benign	7.1%	43.8%	94.7%
Suspicious	6.9%	62.5%	99.6%
Positive	35.7%	91.4%	99.4%

From Donegan WL. N Engl J Med 1992;327:937-942. Need permission

as-needed follow-up appointment, because it is this scenario that often leads to litigation in the rare case that a benign-appearing mass turns out to be a cancer.

In many cases, however, some type of biopsy may be indicated. There are several choices for performing a biopsy of a breast mass, each with relative advantages and disadvantages (Table 3–2). The choice of biopsy depends on the level of suspicion of the mass, the size and location of the mass, the resources available (e.g., an experienced cytopathologist), and the desires of the patient.

Fine-Needle Aspiration

Fine-needle aspiration (FNA) is a quick and technically simple method of diagnosing both breast masses and axillary lymph nodes. However, the procedure does have its limitations. FNA is useful in differentiating between a solid mass and a cystic mass. Aspiration of a cyst is not only diagnostic, but also therapeutic. FNA of a solid mass allows for cytology (Tables 3–3 and 3–4). The reliability of the cytology, however, is dependent upon the experience of the cytopathologist. Reports of sensitivity, specificity, and accuracy vary among reports, with diagnostic accuracy ranging from 77% to 99%. However, in the hands of an experienced cytopathologist, sensitivity can approach 96% and specificity 99%. Thus an individual surgeon's choice of FNA versus core-needle biopsy will depend in part on the level of expertise of the cytopathologist. It is therefore incumbent upon the surgeon to know this information.

It is important to remember that FNA has both false-negative *and* false-positive results. If the mass is suspicious on physical exam or mammography, but the FNA is negative, a more definitive tissue biopsy should be considered. Likewise, a positive FNA should be considered highly suggestive of cancer, but not

TABLE 3–3 • *Fine-Needle Aspiration Biopsy Diagnoses*	
1. Benign	No evidence of malignancy
2. Atypical/ indeterminate	Nondiagnostic cellular findings
3. Suspicious	Significant atypia or architectural distortion suggestive, but not diagnostic, of malignancy
4. Malignant	Cellular findings are diagnostic of malignancy
5. Unsatisfactory	Scant cellularity or artifact precluding diagnosis

absolute. It is not unreasonable to proceed with a lumpectomy and sentinel lymph node biopsy in the face of a highly suspicious lesion and a positive FNA; even in the unlikely circumstance that the FNA results turn out to be falsely positive, the morbidity associated with this procedure is not significantly greater than for an excisional breast biopsy. The most dramatic mistake that can be made is to proceed with a mastectomy on the basis of an FNA. If a patient with a positive FNA desires mastectomy, then either a core biopsy should be performed before proceeding, or an excisional biopsy and frozen section should be obtained in the operating room before mastectomy. Nor can FNA differentiate between in situ and invasive carcinoma. Again, if this information alters your management, a core biopsy or excisional biopsy should be obtained.

What about a negative FNA on a nonsuspicious lesion? Given the false-negative rate associated with FNA, the conventional teaching was that FNA could not be used to rule out cancer. However, when combined with mammography and physical examination, FNA can be quite reliable. The triple diagnosis is more sensitive and specific than each test alone. When the results of all three tests indicate a benign mass,

TABLE 3–2 • *Comparison of Breast Biopsy Techniques*			
	FNA	**Core Biopsy**	**Excisional Biopsy**
Technical ease	Simple	Moderate	Complex
Cost	Inexpensive	More expensive	Most expensive
False-positives	Yes	No	No
False-negatives	Yes	Rare	Very Rare
Complications	Few	Some	Increased
Interpretation	Needs cytopathologist	Routine pathology	Routine pathology
Immunohistochemistry	Difficult	Easy	Easy

TABLE 3-4 • *Benign versus Malignant Features on Fine-Needle Aspiration*

	Benign	Malignant
Cellularity	Hypocellular	Hypercellular
Architecture	Cohesive, orderly cells Few single cells	Dyscohesive, disorderly Several isolated cells
Cell population	Heterogeneous	Homogeneous
Nuclear size	Uniform	Variable and enlarged
Nuclear membranes	Smooth, fine, and evenly distributed chromatin	Irregular, coarse, and clumped chromatin
Nucleoli	Absent	Present
Necrosis	Absent	Present
Myoepithelial cells	Present	Absent

the incidence of cancer is 0% to 0.6%. When the results of all three tests suggest malignancy, the incidence of cancer is 99% to 100%. If the three tests lack concurrence, then the possibility of malignancy is higher and a more definitive tissue diagnosis should be considered. This is particularly true in younger women, in whom mammography may be less sensitive.

Procedure

FNA is typically performed with a 10- or 20-mL syringe and a 21- to 27-gauge needle. Although some physicians prefer it, no local anesthesia is necessary because the injection of lidocaine may be more uncomfortable than the FNA itself. Furthermore, the anesthetic or a hematoma can obscure the mass. The patient should be resting comfortably in the supine position. The arm can be over the head or by the side, whichever is most comfortable for the patient and allows for the best delineation of the mass. The skin should be prepped with alcohol and sterile technique should be used. One hand is used to secure the mass while the other directs the needle. Care must taken so that the needle is not directed toward the chest wall, because pneumothorax is a possible complication. It is better to direct the needle tangentially.

Even though a syringe and needle is all that is necessary, it is technically easier to perform the procedure with a syringe holder that allows for suction to be applied to the syringe (Fig. 3-4). Withdraw the plunger to introduce air into the syringe. Advance the needle into the mass and then place full suction on the syringe. Immediately you may obtain fluid, signaling the presence of a cyst. Continue aspirating until no more fluid can be obtained and the mass has completely disappeared. If the aspirate is bloody or if the mass does not completely

disappear, the fluid should be sent for cytology. Otherwise, the routine cytologic analysis of cyst fluid is not necessary.

If no fluid is obtained, then the mass is solid. Keeping negative pressure on the syringe, the needle should be passed back and forth within the mass. Usually doing this within a single needle tract will give a satisfactory yield, but if no material is seen in the hub of the needle, the needle can be introduced at different angles. While doing this, the wrist should be rotated slightly so that the needle is twisting. Although some advocate keeping negative pressure on the syringe while withdrawing the needle from the mass, this is not necessary and may pull the specimen into the syringe, making it difficult to expel the cells. It is better to return the plunger to the 5-mL mark and withdraw the needle. The specimen can than be blown out onto a glass slide. The needle should touch the surface of the slide. A small drop (no greater than 5 mm in diameter) is expressed onto the slide. The slides are then smeared with a second glass slide. One slide is quickly sprayed with a fixative; the other is allowed to air-dry. A simpler option is to empty the contents of the syringe into CytoLyt solution or tissue culture medium. Tissue medium is preferred if fresh, unfixed cells may be necessary (e.g., for flow cytometry in the case of a potential lymphoma). In the cytopathology laboratory, cells are then collected from the medium with Nuclepore filtration or centrifugation, or they are prepared for a cell block for paraffin embedding. Complications of FNA are rare but can include hematoma, infection (mastitis), and pneumothorax.

Core-Needle Biopsy

Unlike FNA, which removes cells that require a cytopathologist to interpret, a core-needle

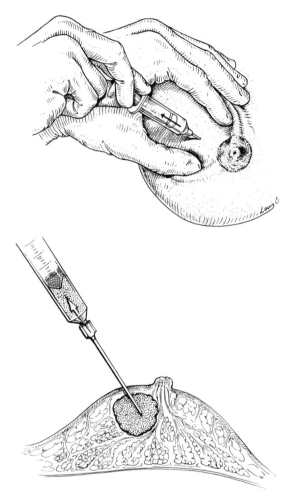

Figure 3–4. Fine needle aspiration of a breast mass. (From Bland KI, Karakousis CP, Copeland EM. Atlas of surgical oncology. Philadelphia: WB Saunders, 1995, Figure 8–3.)

biopsy provides material that can be interpreted by a pathologist. It uses a disposable, hand-held instrument that provides a 1- to 2-cm long specimen (14 to 18 gauge). Automated spring-loaded devices are the most convenient and have essentially replaced the hand-actuated core biopsy needles. The spring-loaded devices are not only simpler but also have a greater diagnostic accuracy. Core-needle biopsy is highly accurate, with false-positive results being rare. Treatment decisions, including mastectomy or neoadjuvant chemotherapy, can thus be based on a core-needle biopsy diagnosis. In addition, core-needle biopsy allows for the immunohistochemical staining of the specimen for hormone receptors, Her-2/neu, or other markers that may be important in clinical decision making (immunohistochemical staining [IHC] can be done on a cell block obtained from an FNA, but this is less reliable and not performed at all institutions). Core-needle biopsy can be

associated with a false-negative rate ranging from 1% to 20%. Much of this is secondary to missing the lesion with the device. This is less common for larger lesions. Some very firm lesions may be difficult to advance the needle into, also leading to a false-negative finding. If the mass is suspicious but the core-needle biopsy shows normal breast parenchyma or other discordant pathology, either an incisional or excisional biopsy is needed to make the diagnosis.

Procedure

Unlike FNA biopsy, core-needle biopsy is a slightly more invasive procedure and requires local anesthetic (Fig. 3–5). Before beginning, it is useful to outline the lesion with a water-soluble pen, then secure the mass with the nondominant hand and mark the location where the needle will be introduced. This site should be chosen so that the needle is not

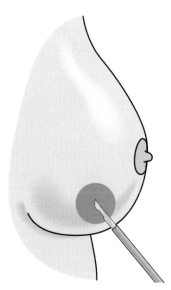

Figure 3–5. Core biopsy. (From Sabel M, Sondak V, Sussman J. Essentials of Surgical Oncology. Philadelphia: Elsevier, 2006.)

heading down toward the chest wall, but tangentially, to avoid pneumothorax. It should also be placed in a location that will be easy to excise if the mass proves to be a cancer. Once this is completed, the breast is prepped with iodine solution and sterilely draped. The skin at the site of entry is anesthetized with 1% lidocaine solution and an 11-blade is used to make a small puncture wound in the skin.

The mass is stabilized with the nondominant hand. The needle is then introduced into the mass and fired. It is withdrawn, opened, and the specimen retrieved and placed into fixative. This is repeated 2 to 5 times until an adequate specimen has been obtained. Hemostasis is then achieved by holding direct pressure for 5 minutes. The skin is reapproximated with a sterile adhesive dressing. The specimen container is immediately labeled with the patient's name, medical record number, and the site of the biopsy to avoid any chance of error. Complications include infection (mastitis), hematoma, and rarely pneumothorax.

Excisional Biopsy

Often, an excisional biopsy is necessary to diagnose a palpable mass. An excisional biopsy refers to the surgical removal of the entire mass, sometimes with a small rim of normal tissue around it. In many cases, this is driven by the patient, who wants the mass removed even if it is benign. Excisional biopsy is also indicated in patients for whom FNA biopsy

or core-needle biopsy was indeterminate or was unable to be performed. If the mass is small, or located in such a way that the surgeon cannot be confident that the biopsy device will truly sample the abnormality, an excisional biopsy might be a better option. Likewise, if the results of the biopsy of a suspicious mass are returned as "normal breast parenchyma," then this might indicate a missed biopsy and an excisional biopsy is indicated.

Excisional breast biopsies can be performed on an outpatient basis under local anesthesia alone or with intravenous (IV) sedation. General anesthesia is rarely necessary. A mixture of long-acting and short-acting local anesthetic is recommended, which greatly reduces the need for narcotics postoperatively. A combination of 5 mL of 1% lidocaine, 4 mL of 0.5% Marcaine, and 1 mL of 8.5% sodium bicarbonate provides excellent local anesthesia, extended pain control, and minimal discomfort during infiltration. Continued infiltration of the tissues throughout the procedure, especially posterior to the mass because this area does not typically get anesthetized initially, keeps the patient comfortable throughout the procedure.

It is imperative to remember that this mass could be cancer. Incisions should be placed with a subsequent reexcision lumpectomy or mastectomy in mind (Fig. 3–6). Circumareolar incisions are cosmetically pleasing and should be used whenever feasible, but excessive tunneling to get to the mass should be avoided. If the lesion is a cancer, excessive tunneling would make a reexcision lumpectomy difficult and negatively impact the final cosmetic result. Likewise, incisions placed at the very periphery of the breast may hide the incision, but they might be very difficult to incorporate in a standard mastectomy incision if that is ultimately required. If a circumareolar incision is not appropriate, a curvilinear incision along Langer lines is the best choice. Many surgeons prefer a radial incision when performing a lumpectomy for a cancer in the inferior half of the breast, particularly in the 6-o'clock position (see Chapter 12). This may be associated with a better cosmetic result after radiation therapy. If there is a high suspicion of cancer for a mass located in this position, it may be reasonable to use a radial incision for the excisional biopsy.

If there is even a minimal suspicion of cancer, a ridge of normal tissue should be taken with the mass. The specimen should be oriented for the pathologist. Using a long stitch to mark lateral, a short stitch to mark superior,

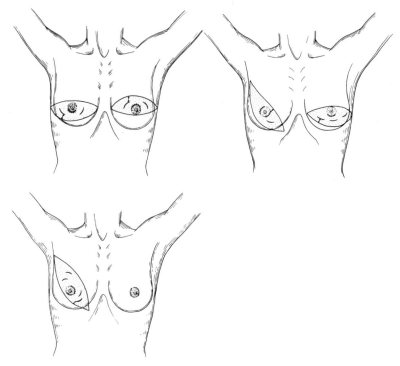

Figure 3-6. When marking out an incision for a breast biopsy, a subsequent reexcision lumpectomy or mastectomy should be kept in mind. Excessive tunneling should be avoided. Radial incisions in the inferior hemisphere of the breast may yield a better cosmetic outcome if cancer is highly suspected. (From Bland KI, Karakousis CP, Copeland EM. Atlas of surgical oncology, Philadelphia: WB Saunders, 1995, Figure 8–4.)

and a double stitch to mark deep will allow the pathologist to use a six-color inking system so that if it is cancer, the location of any close or positive margin can be identified (Fig. 3–7).

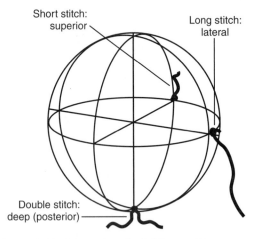

Figure 3-7. Orientation of a left breast biopsy specimen. The specimen should be oriented in three planes so that the pathologist can use a multicolor staining system to identify close or positive margins in case in situ or invasive cancer is diagnosed.

After hemostasis is assured, the wound is closed. No attempt to approximate the edges of the cavity should be attempted, nor should a drain be placed. Two layer closure with deep dermal sutures followed by either a subcuticular stitch or tissue adhesive is recommended for reapproximating the skin.

Incisional Biopsy

Incisional biopsy involves removing only a small part of a breast mass. In essence, a core-needle biopsy is a form of incisional biopsy, and for this reason true operative incisional biopsies have become much less common. Today, the only indication for performing an incisional biopsy are when a core-needle biopsy of a large breast mass fails to demonstrate a suspected malignancy, or demonstrates in situ disease for a suspected invasive cancer. In these cases, excision of the mass is not recommended as if it is invasive disease, and the patient may benefit from neoadjuvant chemotherapy and an attempt at breast conservation, whereas an excisional biopsy may commit the patient to mastectomy if it is cancer (see Chapter 18).

The same principles of excisional biopsy are applied to incisional biopsy. The site of the incision should be placed in a curvilinear fashion paralleling Langer lines in a way that it is easily reexcised with a subsequent lumpectomy or mastectomy. Hemostasis is crucial because a hematoma may not only complicate subsequent surgery, but also may spread malignant cells. Despite the need for hemostasis, it is better to perform the biopsy of the lesion with a scalpel because excess electrocautery artifact will distort the histology. Once the lesion is removed, electrocautery is used to obtain hemostasis, which may be difficult because open tumor surfaces tend to bleed quite a bit.

Breast Biopsies of Nonpalpable Lesions

With increased screening and improved detection of small abnormalities, the need for image-guided biopsies of nonpalpable lesions is increasing rapidly. Several methods exist for biopsy of nonpalpable lesions, and while these have typically been the domain of radiologists, breast surgeons are increasingly performing their own image-guided biopsies.

Ultrasound-Guided Biopsy

Ultrasound can be used to guide the placement of a biopsy needle into a sonographically evident mass. This is useful not only for nonpalpable ultrasound visible lesions, but also those lesions that are only vaguely palpable on physical examination, or have indiscrete margins, such that the surgeon is not confident that the biopsy device is within the abnormality. Ultrasound-guided biopsies is advantageous in that the patient does not need to lie on her stomach or have her breast compressed, and there is no associated radiation. Many radiologists feel that it is faster and easier than stereotactic biopsy. Today many surgeons, especially breast surgeons, have incorporated ultrasound into their practice. This allows for immediate, additional diagnostic information for the patient with a breast mass, as well as guidance for biopsies. Use of ultrasound to guide a biopsy, by allowing real-time visualization of the needle within the lesion, assures adequate sampling and improves accuracy.

A linear array transducer of at least 7.5 MHz or 10 MHz is recommended. The linear shape of the ultrasound beam allows for better visualization of both the needle and the lesion during the procedure. Before beginning the procedure, the surgeon should image the lesion and plan the approach. It is useful to mark the breast accordingly. The breast is prepped and then anesthetized. This should include both the site of the skin incision and the track that the needle will travel toward the mass. An 11-blade is used to make a small incision in the skin and the core biopsy device is introduced into the breast. With the lesion visualized, the needle is identified in the longitudinal plane and slowly advanced toward the lesion (Fig. 3–8). As with palpable biopsies, the needle should remain parallel to the chest wall

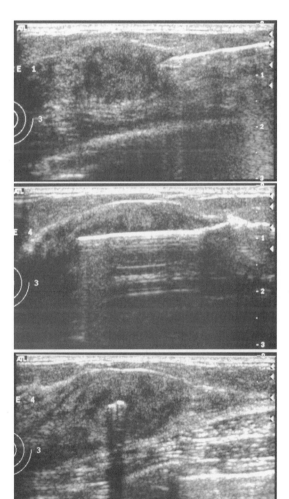

Figure 3–8. A, Image demonstrates predeployment of core-needle biopsy device. **B**, Postdeployment image demonstrates device in mass. **C**, Orthogonal projection documents biopsy device in mass. (Images courtesy of Dr. Alexis Nees, Department of Radiology, University of Michigan.)

to avoid pneumothorax. Once the needle is within the mass, its three-dimensional position in the mass can be assessed by turning the transducer 90 degrees to the trajectory. Once assured that it is in good position, the device is fired and withdrawn, and the specimen is retrieved. As with palpable masses, two to five specimens are taken, all through the single skin incision.

Stereotactic Core-Needle Biopsy

Stereotactic core-needle biopsy is indicated for any mammographically detected lesion that is not easily seen on ultrasound. Stereotactic mammography was introduced in Sweden in the 1970s and introduced in the United States in Chicago by Dr. Kambiz Dowlatshahi in 1980. At that time, stereotactic mammography was used to guide FNA biopsies and was accurate but limited by inadequate specimens. In the late 1980s, stereotactic biopsies using biopsy guns and large-gauge needles greatly increased the success rate, and this approach rapidly became accepted as an alternative to surgical excision. The use of stereotactic mammography to guide core-needle biopsies has greatly reduced the need for surgical biopsies of benign lesions and has minimized the number of operations needed for cancer patients. The ease and low morbidity of stereotactic biopsy has also increased the number of biopsies for BI-RADS 3 lesions, decreasing the chance of missed cancers. Overall, the procedure can be done in 30 minutes with a false-negative rate of less than 2%. Not all patients are candidates for stereotactic core-needle biopsy and may be better served by wire localization biopsy (Box 3–3).

The procedure may be performed with the patient upright or prone, but prone is preferred for keeping the patient stable during the procedure. The patient lies down on the table and the breast to be biopsied is placed through an opening (Fig. 3–9). Stereotactic localization is based on the principle of parallax. Two angled radiographic views acquired 15 degrees on either side of the center are used to determine the location of the lesion based on the "shift" between the two acquired views (Fig. 3–10). The breast is compressed between a compression paddle and a charge-coupled (CCD) plate. A scout image is taken to confirm the lesion is within the working window. The two angled views are taken and the computer then generates the three-dimensional coordinates of the target chosen by the radiologist. Small motors in the

BOX 3–3 CONTRAINDICATIONS TO STEREOTACTIC CORE BIOPSY

- Patients who cannot lie prone for up to 45 minutes (patients with back, neck, or shoulder problems)
- Patients who cannot keep still for up to 45 minutes (anxiety, chronic cough, neurologic or musculoskeletal problems)
- Weight greater than tolerated by the stereotactic machine (typically more than 300 lb)
- Lesions too close to the chest wall or axilla to be accessed by the biopsy needle
- Indiscrete lesions or faint microcalcifications not seen clearly on stereotactic imaging
- Lesions uncomfortably close to blood vessels or breast implants
- Breast compresses to less than 2 cm from the chest wall

table align the vertical and horizontal positions of the biopsy sled. The depth is set by the radiologist using information from the computer.

Once the target is set, the skin and the projected path of the needle are anesthetized. A small incision in the skin is made and the needle is inserted to the determined depth. Two more offset images are taken to confirm placement and the device is fired. There are a number of biopsy instruments available for stereotactic biopsy, including spring-loaded and vacuum-assisted devices and axial coring devices. Several specimens are obtained. Some radiologists have recommended that for spring-loaded devices, at least five 14-gauge cores should be taken for accurate sampling, more for microcalcifications or if a smaller gauge needle is used. The vacuum-assisted devices are typically larger; most operators use an 11-gauge needle, although the same minimal number of cores should be taken. When the target of the biopsy is the microcalcifications, these are radiographed to confirm their removal. Once assured that an adequate biopsy has been performed, a tissue marking clip should be placed at the site of the biopsy so that the area can be easily targeted in the future in case the lesion requires reexcision. Postprocedural mammograms (craniocaudal and mediolateral oblique) confirm that the correct site was sampled and the clip is in the correct spot. Complications include infections, hematoma, and bleeding,

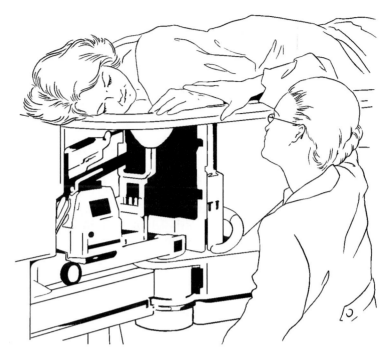

Figure 3–9. Patient undergoing a stereotactic core breast biopsy.

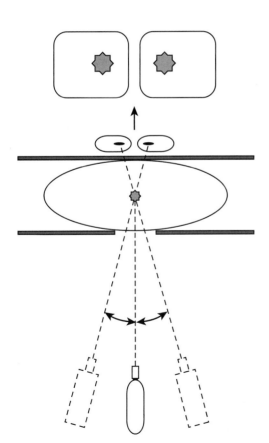

Figure 3–10. Triangulation of the depth of a lesion using two views. (From Bland KI, Copeland EM III. The breast, 3rd ed. Philadelphia: WB Saunders, 2004.)

There are several pathologic results obtained by stereotactic core-needle biopsy that require a follow-up wire-localized excision of the area (Box 3–4). A biopsy demonstrating atypical ductal hyperplasia (ADH), atypical lobular hyperplasia (ALH), or LCIS may harbor an in situ or invasive component missed by the core-needle biopsy (Chapter 8). The chance of this occurring ranges from 4% to 40% depending on the size of the needle and the number of biopsy specimens obtained. Papillary lesions diagnosed as benign papillomas by image-guided biopsy may in fact be a papillary carcinoma. Likewise, radial scars may harbor unrecognized atypical hyperplasia or malignancy. Some radiologists recommend routine excision of these lesions when

BOX 3–4 BENIGN LESIONS FOR WHICH A WIRE-LOCALIZED BIOPSY AFTER STEREOTACTIC CORE-NEEDLE BIOPSY IS RECOMMENDED

- Atypical ductal hyperplasia
- Atypical lobular hyperplasia
- Lobular carcinoma in situ
- Sclerosing adenosis (selective)
- Papillary lesions (selective vs. routine)
- Radial scar (selective vs. routine)
- Discordant finding

diagnosed by core-needle biopsy, whereas some suggest selective excision based on the degree of suspicion. Another indication for a follow-up excisional biopsy is that of a discordant finding, meaning the histologic findings do not correlate with the appearance of the lesion on mammography. These topics will be discussed later in the chapter.

Wire-Localized Excisional Biopsy

As discussed, not all nonpalpable lesions are amenable to an image-guided biopsy, and some needle biopsies will need follow-up excisional biopsies to confirm the diagnosis. This is typically accomplished by a using wire localization to guide the biopsy. Wire-localized biopsy (also referred to as a needle-localized biopsy) requires a coordination of radiology and surgery, although more breast surgeons are performing their own localizations. Localization involves placing a rigid introducer needle with a flexible hooked wire inside of it at the site of the abnormality (or of a clip left after a prior core-needle biopsy) using either biplanar mammography or ultrasound. Ultrasound is relatively simpler and more comfortable for the patient, so if the lesion is ultrasound visible, this method is preferred. Sometimes it is difficult to perform a specimen ultrasound and confirm removal of the lesion, so it may be wise to place a small clip in the lesion under ultrasound guidance before needle localization. In this manner, the specimen may be radiographed to confirm removal of the clip and lesion.

Once the rigid needle is in place, it is withdrawn, leaving the hooked wire in place. The hook keeps the wire in place so it is not easily moved. Even so, the external wire should be secured to the skin so that it is not dislodged as the patient travels from radiology to the operating room. The craniocaudal and mediolateral views of the wire in place accompany the patient to the operating room.

The procedure can be performed under local anesthesia alone or with local anesthesia and IV sedation. Care should be taken not to dislodge the wire when removing the covering dressing and prepping and draping the breast. The same principles of incision placement that hold true for other types of biopsy are in play when performing a wire-localized biopsy. The incision should be curvilinear in Langer lines and created with a subsequent lumpectomy or mastectomy in mind. The incision should be placed over the abnormality and not routinely made at the site of wire entry (Fig. 3–11). Although this may be acceptable for a superficial lesion, in other cases this may lead to excessive tunneling to reach the lesion. This not only results in the removal of excess tissue but complicates a subsequent reexcision if cancer is detected. Instead, the surgeon should use the wire and images to determine the site of the abnormality and place the incision directly over this.

The direction of the dissection is determined by the lesion size, direction of the wire, and the relative proximity of the wire to the lesion. Wires placed just posterior to the lesion are helpful in that the surgeon is assured removal

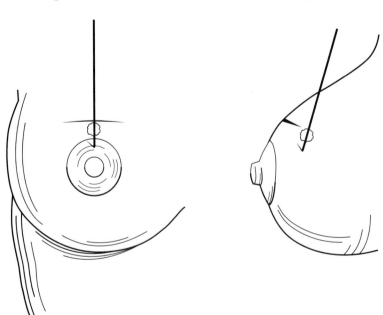

Figure 3–11. Wire-localized excisional biopsy. The placement of the incision and direction of the dissection are determined by the location and direction of the wire and the relative proximity of the wire to the lesion. It is usually best to place the incision over the anticipated site of the abnormality rather than tunneling a long distance along the wire.

of the lesion by staying just deep to the localization needle. Once the incision is made, it is then necessary to identify the shaft of the lesion and retract it into the wound. Dissection in the plane facing the wire entry site allows for simple detection of the wire. Once identified, it is secured at the site of the parenchyma and the distal end of the wire is brought out into the wound. Failure to adequately secure the wire may result in accidental dislodgement. Once out, the tissue is grasped with an Allis clamp. It is preferable to grab the tissue near the wire but not the wire itself, because pulling too hard on the clamp may pull the wire from the specimen. Resection of the tissue surrounding the wire proceeds. The relationship between the wire and the lesion, as demonstrated on mammography, will help guide how much tissue to take. Because the purpose of this operation is solely diagnostic, every attempt is made to remove just enough tissue to make the diagnosis. Staying approximately 1 cm around the wire and going just past the hook of the wire should accomplish this, although this depends on the position of the wire relative to the lesion.

Immediately upon removal of the specimen, it is held in anatomic position and marked with orientation sutures. It is also helpful to place clips at the periphery of the specimen to allow for orientation of the specimen radiograph. These may help guide the excision of additional tissue if the lesion is not present or if margins are a concern. Before sending the specimen to radiology, it is prudent to examine it along with the specimen cavity, so that you may gain an idea of where the lesion might be if it has not been excised. For example, if on examining the specimen you appear to be close to the wire inferiorly, you can place a small clip at the corresponding area in the cavity. If the radiograph fails to show the lesion, you can reexcise that area and send the second specimen to radiology.

As stated, the specimen is sent to radiology for confirmation that the lesion in question was removed. If the wire was dislodged from the specimen, it should still be sent for confirmation that the entire wire was removed. During this time, hemostasis is assured and the skin closed (it can easily be reopened if additional tissue needs to be removed). If the abnormality has been removed, the procedure is over. If the specimen radiograph does not show the lesion, then additional tissue can be excised and sent for radiography. As stated, this may be greatly facilitated by examining the specimen and the cavity before sending it, and by placing clips on the specimen to orient the tissue on the x-ray films. If the surgeon does not know where to reexcise or if a repeated attempt at reexcision failed to excise the lesion, intraoperative ultrasound may be used to identify the lesion, assuming it is ultrasound visible. If not, it may be prudent to end the case and plan on a repeat localization and biopsy in the future. Patients should be counseled that, while rare, this possibility does exist.

MRI-Guided Biopsy

The use of MRI in the diagnosis and staging of breast cancer has expanded over the past several years. MRI is being increasingly used to screen high-risk women, stage the extent of established malignancies, and look for synchronous cancers in the ipsilateral or contralateral breast. The pros and cons of MRI for these situations are discussed in Chapter 2. However, the increased sensitivity of MRI means that there will be more lesions detected that are not visible on mammography and ultrasound. Furthermore, the variable specificity of MRI means many of these lesions will be benign, and biopsy is essential before changing surgical management. This has increased the need for MRI-guided biopsy. Unfortunately, many institutions performing MRI do not have the capability to perform MRI-guided biopsy, leaving some women in a difficult situation. As compared with mammography or ultrasound, variances in MRI equipment, imaging protocols, and interpretation criteria make it very difficult for one institution to evaluate and biopsy a lesion seen on MRI at a different institution. For this reason, it is recommended that breast MRI not be performed at institutions that do not have the capability to do MRI biopsies.

The first step when a suspicious lesion is detected on MRI is to repeat mammogram and ultrasound in the area of the lesion to determine whether a lesion can be detected. With directed ultrasound, the lesion can often be identified, which allows for ultrasound-guided biopsy. If imaging fails to demonstrate the lesion, MRI-guided biopsy is indicated. This requires a high-field-strength magnet (1 to 1.5 T), a specialized breast coil for imaging, a breast biopsy coil, and MRI-compatible needles. Before biopsy, an MRI is obtained that incorporates a copper sulfate marker that is visible on MRI. In this way, the lesion's position can be calculated relative to the marker using three-dimensional images of the breast. The patient is positioned prone with slight compression (less than necessary for stereotactic biopsy). Needle placement is performed with the patient outside of the magnet using MRI compatible (titanium) needles. The patient is then returned to the magnet and images are obtained for confirmation of needle placement within the abnormality. Once confirmed, sufficient samples are taken outside of the bore of the magnet and a clip is deployed at the site, which allows for mammogram-directed localization in case excision is necessary.

Management of Benign Breast Masses

As stated earlier, the majority of breast masses evaluated in the clinic will be benign. Benign lesions are typically categorized as those with minimal proliferation, proliferative lesions without atypia, and proliferative lesions with atypia (Table 3–5). Once the diagnosis is made, the management depends on the proliferative nature of the lesion, the concerns of the patient, the implications for future risk of breast cancer, and the possibility of a misdiagnosis. The management of the most common benign lesions is discussed here. The management of proliferative lesions with atypia, which imply an increased risk of breast cancer, is discussed in Chapter 8.

Fibroadenoma

Fibroadenomas are an extremely common condition of early reproductive life. A fibroadenoma is a benign tumor that forms from the stroma of the lobules of the breast. This is why fibroadenomas are most common between the ages of 15 and 25 years, when lobular development is most active. As opposed to other benign tumors, fibroadenomas do not tend to continue to grow progressively. Most reach 1 to 2 cm in size and then remain stable, or in some cases regress. Some continue to enlarge. They are very sensitive to hormones, which accounts for why many women notice that they get larger with the menstrual cycle and quickly shrink at the conclusion of menstruation. At menopause, fibroadenomas may involute, turning into a mass of hyaline fibrous tissue, possibly with coarse popcorn-like calcifications.

The typical presentation of a fibroadenoma is that of a firm, nontender, highly mobile round or lobulated mass. Often, a breast mass in a woman younger than 35 years is highly characteristic of a fibroadenoma on physical examination and breast imaging. On mammography, fibroadenomas may appear as a well-marginated density against a radiolucent background, although the dense breast tissue of young women often occlude the fibroadenoma (Fig. 3–12). On ultrasound, the presence of internal echoes can differentiate between a fibroadenoma and a cyst (Fig. 3–13). If a mass in a woman younger than 40 has all of these characteristics, is a biopsy mandatory? Some studies have shown that this type of lesion is benign more than 99% of the time, and so a small fraction of clinicians opt for careful observation without biopsy. The patient should return for a repeat clinical examination in 4 to

TABLE 3–5 • *Classification of Benign Breast Lesions*		
Proliferation	**Type**	**Risk**
Minimal	Fibrocystic changes Ductal ectasia Nonsclerosing adenosis Periductal fibrosis Hamartoma Lipoma Hematoma Fat necrosis Granuloma Mastitis Diabetic mastopathy	No increased risk of breast cancer
Proliferative without atypia	Fibroadenoma Usual ductal hyperplasia Sclerosing adenosis Papilloma Radial scar Blunt duct adenosis	Small increased risk of breast cancer
Proliferative with atypia	Atypical ductal hyperplasia Atypical lobular hyperplasia Lobular carcinoma in situ	Moderate increased risk (see Chapter 8)

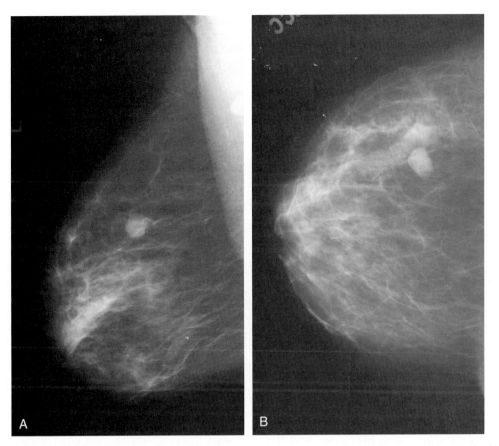

Figure 3–12. Mediolateral-oblique and craniocaudal mammographic views demonstrate circumscribed oval mass in the upper outer quadrant of the left breast. (Images courtesy of Dr. Alexis Nees, Department of Radiology, University of Michigan.)

6 months and consideration should be made for repeat ultrasound to assure stability of the lesion. Most surgeons believe that a biopsy is always warranted. This can be either a core biopsy or FNA, depending mostly on the skill of the cyto-pathologist and the confidence of the surgeon that the biopsy was truly from the mass. Fine-needle aspirates typically contain a high number of ductal and stromal cells. Bare nuclei in stag-horn configurations are characteristic. If a mass is confirmed to be a fibroadenoma, the patient should be followed up with either physical examination or ultrasound to confirm stability. If the mass remains stable in size over 2 years, no further follow-up should be necessary. Although unsuspected cancer can be found within a fibroadenoma, this is quite rare and occurs usually in women older than 50 years of age.

Fibroadenomas either stay stable, decrease in size, completely resolve, or get larger. Occasionally fibroadenomas can grow quite large. These are typically referred to as "giant" or "juvenile" fibroadenomas. Occasionally an enlarging fibroadenoma can in reality be a phyllodes tumor. For these reasons, fibroade-nomas that are rapidly enlarging or that have enlarged more than 20% while being observed should be excised. This can typically be done under local anesthesia, although IV sedation is helpful when the mass is quite large. When excising a fibroadenoma, surgeons may mis-take the dense fibroglandular tissue in a young woman for the fibroadenoma, and begin the excision before the tumor is actually reached. Because there is no need to take a margin of normal tissue (recurrence is very low), dissec-tion should continue toward the mass until the capsule is clearly identified and bulging into the field. After assuring hemostasis, only the skin and subcutaneous tissues need be closed. Closing the defect in the breast paren-chyma will abnormally distort the breast. The defect will close naturally over time, even after the excision of a large fibroadenoma.

Cryoablation has recently been described for the eradication of fibroadenomas after establish-ing the diagnosis by core needle biopsy. This is an office-based, minimally invasive procedure in which a small probe is placed into the center

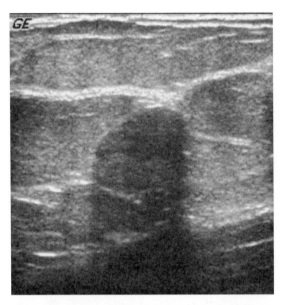

Figure 3-13. Ultrasound demonstrates a circumscribed hypoechoic oval mass with long axis parallel to the chest wall. Note the associated posterior shadowing. Pathology from ultrasound-guided core-needle biopsy confirmed diagnosis of fibroadenoma. (Image courtesy of Dr. Alexis Nees, Department of Radiology, University of Michigan.)

of the fibroadenoma under ultrasound guidance (Fig. 3–14). Argon gas flows through the probe, dropping the temperature of the tip to −196°C, generating an ice ball that encompasses the mass. After thawing, the probe is removed. Over time the fibroadenoma resolves spontaneously.

Adenomas can occur in the breast. These are similar to fibroadenomas (well-circumscribed,

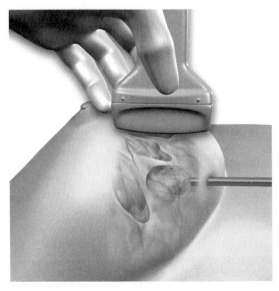

Figure 3-14. Cryoablation of a fibroadenoma (Image courtesy of Sanarus Medical, Inc.)

benign) but differ in that they have sparse, inconspicuous stroma. Tubular adenomas tend to occur in young women and are similar in presentation to fibroadenomas—that of a well-defined, mobile nodule. Lactating adenomas present as a mobile mass during pregnancy or in the postpartum period.

Cysts

Cysts are extremely common, fluid-filled epithelialized spaces. They are usually multifocal and bilateral and vary greatly in size and number. They are typically round with a flattened epithelium surrounding fluid that can range from yellow to green to brown. Whereas most cysts contain 5 to 10 mL of fluid, some cysts can contain more than 75 mL. The surrounding stroma is generally fibrotic and can show an inflammatory infiltrate.

The exact mechanism by which cysts originate is unclear. With the menstrual cycle, the breast stroma and epithelium undergo repeated integrated involution, and cysts appear to be a by-product of abnormalities of this process. Cysts originate from the terminal duct lobular unit or from an obstructed duct. If the stroma surrounding a lobular unit involutes too quickly, the epithelial acini remain and can form microcysts. These are the precursors to macrocysts.

Patients may present with a single or multiple asymptomatic masses or a tender, painful mass. Cysts are easily taken care of through aspiration. When a woman presents with a mass in the breast that is likely a cyst, the first question is whether to proceed directly to breast imaging or to aspiration. If directed imaging is immediately available, many radiologists prefer to image breast masses before aspiration because the aspiration can produce artifacts that make assessment more difficult. After imaging, the patient should return to the office for aspiration if the lesion is a true simple cyst. However, if the cyst is causing discomfort to the patient and obtaining an image can't be done that day, it is reasonable to proceed with aspiration as the first step.

After prepping the breast, a 21-gauge needle on a 10- or 20-mL syringe is placed into the cyst. The opposite hand should be used to secure the mass because it is often quite mobile. This is greatly facilitated by the use of devices that hold the syringe and allow for one-handed aspiration. If the fluid is consistent with a cyst, it should be aspirated until no more fluid is obtained and the cyst has completely disappeared. There is no need to send this fluid for cytology.

If the fluid that returns is bloody, then after aspirating 1 to 2 mL for cytology, the aspiration should be stopped. If no fluid returns, then the procedure can be easily converted to an FNAB. If after aspiration there is still a residual mass, the patient should be sent for imaging (if not already done). If a cystic mass is still present, ultrasound-guided aspiration can complete the process. If there is a solid component, image-guided or open biopsy should be performed as indicated. If not already done, the patient should be sent for imaging and subsequent tissue biopsy of the lesion. The biggest risk in aspirating a mass without preprocedural imaging is that it might be a complex cyst or cystic-solid mass that might be a cancer. Completely aspirating a bloody cyst, leaving no simple method for identifying the lesion on imaging or physical examination if the cytology is atypical, could lead to trouble in making a diagnosis. Likewise, ignoring a residual mass after cyst aspiration could lead to a delay in diagnosis of a malignant lesion.

It is not uncommon for cysts to recur after aspiration. A repeat aspiration is reasonable, assuming the fluid is not bloody and the cyst continues to completely resolve after aspiration. However, cysts that continue to recur should be excised.

Lipoma

Lipomas are soft or semifirm, well-marginated masses that may feel either smooth or lobulated. They are composed of mature fat cells and may occur anywhere on the body, including the breast. The typical physical findings strongly support the diagnosis, especially if the mass has been present for a considerable time or other similar masses are present elsewhere in the breast or rest of the body. If physical examination is consistent with a lipoma, these may be safely observed. Needle biopsy is not usually helpful because the mass provides little resistance to the needle, making it difficult to be sure the biopsy came from the mass. The cytology shows normal fat cells, so it is unclear whether this was a lipoma or the examiner missed the mass. If there is any question about the diagnosis, if the lipoma is enlarging, or if the patient is bothered by its presence, excision is recommended. Lipomas are usually well-circumscribed and can be easily excised through a small incision. However, incomplete excision can be associated with recurrence. Angiolipomas and angiomyolipomas are other benign masses of the breast,

comprised of both fat and mesenchymal tissues, which are also easily taken care of by complete excision. There is minimal distinction between these and lipomas.

Hamartoma

Hamartomas are encapsulated tumors that contain an abnormal mix of normal mammary tissues. They can grow quite large, often presenting as a discrete, mobile mass. On mammograms, hamartomas often have a distinctive appearance; they are smoothly marginated and separated from the surrounding breast by a lucent halo (Fig. 3–15). This has been described as a "breast within a breast." If they are asymptomatic and not bothering the patient, and if a definitive diagnosis can be made based on mammography and biopsy, then observation is an option because these are invariably benign. If the diagnosis is uncertain or if the patient is bothered, excision is recommended.

Trauma/Hematoma/Fat Necrosis

Many women will sustain a trauma to the breast that will leave a mass in the breast, either a hematoma or fat necrosis. Hematomas typically present as the result of trauma or iatrogenic injury. Spontaneous hematomas are extremely rare. The mass is typically painful and associated with ecchymosis. One of the biggest mistakes that can be made is to assume that a mass present in the breast after a trauma is a hematoma and to ignore it. Often a minor trauma will simply alert a patient to the presence of a mass that was there before the event. This is especially true if there is ecchymosis associated with the mass.

If a hematoma is obvious, such as that caused by an iatrogenic injury, the hematoma will resolve with time. Treatment includes a good supportive bra and analgesics. Expanding hematomas require surgical evacuation and hemostasis. Likewise, conservative management of a hematoma after a reported trauma is reasonable if the story matches the physical findings. Immediate imaging can be painful and it is reasonable to avoid it. However, careful follow-up is mandatory to assure that the hematoma is resolving. If there is any question of a residual mass or a failure to resolve, imaging and biopsy is recommended. Likewise, if the story and the findings raise any suspicion of malignancy, a thorough evaluation is warranted.

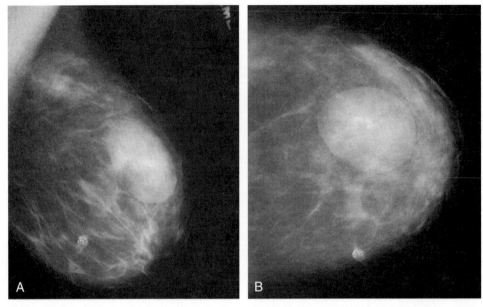

Figure 3–15. Mediolateral-oblique and craniocaudal mammographic images demonstrate circumscribed mixed density fat-containing mass. This is a fibroadenolipoma or breast hamartoma. (Images courtesy of Dr. Alexis Nees, Department of Radiology, University of Michigan.)

Fat necrosis is the result of saponification of fat after trauma. Fat necrosis is relatively uncommon but can often be confused for an invasive cancer. Sometimes, fat necrosis is found in the acute setting, with an identifiable traumatic event associated with it. Biopsy at this time will show the characteristic inflammatory changes with a preponderance of lymphocytes and histiocytes. Often, however, the later stages of fat necrosis may present as a mass in the breast without any recalled trauma by the patient. At this later stage, the predominant histologic finding is collagenous scar, with granular histiocytes surrounding oil cysts. Oil cysts contain the free lipid material released by lipocyte necrosis.

As with hematoma, if there is a strong history for trauma along with characteristic imaging (e.g., an oil cyst), then observation is reasonable. However, if there is any question of possible malignancy, and with fat necrosis it is often difficult to differentiate the two without histology, then biopsy is warranted.

Diabetic Mastopathy

Diabetic mastopathy is a breast mass consisting of fibrous breast tissue associated with long-standing type 1 or type 2 diabetes. The lesion is a combination of connective tissue overgrowth, lobular atrophy, and infiltration of predominately B lymphocytes. A classic histologic feature is fibroblasts set within a keloid-like dense fibrous stroma. The exact mechanism remains unknown and is not related to poor control of the diabetes. In fact, these changes can sometimes be seen in patients without diabetes.

Diabetic mastopathy often presents as a slightly irregular, dense mass. This can be diffuse and bilateral. Mammography is often normal but ultrasound features are worrisome for malignancy. Core biopsy is recommended for definitive diagnosis because surgical excision is not recommended if the diagnosis is confirmed on needle biopsy. Excision is associated with a high rate of recurrence.

Sclerosing Adenosis and Radial Scar

There are several benign findings of the breast that are generally categorized as proliferative lesions without atypia. These include usual ductal hyperplasia, intraductal papillomas, sclerosing adenosis, and radial scars. Although these lesions are all benign, they may be associated with an increased risk of developing breast cancer, approximately 1.5 to 2.0 times that of the general population. *Sclerosing adenosis* is a distortion of epithelial, myoepithelial, and stromal elements arising in a terminal duct lobular unit. It is often an incidental finding but may present as a mammographic finding or occasionally a palpable mass (which is often referred to as an adenosis tumor or nodular adenosis). The stroma of sclerosing adenosis is fibrotic or sclerotic, hence the name. Its appearance and sometimes histology may be confused with invasive cancer, although an experienced pathologist should be able to differentiate the two.

Radial scars may also be incidental findings, but more commonly present as either palpable masses or as a spiculated density on mammography. It is because the lesions are spiculated that they are difficult to differentiate from cancer. They incorporate several very deformed lobular units around a major stem of the ductal system, which is the likely origin of the abnormality. The exact pathogenesis of radial scars is unknown. They are characterized by a central scar from which these elements radiate. On gross examination, they are irregular, gray-white, and indurated with central retraction. This appearance is very similar to scirrhous carcinoma. Histologically, they show focal dense fibrosis associated with centrifugal dispersion of epithelium. They are sometimes fixed to the overlying skin, further raising the suspicion of cancer.

Both radial scars and sclerosing adenosis may be involved by atypical hyperplasia, LCIS or even DCIS or invasive cancer, although this is rare. It is clear that both lesions increase the subsequent risk of breast cancer. However, the presence of a radial scar may be a stronger risk factor than that of sclerosing adenosis, with an increased risk of 3.0 compared with 1.5 for adenosis. Radial scars with atypical hyperplasia have a relative risk of 5.8, which increases to 8.8 if the lesions are greater than 4 mm. Some investigators have suggested that radial scars may be precursors to cancer, citing the similar appearance, the correlation of size with risk, and the occasional finding of atypia, in situ or invasive disease within a radial scar. However, there is no clear evidence that these are premalignant lesions.

Because both of these lesions appear suspicious on mammography, biopsy is mandated. The biggest question is whether needle biopsy is adequate. If a core-needle biopsy is performed and the results show sclerosing adenosis or radial scar, should a subsequent wire-localized excisional biopsy be performed to rule out an underlying atypical hyperplasia, DCIS, or invasive cancer? This depends on the appearance of the lesion on mammography, whether the entire lesion and/or calcifications were removed by the percutaneous biopsy, and the histopathologic evaluation. For sclerosing adenosis, if the mass is circumscribed or indistinctly marginated and the core biopsy demonstrates sclerosing adenosis, then it may be reasonable to watch this. If it is enlarging, however, on short-term follow-up mammogram, excision is warranted. If it is a speculated mass, if there are fine linear or branching calcifications or calcifications in a segmental or linear distribution, or if the biopsy suggests radial scar, excision is recommended. For this reason, when radial scar is suspected at presentation, it is prudent to proceed directly to excisional biopsy, forgoing core-needle biopsy. Although there may be some cases in which a radial scar diagnosed by needle biopsy may be observed, this requires careful review and communication between the radiologist, the pathologist, the surgeon, and the patient.

Although the presence of these lesions does increase the risk of breast cancer, in the absence of atypia, the magnitude of this risk probably does not justify risk reduction counseling. If atypia is present, the patient should be referred for counseling and consideration of chemoprevention.

Papilloma and Papillomatosis

Papillary lesions of the breast are not well understood because they are relatively uncommon and incorporate a spectrum of lesions. These include single benign papillomas, papillomatosis, atypical papillomas, papillary DCIS, and invasive papillary carcinoma. Papillomas appear to be formed from hyperplasia of the duct epithelium supported by a fibrovascular core. This results in a pedunculated, friable tumor within the duct. They grow to about 1 cm in size, dilating the duct, and the friable epithelium often bleeds, causing a spontaneous bloody nipple discharge. Sometimes a palpable mass can be felt near the nipple, and gentle pressure on it causes the discharge. They are primarily in one duct, usually in the major ducts beneath or within a few centimeters of the nipple, but they can be more distant, multiple, or in both breasts. When papillomas are located in the periphery of the breast and are associated with the terminal duct-lobular units, they are usually multiple and are often labeled as diffuse papillomatosis. Whereas papillomas can present clinically as a palpable mass or bloody nipple discharge, they may also be clinically occult, detected as an abnormal density on breast imaging.

For the patient who presents with clinical symptoms, ultrasound can often demonstrate the lesion, as well as the dilated duct (Fig. 3–16). Ductography is the best test, which demonstrates

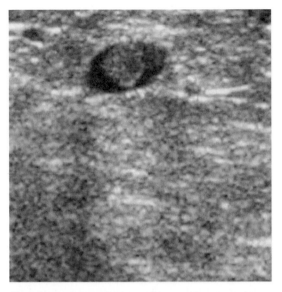

Figure 3–16. Transverse ultrasound image shows dilated duct with intraductal mass. Pathology confirmed papilloma. (Image courtesy of Dr. Alexis Nees, Department of Radiology, University of Michigan.)

a filling defect within the ductal system after cannulating and injecting the duct in question with radiocontrast (Fig. 3–17). They may also be diagnosed by ductoscopy in the patient with a bloody nipple discharge (see Chapter 5).

Even though papillomas are benign, they can be associated with an increased risk of a subsequent breast cancer. The likelihood of a future breast cancer correlates with the degree of atypia. The presence of a single papilloma without atypical hyperplasia carries little risk of cancer. The presence of atypical hyperplasia in the epithelium or the presence of multiple papillomas (for which atypia is more commonly seen) may be associated with a higher risk of cancer. Juvenile papillomatosis (Swiss cheese disease) affects young women (mean age 23) and features atypical hyperplasia and multiple lesions. This is associated with a high risk of cancer; in 4% of patients cancer is found concurrently with the papillomatosis.

Clinically occult papillary lesions diagnosed by core-needle biopsy are rare, representing less

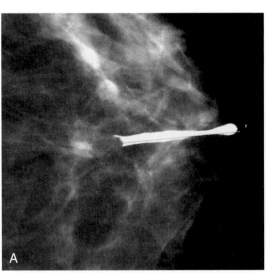

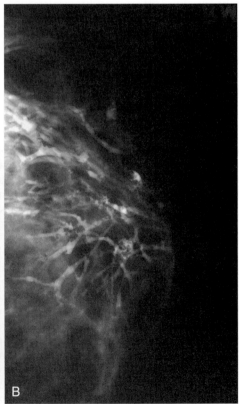

Figure 3–17. A, Image from ductogram demonstrates filling defect with "cut-off sign." Pathology at excision demonstrated papilloma. **B,** Ductogram demonstrates multiple intraductal filling defects. Pathology demonstrated high nuclear grade ductal carcinoma in situ. (Images courtesy of Dr. Alexis Nees, Department of Radiology, University of Michigan.)

than 0.2% of core-needle biopsies. When the lesion was subsequently excised, cancer was revealed in 0% to 50% of cases, usually, but not always, among papillomas containing atypia. For this reason, it is generally recommended that any papillary lesion diagnosed by core-needle biopsy be excised to rule out malignancy.

Likewise, for patients with symptomatic papillomas, treatment is complete excision. If the lesion can be localized by physical examination, imaging, or ductoscopy, then just the duct containing the papilloma can be excised. In the patient with bloody nipple discharge but no identifiable mass, a complete duct excision may be necessary. This will not only secure the diagnosis and rule out malignancy, but also eliminate the discharge. If there is no atypia associated with the lesion, no further treatment is necessary. However, for the patient with associated atypia, risk reduction counseling should be considered. In this case, the benefits of chemoprevention may be comparable to patients with ADH, although there is not enough data to be sure of this.

Suggested Readings

1. Carty NJ, Carter C, Rubin C, et al. Management of fibroadenoma of the breast. Ann R Coll Surg Engl 1995;77:127.
2. Courtillot C, Plu-Bureau G, Binart N, et al. Benign breast diseases. J Mammary Gland Biol Neoplasia. 2005;10(4):325–d335.
3. Gordon PB, Gagnon FA, Lanzkowsky L. Solid breast masses diagnosed as fibroadenoma at fine-needle aspiration biopsy: Acceptable rates of growth at long-term follow-up. Radiology 2003;229:233.
4. Hartmann LC, Sellars TA, Frost MH. Benign breast disease and the risk of breast cancer. N Engl J Med 2005;353:229.
5. Hartmann LC, Sellers TA, Frost MH, et al. Benign breast disease and the risk of breast cancer. N Engl J Med 2005;353:229.
6. Ibarra JA. Papillary lesions of the breast. Breast J 2006;12(3):237–251.
7. Kaufman CS. Office-based cryoablation of breast fibroadenomas: 12-month followup. J Am Coll Surg 2004;198:914.
8. Kudva YC, Reynolds CA, O'Brian T, Crotty TB. Mastopathy and diabetes. Curr Diabetes Rep 2003; 3(1):56–59.
9. Littrup PJ, Freeman-Gibb L, Andea A, et al. Cryotherapy for breast fibroadenomas. Radiology 2005; 234:63.
10. Santen RJ, Mancel R. Benign breast disorders. N Engl J Med 2005;353:275.
11. Sydnor MK, Wilson JD, Hijaz TA, et al. Underestimation of the presence of breast carcinoma in papillary lesions initially diagnosed at core-needle biopsy. Radiology 2007;242:58.
12. Valdes EK, Feldman SM, Boolbol SK. Papillary lesions: A review of the literature. Ann Surg Oncol 2007;14:1009.

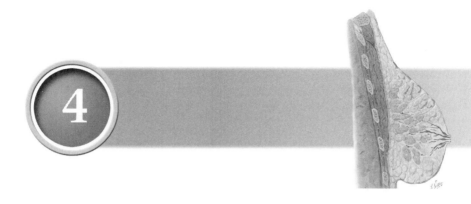

Breast Pain and Fibrocystic Disease

ETIOLOGY OF CYCLIC
MASTALGIA

EVALUATION OF BREAST PAIN

TREATMENT OPTIONS
Reassurance

Nonhormonal Therapies
Hormonal Therapies
Surgery for Mastalgia

Breast Pain and Fibrocystic Disease: Key Points

Understand the various etiologies of breast pain and the differences
in presentation of cyclic mastalgia, noncyclic mastalgia and
extramammary pain.

Appreciate the suggested relationships between fibrocystic disease,
hormones, and dietary factors.

Describe the thorough evaluation of the woman with breast pain.

Develop an algorithm for the treatment of the woman with cyclic mastalgia.

Breast pain is a frequent reason for office visits to family doctors, internists, gynecologists, and surgeons. It is common in women, but occasionally occurs in men. Depending on the population studied and how breast pain is defined, more than half the population has at least mild symptoms of breast pain. Fortunately, only a small percentage of patients with breast pain seek treatment. The role of the diagnostician is to determine whether this pain is pathologic or physiologic, related to hormonal fluctuation, and whether the severity warrants therapy.

Although breast pain is rarely associated with malignancy and is usually self-limited, it is of significant concern to patients. Mild breast pain spontaneously resolves in 9 out of 10 patients, and even severe breast pain resolves in more than half of patients.

There are three categories of mastalgia: cyclic mastalgia, noncyclic mastalgia, and extramammary pain (Box 4–1). Cyclic breast pain is typically an extreme form of the normal breast fullness present in the late luteal phase of the cycle.

BOX 4-1 CATEGORIES OF BREAST PAIN

- Cyclical breast pain
- Noncyclic breast pain
- Extramammary pain

Etiology of Cyclic Mastalgia

The exact etiology of breast pain remains in question. Mastalgia is often referred to as a component of "fibrocystic disease," although this nomenclature is confusing. For one thing, fibrocystic changes in the breast are normal and so it is misleading to refer to this as a disease. Postmortem studies show that fibrocystic changes occur in most if not all women. It also suggests that there is a histologic change that occurs in the breast that triggers the pain. However, findings such as fibrosis, adenosis, and lymphoid infiltration have not correlated with clinical episodes, nor have histologic differences been observed between symptomatic and asymptomatic women.

What is clear is the hormonal nature of cyclic mastalgia. It does not occur until after menarche, usually (although not always) resolves at menopause, and clearly fluctuates with the reproductive cycle. However, the exact hormonal influences that lead to mastalgia remain theoretical at best (Box 4–2). Differences in hormone levels between symptomatic and asymptomatic women have been variable, and in cases where an abnormality is present, symptoms do not necessarily resolve with correction.

Prolactin is a strong suspect in the development of mastalgia because it is involved in growth and secretory differentiation of the breast and is episodic and circadian. In addition, prolactin levels and effects can be influenced by changes in estrogen and progesterone, so that a more complex interaction of these hormones may be a cause, explaining why levels may not always correlate with symptoms. Finally, exogenous factors associated with mastalgia can impact prolactin levels, accounting for their connection.

The association between caffeine and "fibrocystic changes" or mastalgia has been long known, and it is believed that this works through cyclic adenosine monophosphate (cAMP). Increased cAMP leads to increased cellular proliferation in the breast and perhaps pain. Although caffeine does not directly impact cAMP, it can increase catecholamines, which do increase cAMP. Patients with mastalgia may have an increased sensitivity to catecholamines, with higher levels of β-adrenergic receptors. Catecholamine levels can also be increased by nicotine, tyramine, and stress, both physical and emotional.

There may also be an association between fat and breast pain. At first, it was thought that increased body weight led to increased estrogen levels and thus breast pain. However, it may be more related to an imbalance in the ratio of saturated to unsaturated fatty acids. Many women with breast pain have lower levels of the plasma essential fatty acid gamma-linolenic acid (GLA). This may be due to the inhibition of the conversion of linoleic acid and GLA by high levels of saturated fats. This deficiency of essential fatty acids could affect the breast cell membrane receptors, leading to this increased sensitivity. It is for this reason that decreased intake of saturated fats and supplementation of GLA may help manage mastalgia (see Nonhormonal Therapies).

Evaluation of Breast Pain

The evaluation of breast pain should always begin with a thorough history and physical examination. It is important to characterize the pain as carefully as possible, starting with whether it is cyclic or noncyclic in relation to the menses. When is the peak of the pain? Establish the type of pain, its typical duration, the location within the breast, and whether it is unilateral or bilateral. Is the pain generalized throughout the breast or is it focal within one spot. Cancer must be considered in the patient with a persistent, well-localized pain. You should also document the extent to which mastalgia disrupts the patient's normal lifestyle.

It is also critical to determine whether the pain is preceded by any specific movement or

BOX 4-2 THEORIES OF HORMONAL LINKS TO MASTALGIA

- Excessive estrogen
- Deficient progesterone
- Changes in progesterone/estrogen ratio
- Abnormalities in receptor sensitivity
- Abnormalities in follicle stimulating hormone/luteinizing hormone levels
- Low androgen levels
- High prolactin levels

position and if there was a history of trauma or overexertion, specifically of the pectoral muscle group. Is there a concurrent neck problem? Are there any associated symptoms such as fever, cough, shortness of breath, pain radiating down the arm, numbness or tingling, or erythema? The patient's past medical history, including medications, should be obtained. Did the pain begin after a recent birth, pregnancy loss or termination, or beginning of the use of oral contraceptive pills or hormone replacement therapy? It is also important to determine the patient's primary concerns, including concerns about malignancy, how the pain affects her, and what she has done to alleviate the pain to date.

Approximately two thirds of patients will have cyclic breast pain while one third will have noncyclic pain, which may be either related to the breast or to the chest wall (Box 4–3). For women with noncyclic pain, the location of the pain may help elicit the source. Forty percent of women with noncyclic breast pain have a musculoskeletal cause. Pain in the inner quadrants is often related to the chest wall, possibly secondary to an overexertion injury or strain of the pectoral muscle. Sometimes this pain can be reproduced by having the woman place her hand flat on the iliac wing and pushing inward. Other sources of chest wall pain are costochondritis (Tietze's syndrome) or arthritis, all of which can cause peristernal discomfort. Direct pressure on the sternum can reproduce this pain. Most of these patients can be successfully

treated with oral or topical nonsteroidal anti-inflammatory drugs (NSAIDs).

Noncyclic pain located in the lower outer quadrant of the breast may be secondary to vertebral, spinal, or paraspinal problems. A radiculopathy can lead to both pain and hyperesthesia in this area, and women often describe a burning pain. A respiratory infection may cause an intercostal neuralgia. If the pain is on the right, gallbladder disease must be included in the differential, and if it is on the left, a cardiac source must be considered. A careful review of systems can help rule these in or out and the appropriate workup can be initiated.

Cyclic mastalgia is usually first seen during the third decade of life. Many patients describe the pain as dull, burning, throbbing, or aching, usually starting in the upper, outer quadrant of the breast. Even though both breasts can be involved, patients often claim one breast is worse than the other. Sometimes a shooting pain radiating to the arm and axilla may be present. This might be secondary to glandular pressure on the intercostobrachial nerve. The pain usually starts about 5 days before the menstrual cycle, although some women have constant pain, which worsens at this time.

Physical examination should begin with gentle palpation of the breasts because deep palpation may be uncomfortable for the patient and may limit the rest of the examination. The goal of the examination is to identify other signs that may suggest malignancy, such as an associated mass, skin changes, or nipple discharge. If the pain is localized, attention should be focused on this area to exclude a discrete pain. If the pain is reproducible with palpation, it is helpful to have the patient roll to one side so that the breast tissue falls away from the chest wall. It then might be possible to determine whether the pain is arising from the underlying rib.

Radiology has a limited role in the evaluation of breast pain. Because most women are young, mammography is limited. However, women older than age 35 years who have not had a recent screening mammogram should obtain one. Women younger than 35 years with physical findings or a strong family history of breast cancer should also undergo mammography. Ultrasound is helpful in characterizing a mass at the site of the pain, but in the absence of a palpable finding, is rarely of value. It can be considered when the breast pain is focal. Fine-needle aspiration biopsy of a

BOX 4–3 POSSIBLE CAUSES OF NONCYCLIC BREAST PAIN

Breast
  Cysts
Focal or periductal mastitis
  Mondor's disease (sclerosing
    periphlebitis)
  Ill-fitting brassiere
  Trauma
  Hidradenitis suppurativa
Chest wall
  Costochondritis
  Diffuse or localized lateral chest
    wall pain
  Radicular pain from cervical arthritis
Other
  Lung disease
  Hiatal hernia
  Gallbladder disease
  Ischemic heart disease

focal source of pain can theoretically be used, but it is associated with extremely low yield and is probably more beneficial in reassuring the patient. If a spinal source is suspected, x-rays of the neck and back may be helpful. Laboratory tests are rarely useful.

Treatment Options

Reassurance

If the pain seems to be musculoskeletal in nature, further workup and treatment recommendations should be initiated based on the likely source. For primary breast pain, if the clinical examination and imaging studies are negative, then simple reassurance that the pain is unlikely to be secondary to breast cancer will provide adequate relief for most women (Fig. 4–1). It can be helpful to ask women with cyclic pain to record the occurrence and severity of breast pain. By doing so, the woman often notes aggravating factors that she had not previously noted, and she can eliminate them. Cyclic mastalgia will spontaneously resolve within 3 months in approximately one fourth

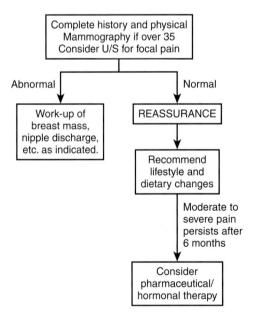

Figure 4–1. Approach to the patient with breast pain. Mammography should be obtained in any woman older than 35 and women younger than 35 if they have a family history or physical finding. Ultrasound may be considered if the pain is focal. If no abnormality is found, reassurance is the first step, followed by simple lifestyle and dietary changes. Patients with severe cyclic mastalgia or mastalgia unresponsive to conservative treatment should be considered for hormonal therapy.

of patients, and noncyclic mastalgia will spontaneously resolve in half. In a study of large referral clinics, 85% of women were comfortable with watchful waiting after their anxiety about malignant disease was alleviated. The other 15% requested treatment. Several minor recommendations may help a significant number of women alleviate the pain.

Nonhormonal Therapies

After assuring women that their pain is unlikely to represent an underlying malignancy, the first steps to alleviate the pain should be simple (Box 4–4). Application of either warm compresses or ice packs may be helpful. A supportive brassiere can be extremely effective. Precise fitting of a brassiere to provide support for pendulous breasts may provide pain relief. The use of a sports bra during exercise or excessive activity has been shown to reduce pain related to breast movement. Analgesics, both acetaminophen and NSAIDs, can help. These may be administered orally or topically.

Dietary changes can also be helpful. Caffeine has often been described as an aggravating factor for fibrocystic disease of the breasts, and avoidance of caffeine is one of the first recommendations made to patients. However, the relationship between methylxanthines and cyclic mastalgia is not quite straightforward. Based on evidence that cAMP levels were elevated when the breasts were swollen and painful, women with "fibrocystic disease" were asked to avoid agents that activate cAMP. Primarily, this involved avoidance of methylxanthine-containing products, such as coffee, tea, colas, and chocolate. Indeed, in many women, the pain begins to resolve after

BOX 4–4 LIFESTYLE AND NUTRITIONAL CHANGES RECOMMENDED FOR MASTALGIA

Lifestyle
  Stop smoking
  Better fitting bra
  Sports bra during exercise
  Weight loss and exercise
  Stress management
  Analgesics, either topical or oral
Nutritional
  Avoidance of methylxanthines (coffee, tea, chocolate, cola)
  Diminish dietary fat intake
  Gamma-linolenic acid (evening primrose oil)

a few months and stays away as long as methyl-xanthine is avoided. It is important to inform women that it may take up to 6 months to see a resolution of symptoms after eliminating methylxanthines. However, in other women, even after total abstention from methylxanthines, the symptoms recur or never resolve. One reason for this may be that women deprived of methylxanthines may eat more foods containing tyramine (e.g., cheese, wine, beer, spices, nuts, mushrooms, and bananas). As discussed earlier, both methylxanthines and tyramines can elevate serum catecholamines. In addition to methylxanthines and tyramines, catecholamines can also be elevated by nicotine, stress, and other hormones. Therefore avoiding all the agents that increase catecholamine levels would be extremely difficult. While avoiding caffeine may help some women control their breast pain and may be recommended as a first step, it may only benefit a minority of patients. Nicotine also increases epinephrine levels and stimulates cAMP. Smoking cessation should always be strongly recommended as a method to reduce mastalgia, as much for palliation of the breast pain as the countless other reasons to not smoke. Emotional and physical stresses can also reactivate symptoms.

There is better evidence that reduction in dietary fat intake can alleviate breast pain. However, it may also take up to 6 months to see the results. In one study, a significant reduction in breast pain was found among women who could reduce their dietary fat content to 15% of total calories. Although this may have additional side benefits to health, long-term dietary changes may be difficult for patients to maintain.

A commonly recommended treatment for cyclic mastalgia is evening primrose oil. Evening primrose oil is one of the richest sources of essential fatty acids. It contains 72% linoleic acid and 7% GLA. Its use is based on the observation that women with mastalgia had increased proportions of saturated fatty acids and reduced proportions of essential fatty acids. In some observational studies, the response rate has been reported between 45% to 97% of women, and one randomized trial of 73 patients showed significant improvement from treatment with evening primrose oil. However, other randomized trials have not shown a benefit. Although the data supporting its use could be stronger, given the relative safety and minimal adverse effects, evening primrose oil should be thought of as first-line

therapy. For evening primrose oil to work best, it should be combined with a diet low in saturated fats. It also takes time to see the benefit, so therapy should be continued for at least 6 months. The usual dose is 1500 to 3000 mg daily in divided doses. Evening primrose oil usually comes in capsules of 500 mg, meaning patients would take three to six pills a day, which can be difficult for patients.

Vitamin E has been promoted as a mastalgia cure; however, a double-blind randomized trial showed no significant effect. Likewise, vitamin B_6 is alleged to improve mastalgia, but a randomized trial with a crossover design failed to find any significant difference between vitamin B_6 and placebo. Other commonly recommended interventions for which there is little evidence include calcium, vitamin A, selenium, rose hips, soy, and diuretics.

Hormonal Therapies

If the cyclic mastalgia is not sufficiently relieved by the aforementioned interventions, pharmaceutical intervention can be considered. This should be a rare situation, however. The first step is to identify a possible exogenous source and modifying it. For premenopausal women, this may involve lowering the dose of estrogen in their oral contraceptives or changing to a formulation containing 19-norprogestogens, which have androgenic properties. For postmenopausal women, this might involve lowering the dose of estrogen in their hormone replacement therapy or switching to raloxifene (Evista), a selective estrogen receptor modifier. Progestins administered during the luteal phase or the addition of an androgen to estrogen-replacement therapy can also be helpful.

Danazol is an attenuated androgen that is effective in relieving breast pain in more than 90% of cases and is the only Food and Drug Administration (FDA)–approved drug for the treatment of "fibrocystic breast disease." It functions by decreasing ovarian function by suppressing gonadotropin release by the pituitary gland. Danazol is used at a dose of 200 to 400 mg daily, or only during the luteal phase of the menstrual cycle in premenopausal women. Relief typically comes within a month of using the drug. However, the side effects at higher doses are often as distressing as the breast pain and include headaches, nausea, depression, muscle aches, menstrual irregularity, weight gain, acne, oiliness of the hair, decreased breast size, hirsutism, voice change, increased libido, and dyspareunia. Almost two thirds of patients experience side effects, many of whom discontinue therapy, and symptoms often recur within 12 months of discontinuing therapy. To help minimize side effects and avoid symptoms from recurring, the drug can be gradually weaned (100 mg twice daily for 2 months, then 100 mg/day for 2 months, then 100 mg every other day or 100 mg/day only during the second half of the menstrual cycle). If the reductions are well tolerated, the drug can be discontinued. If after 2 months there is no resolution, the dose can be increased to 200 mg twice daily. Therapy should not continue longer than 6 months.

Bromocriptine is a long-acting dopaminergic drug that suppresses prolactin and has been studied as a treatment for mastalgia. At a dosage of 7.5 mg/day for 3 months, bromocriptine can improve mastalgia in many women, and this remains after discontinuing the drug. Bromocriptine is not as effective as danazol. Common side effects include nausea and vomiting and dizziness. This often leads to discontinuation, although these side effects can be reduced by using a gradual buildup of doses over 2 weeks. However, recent reports of serious side effects of bromocriptine (when used to stop lactation), including seizures, strokes, and even death, have raised concerns. Bromocriptine is no longer FDA approved for lactation cessation and is not FDA approved for mastalgia. New long-lasting selective dopamine agonists are presently being studied.

Tamoxifen has also been used to treat moderate to severe breast pain. In the International Breast Cancer Intervention study, which examined tamoxifen as adjuvant therapy for breast cancer (see Chapter 17), a side benefit was the efficacy of this drug in relieving mastalgia. Some clinicians recommend a dose of 10 mg daily for 3 to 6 months, or only during days 5 to 25 of the menstrual cycle. Several trials have subsequently shown the benefit of tamoxifen compared to placebo in treating mastalgia. Using a dose of 20 mg, as is done for the treatment of cancer, has not been shown to improve efficacy. The benefits must be weighed against the known risks and side effects of Tamoxifen, which include hot flashes, vaginal discharge, and an increased risk of thrombophlebitis or endometrial cancer.

Gonadotropin-releasing hormone agonists have also been used successfully for severe pain. Goserelin (Zoladex) has been reported as effective in up to 80% of women. However, the menopausal symptoms and effects on bones limit its use to short-term trials and only in severe cases that did not respond to other interventions. Only short courses of luteinizing hormone-releasing hormone analogues should be used for very severe cases of mastalgia not responding to other therapies.

Progesterone cream and oral progestin have been examined, as have oral contraceptives using a combination of estrogen and progestogen, and have been reported to relieve symptoms of mastalgia, but most trials have been disappointing.

Surgery for Mastalgia

Although mastectomy (or quadrantectomy in women with focal symptoms) has been used in the past for the treatment of severe, incapacitating mastalgia that has not responded to other therapies, its use should be strongly discouraged. Most patients will continue to have pain after surgery.

Suggested Readings

1. Bundred N. Breast pain. Clin Evid 2005;14:2190–2199.
2. Carmichael AR, Bashayan O, Nightingale P. Objective analyses of mastalgia in breast clinics: Is breast pain questionnaire a useful tool in a busy breast clinic? Breast 2006;15(4):498–502.
3. Colak T, Ipek T, Kanik A, et al. Efficacy of topical nonsteroidal antiinflammatory drugs in mastalgia treatment. J Am Coll Surg 2003;196:525.
4. Gumm R, Cunnick GH, Mokbel K. Evidence for the management of mastalgia. Curr Med Res Opin 2004;20(5):681–684.
5. Olawaiye A, Withiam-Leitch M, Danakas G, Kahn K. Mastalgia: A review of management. J Reprod Med 2005;50(12):933–939.
6. Plu-Bureau G, Le MG, Sitruk-Ware R, Thalabard JC. Cyclical mastalgia and breast cancer risk: Results of a French cohort study. Cancer Epidemiol Biomarkers Prev 2006;15:1229.
7. Smith RL, Pruthi S, Fitzpatrick LA. Evaluation and management of breast pain. Mayo Clin Proc 2004;79:353.
8. Srivastava A, Mansel RE, Arvind N, et al. Evidence-based management of mastalgia: A meta-analysis of randomised trials. Breast 2007;16(5):503–512.

Management of Nipple Discharge

Management of Nipple Discharge: Key Points

Understand the differences between normal and abnormal discharges from the nipple.

Describe the features of nipple discharge that raise concern for malignancy.

Describe the thorough history and examination of the woman with nipple discharge.

Develop an algorithm for the diagnostic workup of the woman with abnormal nipple discharge.

Describe how a duct excision is performed and when it is indicated.

After breast pain and a breast mass, nipple discharge is the third most common complaint related to the breast for which women seek medical attention. Approximately 5% to 7% of women referred to breast clinics have symptomatic nipple discharge. Although this may be a highly concerning symptom for women, it is very rarely a sign of malignancy. More than half of women in their reproductive years are able to express some fluid from the nipple. The overwhelming majority of women with symptomatic nipple discharge have underlying benign disease. Only a very small percentage of women with nipple discharge are found to have an underlying malignancy. Nipple discharge is present in roughly 10% to 15% of women with benign breast disease. It is very rare for cancer to present only as nipple discharge (less than 1% to 2% of cancers). If nipple discharge is associated with cancer, there is most often an associated mass on physical examination or mammography. The dilemma of the clinician is to determine which patients with nipple discharge can be safely observed, and which require further evaluation and what that evaluation should consist of.

Nipple Aspirate Fluid in the Nonlactating Breast

As stated, most women in the reproductive years can express some fluid from their nipples and this is normal. The breast is a modified apocrine gland whose ultimate function is lactation. However, the nonlactating breast does have secretory activity. This is not clinically appreciated by patients because the lactiferous sinuses are often plugged by keratotic material. However, if the plugs are removed and the nipples aspirated, fluid can be obtained in a large majority of women. Some investigators have thought that this nipple aspirate fluid (NAF) could potentially be used to diagnose breast cancer at an early stage or to assess and individual woman's risk of breast cancer.

NAF varies in color and consistency depending on its composition. The color can range from clear to black, with descriptions of yellow, dark yellow, tan, brown, or green discharge being common. Nipple discharge can also be red or maroon if blood is present, or white if the discharge is milk or infectious. NAF is a secretion of both endogenous and exogenous substances (Box 5–1). In comparing the serum levels of these exogenous substances to the levels in NAF, it is evident that the breast is a true secretory organ. It is possible that the increased concentrations of these agents in NAF may contribute to breast cancer development. Also within the fluid are exfoliated epithelial cells and hematogenous cells.

The cellular components of NAF may be reflective of benign or malignant disease within the breast. For this reason, there has been considerable interest in the evaluation of NAF as a screening or diagnostic test. Some have compared this to a "Pap smear for the breast." This has been limited, however, by difficulties in not only obtaining adequate volumes of NAF to evaluate, but also in the cellularity of the fluid. The cytologic appearance of cells in the NAF can be characterized by a

BOX 5–1 COMPOSITION OF NIPPLE ASPIRATE FLUID

ENDOGENOUS COMPONENTS
Lactose
β-lactalbumin
Immunoglobulin
Cholesterol
Fatty acids
EXOGENOUS COMPONENTS THAT CAN BE FOUND
Nicotine
Caffeine
Pesticides
Technetium
Barbiturate
CELLULAR COMPONENTS
Benign ductal epithelial cells
Squamous epithelial cells (rare)
Transitional cells (rare)
Apocrine metaplastic cells (very rare)
Foam cells
Neutrophils
Lymphocytes
Histiocytes

system similar to that of ductal changes seen on biopsy (Table 5–1). Differences in the cytology of NAF between "normal" women and women with benign disease can be seen. This includes both benign disease that is not associated with an increased risk of cancer (e.g., fibrocystic disease, apocrine metaplasia, duct ectasia, fibroadenomas, and mild hyperplasia) and those diseases that are associated with an increased risk (atypical hyperplasia). These changes include increased cellularity and a

TABLE 5–1 • Terminology for Cytologic Classification of Nipple Aspirate Fluid

Benign, nonproliferative	Ductal epithelial cells or apocrine metaplastic cells within normal limits
Mild hyperplasia	Minimal cellular changes, slight cellular and nuclear enlargement, papillary or apocrine metaplastic changes
Moderate hyperplasia	Moderate cellular changes, increased cell and nuclear size and increased nuclear-to-cell-size ratio, chromatin granularity
Atypical hyperplasia	Marked cellular changes but not frank malignancy
Malignant cells	Unequivocal nuclear features of malignancy

greater prevalence of duct epithelial cells and duct cells in groups. Apocrine metaplastic cells are more common while fewer foam cells are seen. Only rarely does the cytology of NAF from women with benign breast disease correlate with a specific lesion, with the possible exception of a papilloma. However, the cytologic analysis of NAF can often reveal the presence of cells exhibiting signs of moderate or marked hyperplasia. This can possibly be used to assess risk (see Chapter 8).

Abnormal Discharge of the Nipple

Endocrine Causes of Nipple Discharge

Abnormal nipple discharge may be a response to elevated levels of prolactin. In this case, the discharge is commonly bilateral, spontaneous, and white (galactorrhea). Prolactin is significantly elevated during pregnancy and particularly in the postpartum/nursing period. Milk production can continue for up to 1 year following weaning. However, it can also be mildly elevated during sleep and during the later follicular and luteal phase of the menstrual cycle. Prolactin can also be mildly elevated with

BOX 5–2 MEDICATIONS THAT CAN CAUSE NIPPLE DISCHARGE

- Oral contraceptives, estrogen, progestin, danazol
- Tricyclic antidepressants (amitriptyline, desipramine, doxepin, imipramine, nortriptyline)
- Anti-hypertensives (reserpine, methyldopa, verapamil, calcium channel blockers)
- Phenothiazines (acetophenazine, chlorpromazine, ruphenazine, perphenazine, prochlorperazine, promethazine, thioridazine, trifluoperazine, triflupromazine)
- Butyrophenones (droperidol, haloperidol)
- Antiemetics (metoclopramide, sulpiride)
- Opiates, codeine, heroin, marijuana
- Cimetidine
- L-arginine
- Digitalis
- Amphetamines

BOX 5–3 MEDICAL CONDITIONS ASSOCIATED WITH ELEVATED PROLACTIN LEVELS

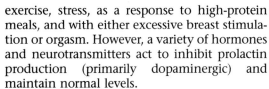

- Chronic renal failure
- Hypothyroidism
- Herpes zoster (shingles)
- Hypernephroma

exercise, stress, as a response to high-protein meals, and with either excessive breast stimulation or orgasm. However, a variety of hormones and neurotransmitters act to inhibit prolactin production (primarily dopaminergic) and maintain normal levels.

If this balance is thrown off, either by excessive prolactin production or diminished inhibition, the end result is galactorrhea. Because the breast lacks the ability to provide efferent feedback to the pituitary, even a small transient elevation in prolactin can lead to galactorrhea. Overproduction may come from a pituitary adenoma (prolactinomas) or ectopic production from other tumors. Because high levels of prolactin can also result in oligomenorrhea or anovulation by suppressing gonadotropin-releasing hormone, patients with a history of galactorrhea and oligomenorrhea should be considered highly likely to have a prolactinoma.

Hypothyroidism results in elevated levels of thyrotropin-releasing hormone, which can result in pituitary lactotroph stimulation and decreased clearance of prolactin. Oral contraceptives have a similar effect. Other drugs that have an antidopaminergic effect can also result in increased prolactin release (Box 5–2). Several medical conditions can lead to increased prolactin levels (Box 5–3). Finally, chronic breast stimulation can cause increased levels of prolactin. These include manipulation by the woman or her partner, contact with clothing, or chest trauma, including burns and herpes zoster.

Breast Conditions Causing Nipple Discharge

As opposed to external stimuli, which usually results in bilateral nipple discharge, a variety of intrinsic breast conditions can cause nipple discharge, which is more commonly unilateral. The three most common lesions are duct ectasia, intraductal papillomas, and fibrocystic changes; however, nipple discharge can be secondary to intraductal or invasive (usually papillary) carcinoma.

Fibrocystic changes, both proliferative and nonproliferative, can result in nipple discharge. This is typically multiductal and more often expressed than spontaneous. The discharge is typically serous or light green. Many of these patients have other symptoms of fibrocystic changes, including dense, "lumpy" breast tissue and cyclic mastalgia.

Duct ectasia is a dilation of the duct wall associated with a loss of elastin within the walls and the presence of inflammatory cells (primarily a plasma cell infiltrate) and fibrosis around the walls. It is found in about 15% to 20% of women with symptomatic nipple discharge. The cause is unknown (see Chapter 6). The peak incidence is in women older than 50 years although it is not uncommon in premenopausal women. The discharge can be white, dark green or black, but can be bloody or purulent. Duct ectasia is a completely benign lesion that has no connection to cancer. Although changes may sometimes be seen on imaging, typically duct ectasia is radiographically occult.

Papillomas are benign lesions of the epithelium, growing within the ducts. Most often these are solitary, growing within the major ducts near the nipple, most located within 1 to 2 cm of the areolar edge within the major ducts. Grossly, this lesion appears as a small, fragile, finger-like growth within the lumen of the duct. The discharge is most commonly spontaneous and easily reproducible. Intraductal papillomas are the most common cause of bloody nipple discharge.

Clinical Evaluation of the Patient with Nipple Discharge

In addition to the standard information regarding breast cancer risk, the history should cover the details of the discharge, including whether it is unilateral or bilateral, whether it is spontaneous or elicited, and the nature of the discharge (Box 5–4). Whether the discharge is spontaneous or not is a crucial question. As the popularity of self breast examination increases, more women will present with discharge that they express themselves. Because nonspontaneous expression of non-bloody nipple discharge is not associated with breast cancer, these patients can be reassured that this is a normal physiologic finding. Whether there is itching or burning pain of the nipple in association with the discharge is important, because this might be associated with infection or duct ectasia, or with a skin

BOX 5–4 HISTORY IN THE PATIENT WITH NIPPLE DISCHARGE

- How frequent is the discharge?
- Is it spontaneous or do you elicit it?
- What color is it (white, green, yellow, brown, red, maroon)?
- What consistency is it (serous, watery, serosanguinous)?
- Is there blood in it?
- Is it unilateral or bilateral?
- Does it come from just one duct or multiple ducts?
- Has there been recent trauma or infection?
- Breast cancer risk factors (age of menarche, menopause, childbearing, estrogen use, family history)
- Thorough past medical history
- Signs and symptoms of thyroid disease (weight gain/loss, cold/heat intolerance, tachycardia)
- Visual field defects (pituitary tumor?)
- Infertility, oligomenorrhea, amenorrhea, acne, facial hair (hyperandrogenism or hyperprolactinemia)
- Polyuria, polydipsia
- Complete list of medications (including over-the-counter and "natural" medications)
- Possibility the patient may be pregnant

process involving the nipple. In regard to the discharge itself, the patient should describe the color (white, green, yellow, brown, red) and consistency (serous, watery, serosanguinous). A complete reproductive and endocrine review of systems and list of current medications should be obtained. The patient should be queried about recent trauma, possible stimulation, and drug use. Other symptoms that may be suggestive of an endocrine source should be elicited on the review of symptoms, including double vision, headaches, polyuria, polydipsia, fatigue, heat/cold intolerance, nervousness or restlessness, weight loss/gain, change in appetite, decreased libido, infertility, amenorrhea, and the likelihood of pregnancy.

Physical examination should begin with examination of the nipples. Sometimes a nipple discharge is actually an exudate related to skin irritation from inverted nipples, eczematoid lesions, trauma, or herpes simplex infections. Even though these are not associated with cancer, it is also important to rule out Paget disease as a source of a nipple exudate (see Chapter 11). Tubular swellings called "varicocele lesions" of the breast may be palpable below the nipple-areolar complex, and are often associated with duct ectasia. The next step is to determine which duct (or ducts) is producing the discharge. Bilateral discharge or discharge from multiple ducts within one breast are very rarely malignant, whereas discharge from a single duct is more worrisome. Single duct discharge can usually be expressed when pressure is applied to a trigger point. With the patient supine and the arm over the head, apply pressure at various points around the areola until discharge is expressed. You should carefully document this point because this may be important in planning subsequent surgery. The discharge can easily be tested for the presence of heme by laboratory test sticks (Hemoccult). In some cases, the discharge can also be easily collected on a glass slide for cytology. The slide is held at the opening of the duct and while applying pressure to cause discharge, the slide is moved across the surface of the nipple to make a thin spread. It can be immediately fixed. If more discharge can be expressed, several smears should be prepared because the last few drops are usually more cellular. The remainder of the breast should be carefully examined for the presence of a mass or other signs of malignancy.

The next step is typically mammography and ultrasound, particularly in age-appropriate patients. Mammogram is indicated in all women with a unilateral, spontaneous nipple discharge, including women younger than 35 years. Ultrasound is recommended in addition to mammogram. However, both studies are usually negative. Ultrasonography may or may not reveal dilated ducts with an intraluminal lesion (Fig. 5–1). The utility of magnetic resonance imaging (MRI) for the patient with a nipple discharge of high suspicion has been suggested, but data are limited on its utility in this situation. It may be a consideration in the high-risk woman presenting with nipple discharge or when the cytology is positive and the remainder of the workup is negative.

The remainder of the workup depends on the findings on history and physical examination (Fig. 5–2). A mass identified on examination or mammography should be biopsied. Patients who likely have discharge associated with fibrocystic changes can be reassured and managed conservatively. These include patients with bilateral or unilateral multiductal discharge that is serous or light green, especially if they have other symptoms of fibrocystic changes on examination (e.g., nodularity, premenstrual lumpiness, and discomfort). Patients with discharge that is multifocal, sticky, and

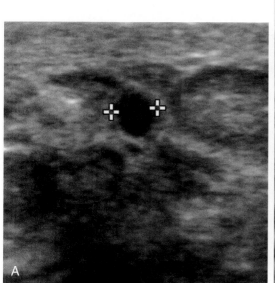
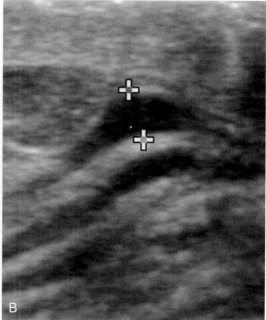

Figure 5–1. Radial and antiradial images demonstrate a mildly dilated duct in axial and longitudinal projections. (Images courtesy of Dr. Alexis Nees, Department of Radiology, University of Michigan.)

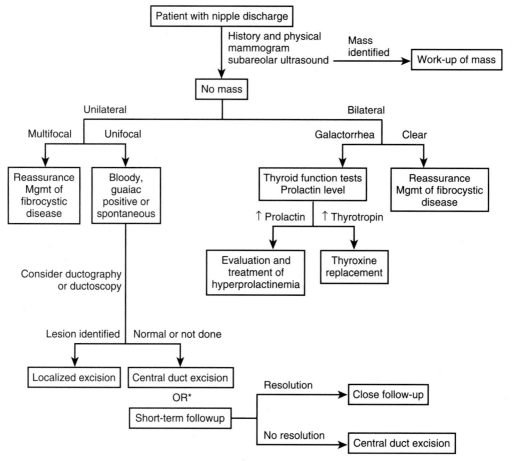

Figure 5–2. Approach to the patient with nipple discharge. Bilateral discharge is rarely malignant and may represent fibrocystic disease or galactorrhea. For the latter, thyroid function tests and a prolactin level should be obtained. Unilateral, single duct discharge is concerning if it is bloody or spontaneous. Whereas cytology, ductography, or ductoscopy may be helpful, duct excision may ultimately be necessary to rule out cancer. Recent studies suggest that if the mammogram and ultrasound are negative, the likelihood of malignancy may be low enough to warrant short-term follow-up rather than proceeding to central duct excision.

multicolored (including dark green or black, but heme-negative) most likely have duct ectasia and can also be safely observed. Surgery in these cases is reserved for palliation because continued discharge can be distressing and inconvenient to many patients. If there is obvious blood in the discharge or if the Hemoccult is positive, patients will require further evaluation and ultimately surgery.

Patients with bilateral white discharge consistent with galactorrhea should have a workup for the source of hyperprolactinemia. Both prolactin levels and thyroid function tests should be obtained. If the patient is taking a medication known to increase prolactin, it should be discontinued if possible. Because transient elevations of prolactin can be seen with trauma or stimulation, the patient may be advised to avoid these to determine whether there is

resolution of the discharge. If hyperprolactinemia is persistent, an MRI of the brain should be obtained to rule out a prolactinoma.

Finally, there is the patient with unilateral, uniductal spontaneous discharge. This is otherwise known as pathologic discharge. It may or may not contain blood. A unilateral, spontaneous clear discharge from one duct is still suspicious, even if no blood is present. However, women with pathologic nipple discharge are still highly likely to have benign disease, with half having an intraductal papilloma, 15% to 20% having duct ectasia, and only about 10% having carcinoma. Although there are many modalities available to evaluate this condition further, most do not have the sensitivity or specificity to completely rule out malignancy, so almost all of these patients ultimately require a duct excision for diagnosis.

Testing the nipple discharge for the presence of occult blood by means of Hemoccult is inexpensive, so it is hard to argue against performing it during physical examination. Any patient with occult blood requires duct excision for definitive diagnosis, although most cases of bloody nipple discharge are secondary to intraductal papillomas and not malignancy. The results of Hemoccult evaluation are useful to rule out occult blood with the dark, multifocal discharge associated with duct ectasia. In this case, a negative result may allow the patient to avoid a duct excision. However, with unifocal, spontaneous discharge, the sensitivity of Hemoccult is not high enough for a negative result to preclude the need for surgery. Cytologic examination of the discharge, as described, may be useful if the fluid shows cancer, but this is rare and the high false-negative rate precludes using cytology to exclude cancer. Thus, cytology may be useful but does not preclude a biopsy if negative.

Ductography is often the next test obtained in the woman with pathologic nipple discharge. This procedure involves anesthetizing the breast (using topical agents such as EMLA cream [2.5% lidocaine and 2.5% prilocaine] or injectable agents) followed by duct cannulation with a small nylon catheter or needle. A water-soluble contrast agent is then injected into the duct and mammograms are obtained immediately (Fig. 5–3). Several studies have shown that an abnormal ductogram does not preclude the presence of cancer, however. Therefore a woman with a suspicious nipple discharge and a normal ductogram still requires biopsy to rule out cancer. One advantage to obtaining a ductogram may be the combination of wire localization and ductography to localize a lesion seen on ductogram. Ductography can also sometimes be used to estimate the extent of a lesion seen on imaging.

Ductal Lavage and Ductoscopy

Newer modalities are playing an emerging role in the evaluation of nipple discharge. Ductal lavage is a procedure that involves eliciting cells from one or more ducts using catheterization and irrigation of the duct followed by cytopathologic evaluation (Fig. 5–4). This technique is currently being evaluated as a screening test for asymptomatic women, and there are minimal data on its sensitivity and specificity in women with pathologic nipple discharge.

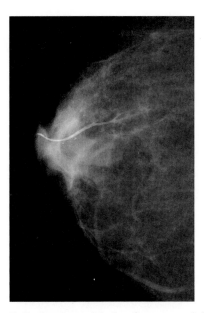

Figure 5–3. Craniocaudal view from normal ductogram. (Image courtesy of Dr. Alexis Nees, Department of Radiology, University of Michigan.)

A more promising technology is that of ductoscopy. Mammary ductoscopy involves the insertion of a microendoscope into the duct to directly visualize the ductal lining of the breast (Fig. 5–5). This also allows for the retrieval of epithelial cells by lavage. Albeit relatively new in the United States, this has been used in Europe and Japan for several years. The newest generation of microendoscope, the ViaDuct mammary ductoscope (Acueity, Larkspur, CA)

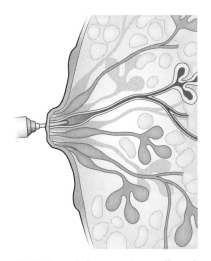

Figure 5–4. Ductal lavage. A small catheter is inserted into one or more ducts, allowing the irrigation of the duct. The retrieved fluid is then sent for cytopathologic evaluation.

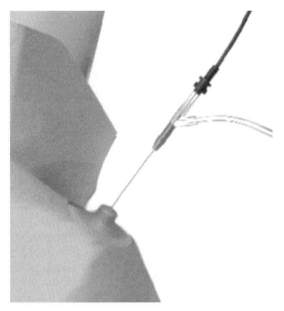

Figure 5–5. The ductoscope is inserted into the duct for both direct visualization and lavage. (Images courtesy of Acueity, Inc.)

advisable to do the procedure in the operating room so that it may be combined with an excision of any pathology identified. After expressing the nipple discharge so that the ductal orifice can be identified, the opening is dilated and the ductoscope advanced under direct visualization (Fig. 5–6). Ductal washings are obtained by aspirating fluid. If any pathology is identified, these can be marked for immediate excision or future image-guided biopsy.

Although ductoscopy has been promoted for use in patients with known cancer undergoing lumpectomy or as a screening test in high-risk individuals, the largest experience has been in the evaluation of pathologic nipple discharge. The ductal dilation associated with pathologic nipple discharge makes it easier to introduce the ductoscope and many of the patients have an intraductal papilloma that is easily localized and excised (Fig. 5–7). If a point of interest is seen, the light can be seen in the skin of the breast (if the room is dark) and can be marked to guide a subsequent excision.

is now approved by the Food and Drug Administration for human use. It has a slim diameter (0.9 mm) consisting of an outer sheath for insufflation and aspiration surrounding a fiberoptic core, which connects to a video system. The procedure can be performed in an office setting with minimal discomfort after performing a nipple block with topical EMLA cream for 30 minutes and either an intradermal injection of lidocaine around the nipple-areola complex or intraductal lidocaine. In the case of ductoscopy for nipple discharge, it may be

Duct Excision

If a lesion is noted on physical examination, mammogram, ductography, or ductoscopy, it should be the target of a biopsy. However, this still leaves many women with a suspicious discharge and no specific area of abnormality. In a patient with a worrisome discharge, duct excision has been considered the gold standard and is generally recommended. This procedure is both diagnostic and therapeutic. This

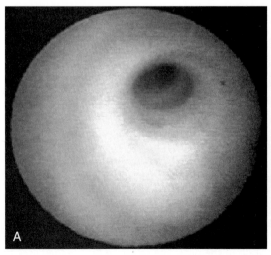

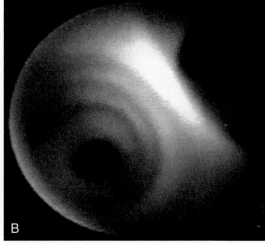

Figure 5–6. Ductoscopic images of normal ducts. (Images courtesy of Acueity, Inc.)

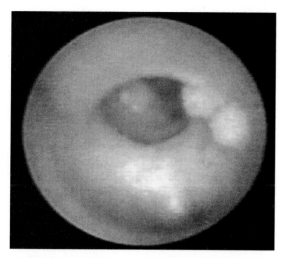

Figure 5–7. Ductoscopic image of an intraductal papilloma. (Images courtesy of Acueity, Inc.)

recommendation is based on the 3% to 10% incidence of finding occult cancer in patients with worrisome discharge. However, much of these data were collected when breast imaging was not as sensitive. With improved mammography and the use of subareolar ultrasound, more recent studies suggest that patients with single duct, spontaneous discharge or guaiac-positive discharge have a very low risk of malignancy when all imaging studies are negative. Close observation with short-term follow-up to determine whether the discharge resolves may be reasonable. However, if the discharge fails to resolve, duct excision should be performed. The procedure may also be considered for palliative reasons, even if malignancy is not suspected.

A circumareolar incision is marked to encompass one-third to one-half the circumference of the areola. When more than 50% is included, one risks devascularization. Placing the incision in the inferior aspect of the areola minimizes the risk of decreasing nipple sensation. Lidocaine is infiltrated into the skin at the site of the incision and underneath the areola. After making the incision, the skin of the areola is elevated with a skin hook so that dissection can be carried out under gentle tension. Dissection with blunt tenotomy scissors elevates the areola to the area directly behind the nipple.

Every attempt should be made to identify the involved duct. A large dilated duct can often be identified during dissection behind the nipple. If not, a small lacrimal duct probe can be placed through the involved duct via the skin opening. If this fails to work, methylene blue can be injected into the duct; this is preferably done before making the skin incision. Once identified, the duct should be dissected free and divided between clamps. This should be done close to the nipple if possible because small papillomas can occur in this location. The duct should then be traced deeper into the breast with a small cone of surrounding tissue, getting slightly wider as the dissection continues. Approximately 3 cm of duct and surrounding breast tissue should be excised. Once the duct is excised, the surgeon should apply pressure to the trigger point and around the areola to confirm that there is no continued discharge. This can also be done from within the wound by milking the other ducts toward the nipple. If the involved duct cannot be identified, a complete duct excision can be performed by encircling all of the major ducts (Fig. 5–8). Approximately 2 to 3 cm of the deep breast tissue should be excised with the ducts. If needed, a purse-string suture can be placed below the nipple to avoid nipple

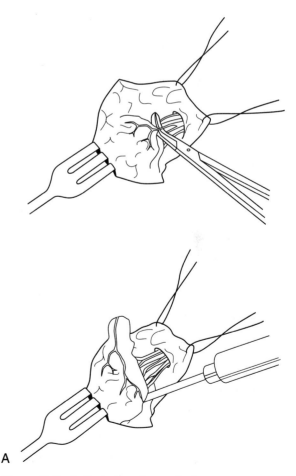

A

Figure 5–8. A, Technique for single duct excision.

(Continued)

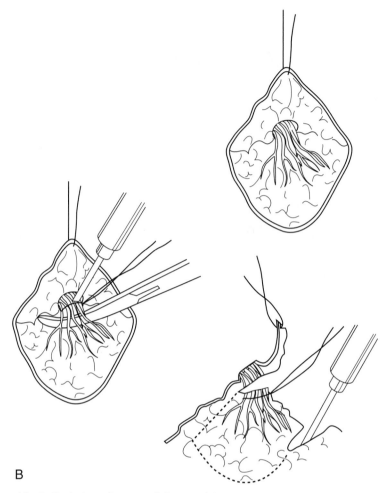

B

Figure 5–8—cont'd B, Technique for central duct excision.

inversion. Once it is assured that there is no further discharge and hemostasis has been achieved, the skin can be reapproximated with small, interrupted absorbable sutures.

Suggested Readings

1. Carty NJ, Mudan SS, Ravichandran D, et al. Prospective study of outcome in women presenting with nipple discharge. Ann R Coll Surg Engl 1994;76:387.
2. Escobar PF, Crowe JP, Matsunaga T, Mokbel K. The clinical applications of mammary ductoscopy. Am J Surg 2006;191(2):211–215.
3. Gray RJ, Pockaj BA, Karstaedt PJ. Navigating murky waters: A modern treatment algorithm for nipple discharge. Am J Surg 2007;194(6):850–855.
4. Hussain AN, Policarpio C, Vincent MT. Evaluating nipple discharge. Obstet Gynecol Surv 2006;61(4):278–283.
5. Nelson RS, Hoehn JL. Twenty-year outcome following central duct resection for bloody nipple discharge. Ann Surg 2006;243:522.
6. Richards T, Hunt A, Courtney S, Umeh H. Nipple discharge: A sign of breast cancer? Ann R Coll Surg Engl 2007;89(2):124–126.
7. Sakorafas GH. Nipple discharge: Current diagnostic and therapeutic approaches. Cancer Treat Rev 2001;27(5):275–282.
8. Santen RJ, Mansel R. Benign breast disorders. N Engl J Med 2005;353:275.
9. Simmons R, Amadovich T, Brennan M, et al. Nonsurgical evaluation of pathologic nipple discharge. Ann Surg Oncol 2003;10:113–116.
10. Vargas HI, Vargas MP, Eldrageely K, et al. Outcomes of clinical and surgical assessment of women with pathological nipple discharge. Am Surg 2006;72(2):124–128.

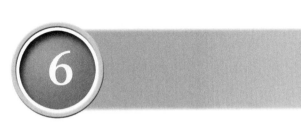

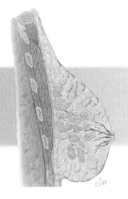

6

Infectious and Inflammatory Diseases of the Breast

MASTITIS
Management
BREAST ABSCESS
RECURRING SUBAREOLAR
ABSCESS

Pathophysiology
Workup
Treatment
GRANULOMATOUS MASTITIS

Infectious and Inflammatory Diseases of the Breast: Key Points

Review the clinical presentation and management of mastitis.

Describe the differences in presentation and treatment of a simple breast abscess versus a recurrent subareolar abscess.

Develop an algorithm for treating the patient with a recurrent subareolar abscess and appreciate when and what type of surgery is indicated.

Describe the differential diagnosis and the diagnostic workup of the woman suspected to have granulomatous mastitis.

Mastitis

Mastitis is an infection of the breast that occurs most commonly among women who are breast feeding. Three percent to 10% of lactating women may develop signs or symptoms of mastitis. Mastitis may be more common in lactating women who have had a previous episode of mastitis, women with cracks or sores on their nipple, older women,

and professional women. When mastitis occurs in lactating women, it is referred to as *puerperal mastitis*. Nonpuerperal mastitis may also occur as a result of trauma, possibly fibrocystic disease or sometimes an unrecognized etiology.

Patients typically present with a hard, warm, red, tender, swollen area of one breast. They may have associated fever, shakes, chills, myalgia, and malaise. *Staphylococcus aureus* is the most common causative organism but streptococci, coagulase-negative staphylococci, and *Escherichia coli* may also be cultured from infected patients.

Management

History and physical examination should focus on identifying a likely etiology for the mastitis, as well as the risk of breast cancer. The possibility of inflammatory breast cancer, though unlikely, must be kept in mind, particularly in women with nonpuerperal mastitis with no clear etiology. Some lactating women present with plugged ducts or galactoceles. These may be hard masses in the breast, with or without erythema or associated pain or fever. Imaging findings are relatively nonspecific. However, ultrasound of the breast is useful in identifying an underlying abscess and possibly guiding intervention (see later) (Fig. 6–1).

If no abscess is detected on either physical examination or ultrasound, then management is conservative. Antibiotics (dicloxacillin or cloxacillin, 250 mg orally four times a day for 10 to 14 days) should be initiated. Culturing the milk or any purulent nipple discharge for

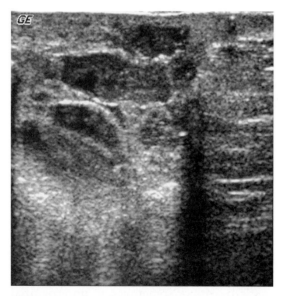

Figure 6–1. This ultrasound image shows a heterogeneous, predominantly hypoechoic mass with thick internal septations and overlying skin thickening. This corresponded to a breast abscess, which was percutaneously drained by the breast surgeon. (Image courtesy of Dr. Alexis Nees, Department of Radiology, University of Michigan.)

antibiotic sensitivities may help guide a change if the patient does not respond. The patient should be advised to rest, continue nursing, and use warm compresses and short-acting nonsteroidal antiinflammatory agents for pain control. If no response is seen within 24 to 48 hours, coverage should be switched to cephalexin or amoxicillin with clavulanate, or should be based on the sensitivities of culture.

Any abscess needs specific attention (see later). If patients fail to respond, or if they respond but mastitis recurs, this may be a sign of lactational problems, but it could also indicate inflammatory breast cancer (see Chapter 19). Breast imaging, biopsy of the skin and of any underlying mass to rule out cancer should be considered.

Breast Abscess

Epidermal inclusion cysts can occur in the skin of the breast because they can occur anywhere. However, because they often present as a "breast mass," they often invoke a higher degree of anxiety. Epidermal inclusion cysts are typically subcutaneous masses fixed to the dermis. Examination usually reveals an overlying pore and keratinaceous material can often be expressed. These show up on mammography as a discrete density, although careful directed imaging with a lead marker over the palpable abnormality can help differentiate this from a suspicious lesion within the parenchyma.

Often these inclusion cysts become infected, typically with *S. aureus*. Clinically, this presents as a tender, warm, erythematous mass. Patients may report a previous spontaneous drainage of the cyst with improvement in symptoms. Management is aimed at resolution of the acute infection followed by surgical resection to prevent recurrence. If only inflammation is present, oral antibiotics with warm soaks is appropriate. If an abscess is present, incision and drainage is indicated with evacuation of the "pasty" contents. Once the acute infection resolves, the patient is often left with a small indurated area with an overlying scar. Because these are susceptible to repeated cycles of inflammation and infection, they should be excised electively.

Peripheral breast abscesses develop in about 5% to 10% of women with mastitis, possibly because of a delay in diagnosis or inadequate therapy. These are different from the subareolar

TABLE 6–1 • *Features of Peripheral Breast Abscess versus Subareolar Breast Abscess*		
	Peripheral Breast Abscess	**Subareolar Breast Abscess**
Preceding history	Lactation, trauma	None; patients are often smokers
Site	Periphery of breast	Periareolar
Organism	*Staphylococcus aureus*	Multiple aerobic and/or anaerobic species
Treatment	High likelihood of resolution with aspiration/antibiotics or incision and drainage	Multiple recurrences after antibiotics or incision and drainage

abscesses discussed below (Table 6–1). The presentation is similar to that of mastitis (pain, erythema, tenderness) but with a palpable fluctuant mass. There is usually a precedent history of lactation or trauma, although this is not always the case. In some cases, the mass may not have been palpable but was detected by ultrasound in a mastitis patient.

Management consists of antibiotics and drainage. However, many of these can be successfully treated by needle aspiration rather than incision and drainage. Ultrasound guidance for the aspiration is preferred to ensure complete aspiration of the abscess. When needle aspiration is not possible, or not effective, incision and drainage may be necessary. The operation should be performed in the operating room with sedation because local anesthesia for an abscess is difficult to achieve. The incision is placed directly over the abscess, where the skin is thinnest. Cultures should be obtained. All loculations should be disrupted and the wound irrigated with saline. A small sample of the abscess wall should be sent for pathology study to rule out cancer, even though this is extremely unlikely, especially among lactating women. The wound is packed with gauze and allowed to heal by secondary intent. Antibiotics need only be continued until the local inflammation resolves and the patient has remained afebrile for 3 days.

Women who are lactating will have questions regarding continued breast-feeding. Most antibiotics are safe during breast-feeding, but this should be confirmed. Nursing should continue on the opposite side. If the incision does not interfere with the ability of the infant to latch on, breast-feeding may also continue on the affected side. If it does interfere, then a breast pump should be used for several days until enough healing has occurred to allow nursing. The patient may notice milk draining from the abscess cavity, but the antiinfectious properties of breast milk may actually accelerate healing.

Recurring Subareolar Abscess

One of the most frustrating entities to deal with in breast surgery is that of the recurring subareolar abscess. The disease is characterized by a recurring abscess not associated with lactation. Over the years, this condition has gone by many names, reflecting a lack of understanding (Box 6–1). Recurring subareolar abscess appears to represent the most extreme form of duct ectasia. Many women have mammary duct ectasia, which can be either asymptomatic or present with nipple discharge, nipple crusting, pain, or induration. It is believed that subareolar abscesses and recurring subareolar abscesses are the result of the introduction of bacteria into the diseased ducts. It is estimated that approximately 30% of women have some degree of disease of the ducts, although much of this is asymptomatic (detected on autopsy or incidentally during biopsies for other findings). Approximately 6% to 7% of women have symptomatic benign duct disease, accounting for approximately 20% of all benign conditions of the breast. The incidence of subareolar abscesses or periareolar fistulae is estimated to be about 1.2%.

BOX 6–1 NAMES USED TO DESCRIBE RECURRENT SUBAREOLAR ABSCESS

Mastitis obliterans
Chronic pyogenic mastitis
Stale milk mastitis
Involutional mammary duct ectasia with periductal mastitis
Comedomastitis
Periductal mastitis
Fistulae of lactiferous ducts
Zuska's disease
Squamous metaplasia of mammary ducts
Mammary duct–associated inflammatory disease sequence (MDAIDS)

The clinical presentation of this form of subareolar abscess is different from that of the typical breast abscess, which occurs primarily in lactating women. These can occur anywhere in the breast and are typically not periareolar (see earlier). In contrast, the abscesses related to duct ectasia are almost always periareolar. It typically occurs in young women, with a mean age of 34 years, most of whom are smokers. Patients usually present initially with the rapid onset of acute breast pain, tenderness, and a palpable mass in the central subareolar region. Although this is thought to be related to duct ectasia, many women may have had subclinical or asymptomatic disease and so a history of nipple discharge or other symptoms may not be present. The patient may present to the surgeon during this acute phase or with a chronic fistula. The fistula is usually an established fistula at the vermilion border, although it may be at the base of the nipple. This usually represents multiple inadequate attempts at treatment.

Many women report a history of symptoms that resolve with treatment or spontaneously, followed by an asymptomatic period lasting months to years, and then recurrence. Patients may be extremely frustrated with the chronic nature of this process, or from being passed from one doctor to another without resolution.

Pathophysiology

As described in Chapter 1, the lobules of the breast drain into minor intralobular ducts, which subsequently drain into 16 to 18 major mammary ducts. As each major mammary duct converges centrally at the base of the nipple, they dilate to form a secretion-storing lactiferous ampulla. These are located immediately below the nipple-areolar complex. From the ampulla, these ducts then exit via an opening at the apex of the nipple. There is a constant discharge from the orifices of these ducts onto the nipple. This is either imperceptible or may dry into a scarcely discernible crust that is usually brushed away by clothing.

The ducts are lined by a double layer of cells, an inner cuboidal (low columnar) epithelium and an outer myoepithelial layer. However, the final few millimeters of the intranipple ducts are lined by a stratified squamous epithelium. It is believed that the underlying problem with duct ectasia and recurrent subareolar abscesses is epidermalization of the ductal columnar epithelium and the obstruction

of the duct secondary to squamous metaplasia. At first, when the ducts begin to epidermalize, there may be discharge from one or more ducts, nipple retraction, or subareolar induration. As the disease progresses, there is increased production of keratin that leads to obstruction of the ducts. This leads to duct dilation secondary to accumulation of the normal secretory material. Ultimately, this can lead to the rupture of the thinned epithelial lining, exposing the surrounding tissues to the luminal contents. Keratin is irritating and can lead to an inflammatory response. The resultant inflammation can lead to a periductal lymphocytic infiltrate (sometimes predominated by plasma cells). This setting is ideal for bacterial growth. The bacteria may be aerobic or anaerobic, coming from skin, endogenous breast flora, or oral contamination of the nipple. As opposed to other forms of breast abscess, which are almost always *S. aureus*, cultures of subareolar abscesses often contain multiple organisms (Box 6–2). If bacteria do colonize this tissue, an abscess or fistula can occur.

So what causes epidermalization of the ducts and squamous metaplasia? Although the exact process by which this occurs is unclear, there are several factors that have been found to be associated with this process. There may be hormonal influences related to prolactin or estrogen levels. Vitamin A deficiency is a likely suspect because this also leads to keratinizing squamous metaplasia on multiple mucosal surfaces. Experimental evidence shows that vitamin A has a significant biologic effect on the epithelial differentiation and proliferation. Vitamin A deficiency also impairs blood clearance of bacteria and phagocytic activity, and thus may also be a contributing factor to infection.

The causative factor with the strongest link to both squamous metaplasia and recurrent

---

BOX 6–2 BACTERIA THAT MAY BE INVOLVED WITH RECURRING SUBAREOLAR ABSCESS

Anaerobic peptostreptococci
Bacteroides
Diphtheroids
Staphylococcus epidermidis
Staphylococcus aureus
Proteus
Lactobacilli
Streptococcus viridans

BOX 6–3 METHODS BY WHICH SMOKING MAY BE ASSOCIATED WITH RECURRENT SUBAREOLAR ABSCESS

- Direct cellular injury of ducts by metabolites in the glandular secretions
- Reduction of bioavailability of estrogen by 2α-hydroxylation of estradiol or inhibition of the aromatase-catalyzed conversion of testosterone to estrogen
- Effect of nicotine on prolactin levels
- Altered composition of endogenous flora in the breast

subareolar abscesses is smoking. The incidence of disease rises dramatically with smoking and with the degree of smoking (heavy versus light). Ninety percent of patients with recurrent breast abscess had been exposed to cigarette smoke for many years before the onset of symptoms. Although the association is extremely strong, the mechanisms by which smoking induces squamous metaplasia remains unclear (Box 6–3).

Workup

When seeing a patient with a subareolar abscess, it is important to document any preceding events and a history of similar symptoms. In addition to finding out whether the patient is breast-feeding, has there been any recent trauma? Does the patient have other disease of the breast, such as fibrocystic disease or previous cancer? How long have the symptoms been present and how has this been treated in the past (antibiotics, incision and drainage)? Has this ever occurred in the opposite breast? It is crucial to document smoking history. On physical examination, there may be an acute abscess with tenderness, erythema, induration, or fluctuation, or there may be a draining periareolar fistula. Compression of the nipple-areolar complex with the finger and thumb may reveal subareolar masses. Both breasts should be examined to assess symmetry. The diagnosis is made primarily by history and physical examination. If a mass is present, then mammography and ultrasound should be obtained. In the absence of a mass, mammography should still be obtained to rule out an underlying cancer, especially in women older than 35 years.

Treatment

The treatment of subareolar abscesses is primarily surgical. Antibiotic treatment alone is rarely effective, resulting in complete response in less than 3% of patients. For the patient being seen acutely, the initial treatment depends on the presenting symptoms. If the patient has an acute abscess as characterized by a fluctuant, tender, erythematous mass, incision and drainage is indicated, followed by a 2-week course of antibiotics consisting of a cephalosporin and metronidazole. Although this can be done in the office, it is best performed in the operating room under anesthesia to ensure complete drainage. If it is to be done in the office, remember that lidocaine is seldom effective for providing analgesia secondary to the low pH of the inflamed tissue. It is important to culture the pus for both aerobic and anaerobic bacteria because the type of bacteria involved helps confirm the diagnosis. The wound should be amply irrigated and wicked open. If the patient presents in the early stages, with an indurated mass without fluctuance, then just the 2 weeks of antibiotics should be given. Heat packs may be applied for comfort.

For many breast abscesses, the use of nonoperative therapy consisting of percutaneous fine-needle aspiration, followed by antibiotics, has been advocated. This is a reasonable approach for nonsubareolar abscesses, but is not indicated for this clinical scenario. It is important to keep in mind that for subareolar abscesses, antibiotics and incision and drainage are only temporizing measures. Because this is primarily a disease process of the ducts, treatment that does not address the ducts is unlikely to work.

Once the acute infectious process has been addressed, definitive surgical treatment will involve excision of either the entire involved duct or multiple ducts. For the patient with an initial presentation, the involved duct should be excised via ductectomy. Using either intravenous sedation with local anesthetic or general anesthesia, a radial incision is made starting in the middle of the nipple and encompassing the abscess cavity or fistula tract (Fig. 6–2). Injecting the fistula tract with 1% methylene blue before beginning can help identify the involved duct. The nipple is splayed open and the duct identified and dissected out. After excising the entire duct, the incision is closed. Subcutaneous sutures are

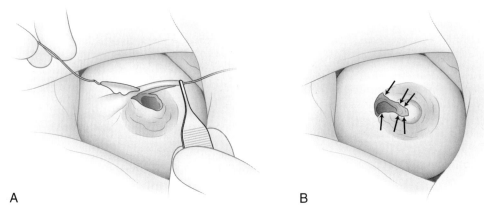

A   B

Figure 6–2. A, The entire abscess, fistula cavity, and involved duct is excised. **B,** After resection, the skin is reapproximated at the crown of the nipple, the base of the nipple, and the periareolar border.

placed at the apex of the nipple, the base of the nipple, and the vermilion border of the areola. Sometimes it is useful to place a purse-string or Z-suture at the base of the nipple to evert it, especially in women who have a retracted nipple. If there is any concern regarding ongoing infection, a wick may be placed in the subareolar defect and brought out beyond the vermillion border. This is then changed daily. The patient should be placed on a 10- to 14-day course of antibiotics postoperatively.

For patients with recurrent disease, it may be necessary to perform a duct excision. This can be performed either through a radial incision or a circumareolar incision. If a chronic abscess or fistula is present at the time of the surgery, this must be excised en bloc with the ducts, and may change the choice of incision. The areola is raised using a knife or Metzenbaum scissors. The major ducts are separated from the base of the nipple by passing a curved forceps around the nipple base and dividing the ducts with a knife. The nipple base is then excised to remove all duct tissue. Although a complete excision of the ducts is the goal, there is a risk in devascularizing the nipple skin. A purse-string or Z-suture should be inserted through the nipple base to maintain eversion, but not so tightly as to cause necrosis. The subareolar duct system is then dissected out from the underlying breast tissue. The subareolar dead space may be obliterated with interrupted absorbable suture and the skin is then reapproximated. Patients should be placed on antibiotics postoperatively (Fig. 6–3).

Granulomatous Mastitis

Granulomatous mastitis is a relatively uncommon disease that involves the development of an inflammatory mass in the breast that may be difficult to differentiate from malignancy. There are several agents that may induce a granulomatous mastitis (Table 6–2). Idiopathic granulomatous mastitis (IGM) is a diagnosis of exclusion, once other sources have been ruled out.

IGM predominantly occurs in women in their third or fourth decade, although it has been reported in older patients. Patients typically present with a firm breast mass, often associated with inflammation of the overlying skin. It may be bilateral. It is readily mistaken for nonpuerperal mastitis, a breast abscess, or carcinoma. The exact pathogenesis is not clear. One hypothesis is an autoimmune reaction to extravasated secretions from lobules. IGM has been associated with other autoimmune diseases such as erythema nodosum, Wegener's granulomatosis, giant cell arteritis, and polyarteritis nodosa, although most women with IGM show no systemic immune abnormalities.

The goal of the clinician is to rule out both cancer and other sources of mastitis. As with any breast mass, this begins with a thorough history, physical examination, and breast imaging. Often prolactin levels are elevated in association with IGM, and these should be measured because antiprolactin therapy may be a consideration. Radiologic findings include nodular opacities on mammography and hypoechoic nodules on ultrasonography. Occasionally imaging shows multiple clustered,

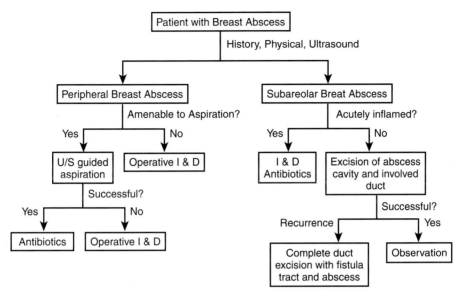

Figure 6–3. Approach to the patient with a breast abscess. A peripheral breast abscess may be aspirated but may require an incision and drainage. Subareolar breast abscesses are slightly trickier. If acutely inflamed, incision and drainage and antibiotics are indicated. Further surgery will then be necessary to prevent recurrence, including excision of the entire cavity with the involved duct. Recurrent disease may require a central duct excision.

contiguous hypoechoic lesions that may suggest GM, but usually the radiologic findings, like the physical findings, are worrisome for malignancy. Ultimately, the diagnosis comes down to a biopsy. Histology shows a predominantly lobular inflammatory process. Core biopsy typically demonstrates a noncaseating granulomatous granuloma, giant cells, chronic inflammation, microabscesses, and necrosis. Tissue should be sent for acid-fast bacillus and fungal stains to rule out tuberculosis or nocardia. An incisional biopsy may be necessary to obtain adequate tissue. Fine-needle aspiration biopsy is useless.

Once cancer has been definitively ruled out, the optimal management is unclear. If the diagnosis is confirmed by core-needle biopsy, excision might not be necessary if the mass is asymptomatic. In this case, careful follow-up to ensure that the area is not getting bigger is necessary. If the mass is painful or enlarging, or if an adequate diagnosis could not be made on core biopsy alone, complete excision may

TABLE 6–2 • *Granulomatous Mastitis*	
Sarcoidosis	Noncaseating granulomas between and within lobules. Histology is diagnostic (epithelioid granulomas and giant cells with no central necrosis). Most often associated with sarcoidosis of the lungs.
Tuberculosis	Caused by *Mycobacterium tuberculosis*. Now quite rare. Acid-fast bacteria can be seen in special stains. Antituberculous therapy is often effective.
Dirofilaria tenuis	A nematode in the United States responsible for breast nodules. Transmitted to humans by insect bites. Can be seen on histologic sections after excision.
Nocardia asteroides	Fungal infection associated with chronic abscess in the breast. Stains for fungi reveal nocardial organisms. Antifungal therapy is often effective.
Foreign material	Paraffin, injected directly into the breast for augmentation, can cause hard masses and chronically draining sinuses. Silicone gel, also injected directly into the breast, can cause hard masses within the breast.

be necessary to both make a definitive diagnosis and obtain the proper stains. This is typically followed by steroid therapy following the idea that this is an autoimmune disease. Prednisolone 60 mg/day is recommended for 6 weeks. If the extent of the IGM precludes excision, then preoperative treatment with steroids, nonsteroidal antiinflammatory drugs, or colchicine may allow for more conservative surgical procedures.

Recurrence after excision, however, is not uncommon and fistula formation is a potential complication. Repeated attempts at excision in patients with chronic granulomatis mastitis is not recommended. In these patients, if prolactin levels are elevated, antiprolactin therapy can be considered. Remission may be achieved with a 12- to 24-month course of low-dose methotrexate and prednisone.

Suggested Readings

1. Baslaim MM, Khayat HA, Al-Amoudi SA. Idiopathic granulomatous mastitis: A heterogeneous disease with variable clinical presentation. World J Surg 2007;31(8):1677–1681.
2. Dener C, Inan A. Breast abscesses in lactating women. World J Surg 2003;27:130.
3. Foxman B, D'Arcy H, Gillespie B, et al. Lactation mastitis: Occurrence and medical management among 946 breastfeeding women in the United States. Am J Epidemiol 2002;155:103.
4. Karstrup S, Solvig J, Nolsoe CP, Nilsson P. Acute puerperal breast abscesses: US-guided drainage. Radiology 1993;188:807.
5. Katz U, Molad Y, Ablin J, et al: Chronic idiopathic granulomatous mastitis. Ann N Y Acad Sci 2007;1108:603–608.
6. Li S, Grant CS, Degnim A, Donohue J. Surgical management of recurrent subareolar breast abscesses: Mayo Clinic experience. Am J Surg 2006;192(4):528–529.
7. Meguid MM, Oler A, Numann PJ, Khan S. Pathogenesis-based treatment of recurring subareolar breast abscesses. Surgery 1995;118(4):775–782.
8. O'Hara RJ, Dexter SP, Fox JN. Conservative management of infective mastitis and breast abscesses after ultrasonographic assessment. Br J Surg 1996;83:1413.
9. Schafer P, Furrer C, Mermillod B. An association of cigarette smoking with recurrent subareolar breast abscess. Int J Epidemiol 1988;17(4):810–813.
10. Schwarz RJ, Shrestha R. Needle aspiration of breast abscesses. Am J Surg 2001;182:117.
11. Taghizadeh R, Shelley OP, Chew BK, Weiler-Mithoff EM. Idiopathic granulomatous mastitis: Surgery, treatment, and reconstruction. Breast J 2007;13(5):509–513.
12. Wilson JP, Massoll N, Marshall J, et al. Idiopathic granulomatous mastitis: In search of a therapeutic paradigm. Am Surg 2007;73(8):798–802.

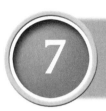

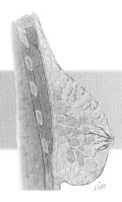

Gynecomastia

ETIOLOGY
Genetic Disorders
Malignancy
Thyroid Disorders
Liver Disease
Renal Failure
Drugs
HIV-Positive Men

EVALUATION
History and Physical

TREATMENT
Medical Therapy
Surgery

Gynecomastia: Key Points

Understand the pathophysiology and risk factors for gynecomastia.

Be familiar with the medications that can cause gynecomastia.

Describe a thorough history, physical, and laboratory evaluation of the patient with gynecomastia.

Describe the risk factors for male breast cancer and the indications for biopsy of a male with a breast mass.

Know the treatment options for gynecomastia, including medical and surgical.

Gynecomastia is a benign proliferation of the glandular tissue of the male breast. While it is a common condition, it can not only be painful for the patient, but can also be an obvious source of psychological distress. Before adulthood, there are two stages of physiologic gynecomastia. Between 60% and 70% of infants have a transient development of breast tissue due to estrogenic stimulation from the mother. Once the estrogens are cleared from the neonatal circulation after delivery, the breast tissue gradually regresses over 2 to 3 weeks. The second stage comes at puberty, when 30% to 60% of boys

may exhibit gynecomastia. This usually resolves by age 16 to 17.

In adulthood, the incidence of gynecomastia increases with age, with a sharp increase after age 50. The prevalence can be as high as 50% to 60% depending on the criteria for defining gynecomastia and the population studied. Most of these patients were unaware that they had any degree of gynecomastia, denying pain or the presence of any palpable breast tissue.

It is important to differentiate gynecomastia from *lipomastia*, which is excessive breast adipose tissue but not enlargement of the ductal elements. This is usually easily differentiated on physical examination. Most patients with gynecomastia present with complaints of a unilateral swelling underneath the areola, which is often tender. In many cases, this might be a firm disc of retroareolar tissue, easily demarcated from the surrounding fat. In other cases, there might be a dramatic increase in the size of one breast over the other, or of both breasts. The goal of the clinician is to rule out a serious underlying endocrine or systemic disease as the cause of the gynecomastia, and if none is present, to guide treatment choices for idiopathic gynecomastia.

Etiology

Examination of the subareolar tissue in normal men reveals the presence of major ductal systems with rare secondary ductal branching. This male breast tissue has estrogen receptors and androgen receptors. With proliferation of this secondary branching and the surrounding stroma, gynecomastia occurs. Estrogens exert a trophic and stimulatory effect on mammary epithelial tissue growth while androgens inhibit this effect. The major androgens include testosterone (synthesized by the testes) and dihydrotestosterone, which is converted from testosterone by several tissues including the skin, adipose tissue, the prostate and others. Estrogen is primarily present in men as estradiol, which is synthesized from peripheral aromatization of testosterone or androstenedione (a weak androgen secreted by the adrenals). Increased levels of estrogen or decreased levels of androgens can tilt the equation toward the growth of ductal breast epithelium.

There are many underlying processes that can lead to gynecomastia. As stated, gynecomastia is not unusual in neonates because of placental estrogens. Around puberty, there can also be a point where the synthesis of plasma estradiol increases before the maximal synthesis of testosterone. This shift in the ratio can lead to temporary gynecomastia. This may occur in 30% to 60% of boys and may be more common in boys with greater body mass. The gynecomastia may be associated with asymmetry, cosmetic concerns, pain, and tenderness, however this almost always resolves. Finally, older men also have an increased incidence of gynecomastia secondary to declining plasma testosterone concentrations. Again,

this appears to be more common in heavier individuals.

There are, however, other causes of changes in the estrogen/androgen ratio that not only lead to the development of gynecomastia but may be significant of a more serious health condition. These include disease processes that result in excess estrogen (either by increased production or decreased clearance), those that lead to decreased androgens, or those caused by exogenous agents (medications, drugs).

Genetic Disorders

Several genetic disorders can be associated with gynecomastia (Table 7–1). The familial aromatase excess syndrome is caused by overexpression of the gene coding for aromatase, leading to increased aromatization of androgens to estrogens. Affected male patients present with precocious puberty and gynecomastia. Absent

TABLE 7–1 • Conditions Associated with Gynecomastia

Physiologic (pubertal, aging)
Obesity
Exogenous estrogen (topical creams or ingested)
Malignancy
Increased estrogen
Sertoli cell (sex cord) tumors
Testicular germ cell tumors (choriocarcinoma, seminoma, teratoma, embryonal carcinoma)
Leydig's cell tumors
Adrenocortical carcinoma
Increased hCG production
Lung carcinoma
Liver carcinoma
Gastric carcinoma
Kidney carcinoma
Choriocarcinoma
Decreased testosterone synthesis
Anorchia, trauma, castration, viral orchitis, irradiation
Hydrocele, varicocele, spermatocele
Testicular failure from hypothalamic or pituitary disease
Klinefelter's syndrome, hermaphroditism
Liver failure
Chronic renal failure
Hyperthyroidism
Refeeding syndrome

or defective androgen receptors may lead to gynecomastia. Klinefelter syndrome (KS) is the most common chromosomal deficiency associated with hypogonadism and thus gynecomastia. KS has a 47, XXY karyotype, which is not only a risk for gynecomastia but also for male breast cancer.

Malignancy

One of the most concerning sources of excess estrogen comes from testicular tumors (Table 7–2). These can include gonadal stromal (nongerminal) neoplasms and germinal cell tumors. Nongerminal neoplasms include Leydig's cell (interstitial) tumors, Sertoli's cell tumors, and granulosa-theca cell tumors. Germ cell tumors include choriocarcinoma, seminoma, teratoma, and embryonal cell carcinoma. For this reason, a testicular examination is a mandatory part of the workup for gynecomastia. Any question of a mass should prompt an ultrasound and referral for urology consultation. Some of these tumors, however, may be nonpalpable, small focal lesions within the parenchyma of the testes. Any young patient with gynecomastia that cannot be explained, is associated with other symptoms such as loss of libido or sexual dysfunction, or is associated with abnormal endocrine laboratory studies should also undergo a testicular ultrasound and be referred for urology consultation.

Other tumors can also lead to an excess estrogen state. Tumors of the adrenal cortex, both adenomas and adrenocortical carcinoma, have been associated with gynecomastia, but this is rare. Adrenocortical carcinoma is a concern in the patient with gynecomastia and symptoms of Cushing's disease or other mixed syndromes, or with other signs of feminization.

Lung carcinoma can lead to an increase in plasma chorionic gonadotropin and a simultaneous escalation in estrogen secretion. Rare cases of malignant mesothelioma, kidney cancer, or gastric cancers producing human chorionic gonadotropin (hCG) have also been reported, but again are rare. Finally, hepatocellular carcinoma can be associated with gynecomastia, the

TABLE 7–2 • *Malignancies Associated with Gynecomastia*		
Tumor	**Characteristics**	**Association with Gynecomastia**
Leydig cell tumors	Rare tumors of testis, mostly benign May occur at any age, but is most common in young and middle-aged men	Secrete estradiol, raising estrogen and suppressing LH, leading to reduction in testosterone
Sertoli cell tumors	Rare tumors of testis, mostly benign	Overexpression of aromatase, increasing conversion to estrogens
hCG-secreting tumors	Germ cell tumors of testes, nontesticular tumors such as lung, liver, gastric, or kidney	Tumors produce hCG, which stimulates normal Leydig cells to secrete estradiol preferentially Take up steroid precursors from circulation and aromatize them into estrogens
Feminizing adrenal tumors	Malignant, poorly differentiated tumors with a poor prognosis Peak incidence among young, middle-aged men	Direct secretion of estrogen
Pituitary tumors		Secretion of LH or interference with secretion of LH leading to a decrease in androgen levels Secretion of prolactin
Prostate cancer	Androgen-dependent tumor often treated by androgen deprivation or blockade	Treatment with estrogen, LHRH analogues, nonsteroidal antiandrogens or bilateral orchiectomy

hCG, Human chorionic gonadotropin; LH, luteinizing hormone; LHRH, LH-releasing homone.

consequence of increased aromatase activity in the hepatic neoplasm.

As androgen deprivation or androgen blockade is a primary treatment of prostate cancer, gynecomastia is often a result of therapy. Treatments such as systemic estrogens, luteinizing hormone-releasing hormone (LHRH) analogues, nonsteroidal antiandrogens (flutamide, bicalutamide), and bilateral orchiectomy can all lead to the development of gynecomastia. Prophylactic radiation therapy has been effective in decreasing the risk of developing gynecomastia, but there is concern regarding the long-term risks. Tamoxifen has also been shown to be effective at preventing gynecomastia in men about to begin antiandrogen therapy.

Thyroid Disorders

Approximately 10% to 40% of men with thyrotoxicosis may develop gynecomastia, although the reasons are not clear. In hyperthyroid individuals, it may be direct mammotrophic effects of thyroid hormone on ductal epithelium, although many people believe it may be mediated through alterations in estrogen metabolism, specifically the increased peripheral conversion of androgens to estrogens and increased levels of sex hormone-binding globulin (SHBG). Regardless, the gynecomastia almost always resolves once the hyperthyroidism is treated.

Liver Disease

Several chronic diseases of the liver can result in gynecomastia, although the incidence may be less than originally suspected. Gynecomastia is present in up to 40% of cirrhotic men, but may also be present in age-matched controls. However, there are some physiologic reasons for gynecomastia among cirrhotic patients. These patients have not only a decreased production of testosterone (alcohol has a direct toxic effect on gonadal function), but also a decreased clearance of androstenedione, leaving more substrate available for aromatization. Patients with liver disease also have an increased concentration of SHBG, resulting in an increase in protein bound testosterone and a corresponding decrease in the free, biologically active fraction of plasma testosterone. Gynecomastia has also been documented in other chronic liver diseases such as idiopathic hemochromatosis and fatty metamorphosis of the liver.

Renal Failure

Gynecomastia can be a common result of uremia and can be seen in up to half of patients undergoing dialysis. This may be secondary to histologic damage to the testes. In addition, decreased metabolic clearance by the kidneys may result in increased levels of luteinizing hormone (LH) and subsequent increased estradiol secretion. Many of these men may be nauseated and anorexic, which improves after initiating dialysis, leading to a refeeding syndrome (see later text).

Drugs

Several drugs can lead to the development of gynecomastia. Some of these do so because they have direct estrogenic activity. These include not only drugs such as estrogens, oral contraceptives, and tamoxifen, but also anabolic steroids, heroin, digitalis, and tetrahydrocannabinol, which is found in marijuana. Other drugs inhibit testosterone or decrease its synthesis. These include drugs such as cimetidine, diazepam, flutamide, phenytoin, or spironolactone. Several other drugs have been linked to gynecomastia, although the mechanisms are unclear. Table 7–3 includes a list of medications associated with gynecomastia. It is estimated that approximately one in four cases of gynecomastia is related to drugs.

Estrogens can clearly lead to gynecomastia, but estrogen is rarely taken intentionally by men (except in the case of prostate cancer treatment or among male-to-female transsexuals). However, some men may be getting unintentional exposures to estrogens. There may be estrogen in certain skin creams or antibalding lotions. It can sometimes be absorbed by men after intercourse with a woman using a vaginal estrogen cream. Estrogen exposure may also occur at work or through the diet, although large amounts are typically needed to develop gynecomastia (except in boys and young men, in whom smaller exposures may lead to gynecomastia) (Box 7–1).

HIV-Positive Men

Gynecomastia is being increasingly seen in men with human immunodeficiency virus (HIV) disease, although the reasons are unclear and likely multifactorial. Many of the antiretroviral medications used to treat HIV are associated with gynecomastia. Some HIV-positive men use illicit drugs (marijuana, heroin) or have concomitant

TABLE 7–3 • *Hormones or Regulators of Hormone Synthesis*

- Anabolic steroids (nandrolone, testosterone cypionate)
- Estrogens and estrogen agonists (oral contraceptives, hormone replacement, tamoxifen)
- Human growth hormone
- Goserelin acetate or leuprolide acetate (gonadotropin hormone-releasing hormones)
- Flutamide
- Nilutamide
- Antibiotics
  - Metronidazole
  - Ketoconazole
  - Isoniazid
  - Ethionamide
  - Minocycline
- Antiulcer medications
  - Cimetidine
  - Omeprazole
  - Ranitidine
- Cardiovascular drugs
  - Spironolactone
  - Bumetanide
  - Digitoxin
  - Digoxin
  - Amiodarone
  - Diltiazem
  - Enalapril
  - Methyldopa
  - Nifedipine
  - Reserpine
  - Verapamil
- Psychoactive agents
  - Diazepam
  - Haloperidol
  - Phenothiazine
  - Tricyclic antidepressants
- Chemotheraputic agents
  - Alkylating agents
  - Methotrexate
  - Vinca alkaloids
  - Busulfan
- Drugs of abuse
  - Alcohol
  - Amphetamines
  - Heroin
  - Marijuana
  - Methadone
- Auranofin
- Calcitonin
- Diethylpropion
- Domperidone
- Etretinate
- Metoclopramide
- Penicillamine
- Phenytoin
- Sulindac
- Theophylline

liver disease. Some HIV-positive patients have hypogonadism. There may also be a refeeding mechanism at play. This phenomenon was first seen after World War II when men liberated from prison camps developed gynecomastia after

BOX 7–1 UNINTENTIONAL EXPOSURE TO ESTROGEN

Medications
  Skin creams
  Antibalding lotions
  Vaginal estrogen cream (through intercourse)
Occupations
  Barbers (who apply estrogen-containing creams into the scalp)
  Morticians (who apply estrogen-containing creams onto corpses)
  Factory workers involved in manufacturing estrogens
Diet
  Milk or meat from estrogen-treated cows
  Phytoestrogens in plants or animals

resuming a normal diet. During starving, men may develop hypogonadotropic hypogonadism, and when these men eat normally and begin to gain weight, there is a transient imbalance of estrogens to androgens. This can also be seen in refugees, in impoverished individuals, or after dieting.

Evaluation

History and Physical

The patient should be queried as to the duration and timing of the breast enlargement (Box 7–2). A thorough family history should be obtained. A review of symptoms focusing on signs and symptoms associated with hypogonadism should be obtained, including erectile dysfunction or decreased libido. Signs and symptoms of systemic diseases associated with gynecomastia should also be reviewed. Finally, an extremely thorough medication history and social history should be obtained. It is usually best to have family members wait outside the examining room during the history and physical to diminish the patient's reluctance to divulge potentially important information.

On physical examination, the breast tissue can be elevated up off of the chest wall by pinching, allowing for accurate measurement. Tenderness should be noted and an attempt should be made to elicit nipple discharge. Bilateral breast examination should be performed to compare symmetry, and a thorough examination for adenopathy should be performed. In addition, percussion and palpation of the liver should be performed, as should be a testicular examination.

BOX 7–2 DETAILED HISTORY IN
PATIENT WITH GYNECOMASTIA

- Onset and duration of breast enlargement
- Associated symptoms (breast pain, tenderness, skin involvement, nipple discharge)
- Systemic symptoms (weight loss, fatigue)
- Family history of cancer
- Symptoms of hyperthyroidism (heat intolerance, nervousness, tachycardia, weight loss, increased appetite)
- Symptoms of liver disease
- Changes in libido, impotence
- Complete past medical history
- Full list of medications (including over-the-counter and "natural" medications)
- Possible occupational or accidental exposures to estrogens

The thickening should be concentric in the breast. Asymmetric thickening or masses should raise the possibility of malignancy. Other worrisome features include ulceration, immobility, bloody nipple discharge, and palpable adenopathy.

Mammography

Mammography is extremely useful in imaging gynecomastia. Gynecomastia appears as a flame-shaped opacity extending into the surrounding fat. Mammography can effectively distinguish between malignant and benign breast disease (Fig. 7–1). If the history, physical, and mammography all suggest simple gynecomastia, biopsy may be avoided.

Biopsy

If at this point in the evaluation there is any concern that an underlying malignancy might be present, then a biopsy is indicated. Biopsy is

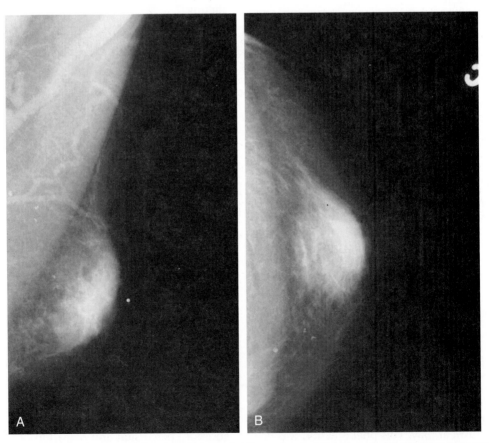

Figure 7–1. A and **B,** Craniocaudal and mediolateral oblique views of right breast demonstrate gynecomastia.

(Continued)

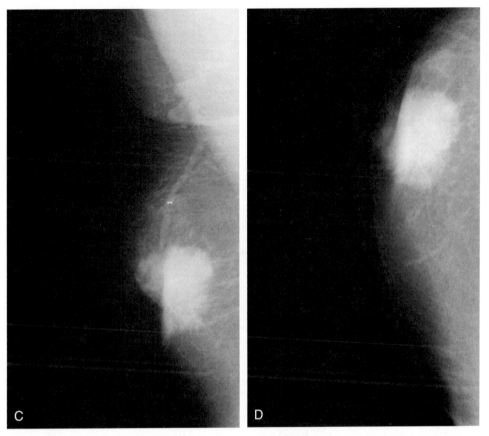

Figure 7–1—cont'd   C and **D,** Craniocaudal and mediolateral oblique views of left breast demonstrate a spiculated retroareolar mass with associated nipple retraction. Patient underwent mastectomy for treatment of invasive breast cancer. (Images courtesy of Dr. Alexis Nees, Department of Radiology, University of Michigan.)

not necessary in every patient with gynecomastia, but patients with worrisome features such as an asymmetric or hard mass, fixed mass, skin ulceration, bloody nipple discharge, or an abnormality on imaging should have a biopsy performed. Core-needle biopsy has been the biopsy method of choice in this situation, although now that the cytologic features of gynecomastia have been well described, fine-needle aspiration biopsy is an option if an experienced cytopathologist is available (Fig. 7–2).

Laboratory Evaluation

If the history does not suggest a drug as the inciting agent, then several laboratory tests may help find the cause (Table 7–4). Biochemical assessment of the liver (liver function tests), kidney (BUN/Cr), and thyroid (T_3, T_4, thyroid-stimulating hormone) should be performed because gynecomastia may be the result of underlying liver disease, chronic renal failure, or thyroid disease. A chest x-ray study, if one has not been done recently, should be obtained. This is particularly true in older individuals. In addition to these tests, measurements of serum concentrations of several hormones may be obtained. These include serum estradiol (or estrone), testosterone, LH, SHBG, hCG, and prolactin. These tests do not need to be obtained routinely in every patient with gynecomastia, but their use should be guided by the clinical situation. If any abnormalities are discovered, further workup and treatment should proceed accordingly. However, the majority of cases will have a normal laboratory evaluation and will be labeled as idiopathic gynecomastia.

Treatment

The treatment of gynecomastia depends on the severity (Table 7–5) and whether an identifiable cause is present. If a possible cause has

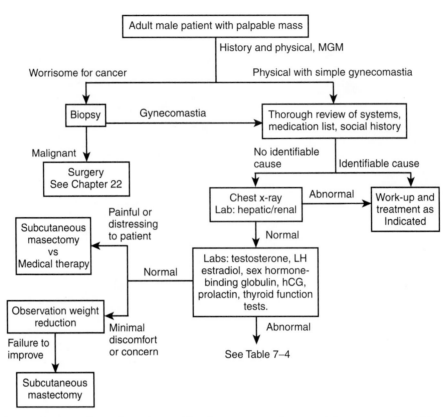

Figure 7–2. Approach to the male patient with a breast mass. Any suspicious mass should be biopsied. A mass consistent with gynecomastia on history, physical, and mammogram may be observed, with a thorough search for possible causes. How extensive of a biochemical evaluation should be undertaken in the asymptomatic patient is controversial because there is a very low yield for identifying any abnormality.

TABLE 7–4 • *Laboratory Workup of Gynecomastia*		
Lab Results	**Consider**	**Further Workup**
↑hCG	Germ cell tumor or hCG-secreting nontrophoblastic neoplasm	Testicular ultrasound (testicular germ cell tumor) CT of chest and abdomen (bronchogenic, renal, gastric, or hepatic carcinoma)
↑ LH, ↓ T	Primary hypogonadism	
↓ LH, ↓ T ↑ P	Prolactin-secreting pituitary tumor	MRI of brain
↓ LH, ↓ T normal P	Secondary hypogonadism	
↑ LH, ↑ T ↑T4, ↓ TSH	Hyperthyroidism	
↑ LH, ↑ T normal T$_4$, TSH	Androgen resistance	
↓ LH, ↑ E2	Nongerminal testicular tumor, adrenal tumor, increased aromatase activity	Testicular ultrasound (rule out Leydig or Sertoli cell tumor) Abdominal CT or MRI (rule out adrenal neoplasm)

CT, Computed tomography; E2, estradiol; hCG, human chorionic gonadotropin; LH, serum luteinizing hormone; MRI, magnetic resonance imaging; P, prolactin; T, testosterone; T$_4$, thyroxine; TSH, thyroid-stimulating hormone.

TABLE 7–5 • *Clinical Classification of Gynecomastia*

Grade	Definition
I	Mild breast enlargement without skin redundancy
IIa	Moderate breast enlargement without skin redundancy
IIb	Moderate breast enlargement with skin redundancy
III	Marked breast enlargement with skin redundancy and ptosis

been identified, then therapy should be directed at correction of that cause. Gynecomastia will almost always resolve with the treatment of the underlying disorder or withdrawal of the causative medication. Resolution can be seen within a few weeks.

If no cause is identified, if the underlying disease cannot be treated, or if the causative medication cannot be discontinued, then the goal of treatment depends on the severity of the condition. Because most cases of gynecomastia are associated with hormonal imbalances or drugs and because gynecomastia itself carries no serious significance (assuming serious causes have been ruled out), reassurance is the first line of therapy, and in many cases patients desire no further intervention. The risk of male breast cancer does not appear to be increased in patients with gynecomastia, except in patients with KS. For patients who have symptomatic gynecomastia, treatment is primarily surgical, although some medical therapies have been proposed. Unfortunately there are few well-designed prospective trials of medical therapies for gynecomastia.

Medical Therapy

Clomiphene citrate is an antiestrogen that acts at the level of the hypothalamic-pituitary axis to increase gonadotropin secretion. Although it may be successful, particularly in the adolescent population, the side effects may be severe (gastrointestinal reactions, rashes, visual disturbances), and in this population spontaneous resolution often occurs. It is therefore not indicated in the treatment of gynecomastia. Likewise, percutaneous dihydrotestosterone heptanoate has been shown to reduce gynecomastia in pubertal patients but has never been tested in prospective

randomized trials and again, spontaneous resolution is common in this population, so its true efficacy is unknown.

Danazol (Danocrine) is the 2,3,isoxazol derivative of 17α-ethyl testosterone and has been tested in patients with gynecomastia of varying causes with response rates of 77% to 100%. Treatment lasts for 3 to 16 weeks with dose schedules of 100 to 400 mg/day for adults or 200 to 300 mg/day for adolescents. Side effects include acne, weight gain, fluid retention, muscle weakness, and cramps. Finally, tamoxifen can be effective in treating gynecomastia, but the long-term effects of tamoxifen in men are not well studied. Doses of 10 to 20 mg/d for 3 to 9 months have been used, with resolution in up to 90% of men. It can be considered in patients who have severe idiopathic gynecomastia after a thorough, exhaustive workup has failed to identify any underlying causes. If the gynecomastia recurs upon stopping the tamoxifen, a second course of therapy may be attempted.

Medical therapies are most effective in men with new-onset gynecomastia. With long-standing gynecomastia, the stroma is more fibrotic and less likely to resolve. Surgery is the preferred treatment in these patients, as well as in patients who decline or fail medical therapy.

Surgery

Most patients with gynecomastia prefer surgical therapy given the rapid cosmetic improvement and the avoidance of medications (many patients are taking several other medications already for their underlying conditions). The primary treatment of gynecomastia is surgical, consisting of a subcutaneous mastectomy. Simple mastectomy is not indicated. Patients must be aware that they may be trading one cosmetic deformity for another.

For most patients with a small amount of gynecomastia, a periareolar incision can be used to excise the breast tissue. A small disk of breast tissue should be left underneath the nipple to prevent the sunken nipple deformity. For patients with more extensive gynecomastia, excess skin may need to be removed to restore the contour of the breast. Several techniques have been described to accomplish this. However, in these more extreme cases, or in cases in which there is both an excess of breast tissue and fat, liposuction may be a useful alternative to surgery.

Suggested Readings

1. Braunstein GD. Clinical practice. Gynecomastia. N Engl J Med 2007;357(12):1229–1237.
2. Gikas P, Mokbel K. Management of gynaecomastia: An update. Int J Clin Pract 2007;61:1209–1215.
3. Narula HS, Carlson HE. Gynecomastia. Endocrinol Metab Clin N Am 2007;36:497–519.
4. Patterson SK, Helvie MA, Aziz K, Nees AV. Outcome of men presenting with clinical breast problems: The role of mammography and ultrasound. Breast J 2006;12(5):418–423.
5. Wise GJ, Roorda AK, Kalter R. Male breast disease. J Am Coll Surg 2005;200:255–269.

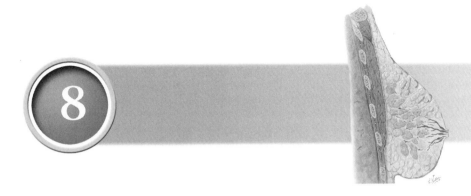

Identifying and Managing the High-Risk Patient

Identifying and Managing the High Risk Patient: Key Points

Know the genetic syndromes associated with an increased risk of breast cancers, as well as the other malignancies also at elevated risk.

Understand the impact of family history and menstrual and reproductive factors on the individual woman's risk of breast cancer and the strengths and limitations of predictive models.

Describe dietary and environmental factors that may increase or decrease the risk of breast cancer.

Understand the implications and management of atypical hyperplasia.

Describe the management options for the woman diagnosed with lobular carcinoma in situ.

Know the risks and benefits of tamoxifen and raloxifene for the chemoprevention of breast cancer.

Recognize the options for the woman with a known or suspected BRCA1 or BRCA2 mutation.

All women are at risk of breast cancer, with one in eight developing the disease within their lifetime. The breast surgeon is going to see a wide array of women, each one at a different risk of developing cancer, or in some cases a second cancer. Knowing that risk will impact several decisions, including when and how to begin screening, whether an abnormal finding should be biopsied or observed, the best course of treatment for a woman diagnosed with cancer, implications for family members, and when a woman without breast cancer may benefit from chemoprevention or prophylactic surgery. In addition, many patients concerned about cancer will have many questions regarding things they can do to decrease their risk.

It is also up to the surgeon to allay patient's concerns and misconceptions regarding their risk of breast cancer. Most women have been inundated with media reports regarding the importance of family history. Women with a single, second-, or third-degree relative who had breast cancer in her 70s may present overly worried about her risk of breast cancer. The emphasis of family history and breast cancer also has the effect of convincing women that if they do not have a family history, they cannot get breast cancer. A large majority of breast cancer cases are not associated with a positive family history. In fact, nearly half of breast cancers patients have no identifiable risk factor.

Discussing risk with a patient is not easy. Telling the patient that she has a 1 in 8 risk over her lifetime or that her risk of developing breast cancer is 4% over the next 5 years is a difficult concept for patients to interpret. It is also important not to overly frighten patients.

Risk Factors for Breast Cancer

The biggest risk factor for developing breast cancer is gender. Breast cancer is 100 times more common in women than in men. The second strongest risk factor is age. The incidence of breast cancer rises sharply with age, although the rise is less steep after age 50, reflecting the impact of hormonal changes. At 75 to 80 years of age, the risk starts to decrease slightly. There are multiple other risk factors for breast cancer, with varying prevalence in the population and varying relative risks.

Certain risk factors may be surrogates for true risk factors. For example, several studies have demonstrated that women of higher socioeconomic status are at greater risk for breast cancer, whether one categorizes this as economic status, education, occupation, or other measures of status. This may be as great as a two-fold difference between the highest and lowest classes. The reasons for this are not entirely clear, but it is hard to believe that higher education directly leads to the development of breast cancer. A more likely explanation is that women of varying socioeconomic factors have differences in their menstrual history. For example, women who spend more time in school or who are dedicated to their career may be delaying their first pregnancy until later in life or have fewer pregnancies. Another possibility is that female infants who have better nutrition may develop menarche at an earlier age.

Another risk factor for breast cancer is the area of the world in which the woman lives. For example, breast cancer incidence and mortality is much higher in the United States and Northern Europe than it is in Asia. The incidence and mortality rates also vary throughout the United States. The incidence is highest in Hawaii and the lowest in Utah. Again, this increased risk may be related to factors such as genetics or differences in the number of children, age at first live birth, or age at menarche. They may also represent differences in environment or diet. For example, studies of first-generation daughters of Japanese American women suggest that risk increases in Japanese women when they move to the United States, suggesting a lifestyle factor.

Hereditary Risk Factors

Race

There are considerable interracial differences in the risk of developing breast cancer. The rates in African-American women, Latina women, and Asian-Americans are all lower than those in Caucasians. The reasons for this are not clear. Some of this might be genetic, but some may be attributable to lifestyle, diet, or environment. As an example, some of the lowest rates of breast cancer were seen in Asia, particularly in the 1970s and 1980s. However, the incidence of breast cancer in Asia has been increasing, and Asian women living in the United States have an increased risk of breast cancer, suggesting environmental causes. This is discussed in more detail in Chapter 22.

Family History

Family history is clearly an important risk factor. Familial clustering of breast cancer has long been recognized, with the greatest risk in women with a first-degree relative with early-onset breast cancer. However, only 10% of women diagnosed with breast cancer have a positive family history. It should be emphasized with women that the absence of a family history does not mean that breast cancer is not a concern. Likewise, not all women with a relative who had breast cancer are at the same increased risk. The risk increases with the age of the patient, the age of the relative, the number of relatives with cancer, and the relation between the subjects (e.g., first degree, second degree). For example, in a metaanalysis using data from 150,000 women, the risk of breast cancer was increased three times for a woman who had a relative with breast cancer before age 30, but only 1.5 times if the relative was diagnosed after age 60. As another example, women with one affected first-degree relative had a risk 1.8 times that of their counterparts, whereas women with two affected first-degree relatives saw risk increase threefold.

Genetic Mutations

One of the strongest risk factors for the development of breast cancer is the family history. However, the number of breast cancers that are due to the inheritance of a specific genetic mutation is relatively low. It is believed that only 5% to 10% of all breast cancers are associated with the inheritance of a high penetrance autosomal dominant cancer predisposing gene such as BRCA1, BRCA2, p53, ATM, PTEN, MLH1, or MSH2.

Breast cancers associated with germ line mutations tend to occur at younger ages. Genetic mutations may be responsible for more than 25% of breast cancers in women younger than 30, compared to less than 1% for women older than 70. There may also be multiple cancers (e.g., bilateral breast cancers) or associations with other malignancies such as ovarian cancer (in the case of BRCA1/2 mutations) or sarcomas (as with p53 mutations). The likelihood that a breast cancer may be secondary to a genetic mutation is more likely when multiple family members have early-onset or bilateral breast cancers, or other malignancies (Table 8–1).

BRCA1 and BRCA2

With the discovery of BRCA1 and BRCA2 in 1994 and 1995, respectively, the management of breast cancer changed dramatically. Physicians caring for all women now need to understand the benefits and pitfalls of genetic testing and which populations should undergo testing. This is particularly true for surgeons seeing patients with signs or symptoms suggestive of cancer, or women already diagnosed with breast cancer. If these patients harbor a BRCA1 or BRCA2 mutation, they have a risk of developing breast cancer as high as 70% to 80% in their lifetime. How mutations in BRCA1/2 predispose to cancer is not well understood, although the evidence suggests that BRCA genes act as tumor suppressor genes.

It should be obvious how the identification of such a mutation may alter the surgical management of the breast cancer patient, increase suspicion in a patient with a breast complaint, as well as impact family members. However, genetic testing should not be obtained indiscriminately. BRCA mutations are rare, occurring in approximately 0.1% of the general population and at a

Gene (Syndrome)	Breast Cancer Risk by Age 70 (%)	Other Associated Cancers
P53 (Li-Fraumeni)	>90%	Sarcoma (soft tissue and osteo), brain tumors, adrenocortical carcinoma, leukemia, colon
PTEN (Cowden's)	25% to 50%	Thyroid, enodmetrial, genitourinary
STK11/LKB1 (Peutz-Jeghers)	45% to 50%	Small intestine, colorectal, uterine, testicular, ovarian sex cord
CDH1 (hereditary diffuse gastric carcinoma)	39%	Diffuse gastric cancer
BRCA1 (HBOC)	39% to 87%	Ovarian, pancreatic
BRCA2 (HBOC)	26% to 91%	Ovarian, prostate, pancreatic, male breast cancer

TABLE 8–1 • *Genes Associated with an Increased Risk of Breast Cancer*

Other genes associated with an increased risk: ATM (ataxia-telangiectasia), BRIP1 (Fanconi's anemia), PALB2

slightly higher rate in certain other populations. For example, Ashkenazi Jewish women (meaning of Eastern European descent) have a higher incidence of BRCA mutations, about 2%. There are substantial psychological and social risks associated with genetic testing. In addition, one must be cognizant of the fact that genetic testing is not perfect. No single technique for genetic testing is able to detect all mutations. Even when the entire gene is sequenced, the detection rate is not 100%. A negative test may give a woman false reassurance about her subsequent risk of breast cancer. Genetic testing can also produce indeterminate or false-positive findings.

When considering a patient for genetic counseling and testing, it is important to assess the likelihood of finding a mutation. The great majority of women do not have a family or personal history suggestive of a BRCA mutation. Overall about 5% of women with breast cancer will be found to have a BRCA mutation. This risk increases with a decrease in the age of diagnosis. As mutations in these genes are inherited in an autosomal dominant fashion, several generations of women in affected families may have breast and possibly ovarian cancer.

The chance of finding a mutation in BRCA1 or BRCA2 increases with the number of family members who have had breast or ovarian cancer, the number of relatives who have had multiple cancers, and the younger age when family members developed cancer (Table 8–2). A detailed family history on both the paternal and maternal sides should be obtained, recording any malignancies (not just breast or ovarian cancer), the age when the malignancy occurred, and in the case of breast cancer, whether the cancer was bilateral. A useful tool to predict the likelihood of an individual having a deleterious BRCA mutation is a computerized program BRCAPRO, which incorporates six predictive models for inherited breast cancer. This program is available free of charge at http://www.cancerbiostats.onc.jhmi.edu/BayesMendel/.

In women with breast cancer, other clues that a BRCA mutation may be responsible may be in the histology, because cancer secondary to BRCA1 mutations is more likely to be poorly differentiated, estrogen receptor (ER)/progesterone receptor (PR)–negative, and may have a medullary-like histology.

TABLE 8–2 • *The Likelihood of Finding a BRCA Mutation Based on Family History*	
Family History	**Chance of BRCA Mutation**
1 Breast cancer younger than 30 years of age	12%
1 Breast cancer younger than 40 years of age	6%
1 Breast cancer between 40 and 49 years of age	3%
2 Breast cancers younger than 50 years of age	15%
2 Sisters with breast cancer younger than 40 years of age	37%
3 Breast cancers younger than 50 years of age	28%
4 Breast cancers younger than 50 years of age	47%
5 Breast cancers younger than 50 years of age	60%
Ovarian cancer younger than 50, not Ashkenazi Jewish	10%
Ovarian cancer older than 50, not Ashkenazi Jewish	3%
Ovarian cancer younger than 50, Ashkenazi Jewish	60%
Ovarian cancer older than 50, Ashkenazi Jewish	30%
1 Ovarian cancer and 1 breast cancer younger than 50 years of age	33%
1 Ovarian cancer and 2 breast cancers younger than 60 years of age	60%
1 Ovarian cancer and 3 breast cancers younger than 60 years of age	90%
2 Ovarian cancers, average age younger than 60 years of age	40%
2 Sisters with ovarian cancer younger than 50 years of age	61%
2 Ovarian cancers, average age older than 60 years of age	20%
2 Ovarian cancers and 1 breast cancer younger than 60 years of age	80%
2 Ovarian cancers and 2 breast cancers less younger than 60 years of age	95%-100%%
3 Ovarian cancers	90%
More than 3 ovarian cancers	100%

If after a careful history a BRCA mutation is suspected (at least a 10% chance), the patient should be referred to a genetic counselor. Genetic testing should not be initiated by the clinician without pretest counseling. Women need to consider the implications of either a positive or negative result. The implications of both are complex enough, and the potential psychosocial, medical, and legal ramifications severe enough, that counseling is necessary to help women make an informed decision and plan how they and their family are going to use the information. There are implications regarding insurance and employment discrimination. Although federal legislation (the Health Insurance Portability and Accountability Act of 1996) and state laws prohibit insurers from excluding an individual from health coverage based on genetic testing, there are still some areas where the law fails to fully extend this protection. Furthermore, genetic testing is not inexpensive and not always fully covered by insurance.

Interpreting the results of genetic testing is not straightforward. When dealing with a woman with a strong family history, the ideal situation is one in which there are family members alive who had or have breast cancer. In this situation, if a deleterious mutation has been identified in the family member, genetic testing would be extremely helpful for the patient. In this case, a true positive result would occur when the individual being tested has the same mutation as the affected family member. In the case of a positive result, the patient would know her increased risk and this would allow her to consider prophylactic measures. A negative result would inform the woman that, despite her family history, she does not carry this elevated risk.

However, if a specific cancer-associated mutation has not or cannot be identified in an affected family member, genetic testing for the patient may not be as helpful. A negative test does not rule out an increased risk secondary to genes other than BRCA1 and BRCA2. Or, there could be a mutation in BRCA1/2 that was not detected by the available methods. A positive result may also be uninformative. Although it may represent a newly identified mutation, it could also simply be a benign polymorphism. It is also unclear what the exact range of cancer risk might be for different mutations.

p53 (Li-Fraumeni Syndrome)

Li-Fraumeni syndrome is an autosomal dominant condition characterized by the development of multiple tumors. Families have identifiable mutations in the p53 gene. In addition to early-onset breast cancer, carriers have an increased risk of soft tissue sarcomas, osteosarcomas, brain tumors, leukemias, and adrenocortical malignancies. Half of Li-Fraumeni patients develop some type of cancer by age 30.

ATM (Ataxia Telangiectasia)

An autosomal recessive disorder, ataxia telangiectasia (AT) results from a mutation in the ATM gene, mapped to chromosome 11q22.3. It is quite rare (between 1 in 20,000 and 1 in 100,000 live births) and is characterized by progressive cerebellar ataxia and other neurologic abnormalities, oculocutaneous telangiectasias, immune deficiencies, diabetes mellitus, and a predisposition to malignancy, including breast cancer Although the disease is rare, it is estimated that as many as 1% to 2% of Caucasians in the United States may carry one defective gene. Several studies support an increased risk of breast cancer in AT carriers (as high as 4 times that of noncarriers).

PTEN (Cowden Syndrome)

Mutations in the PTEN gene (phosphatase and tensin homologue), also referred to as MMAC1, can lead to Cowden syndrome, characterized by hamartomas in the skin, oral mucosa, breast, and intestine. PTEN is a tumor-suppressor gene, and Cowden syndrome is inherited in an autosomal dominant fashion. In addition to the hamartomas, carriers are at an increased risk of both breast and thyroid cancers. Up to 75% of women with Cowden syndrome will manifest benign breast conditions (fibroadenomas, papillomas), whereas cancer will develop in 25% to 50%. Benign thyroid conditions (adenomas, goiter) will develop in half of those affected, whereas thyroid cancer develops in about 10% of individuals. Endometrial and renal cancers may also be associated with Cowden syndrome.

STK11 (Peutz-Jeghers Syndrome)

Peutz-Jeghers syndrome (PJS) is a result of mutations in STK11, a serine threonine kinase, and is characterized by hamartomatous polyps in the gastrointestinal tract. Affected individuals are at increased risk of many malignancies including gastrointestinal (gastric, pancreatic, colon) and cancers outside the gastrointestinal tract (breast, ovarian, endometrial). PJS is also associated with mucocutaneous pigmentation in the buccal mucosa, lips, fingers, and toes.

Menstrual and Reproductive Factors

Prolonged exposure to both exogenous and endogenous estrogen will increase the risk of breast cancer. For premenopausal women, estrogen subtypes (estradiol, estriol, estrone) come from the ovaries. After menopause, the main source of estrogen is dehydroepiandrosterone (DHEA). Produced in the adrenal gland, DHEA is metabolized in peripheral fat tissue to estradiol and estrone. The exposure to estrogen, and thus the risk of breast cancer, can therefore be estimated by assessing key reproductive factors.

Age at Menarche

The later the onset of regular menstrual cycles, the later the exposure to estrogen and less lifetime exposure. Therefore the older a young woman is when she begins the menstrual cycle, the lower the risk of developing breast cancer. There is an approximately 10% reduction in breast cancer risk for every 2-year delay in the onset of menarche.

Age at Menopause

In contrast to the age of menarche, the later a woman undergoes menopause, the higher her risk for breast cancer, which is thought to reflect longer exposure to endogenous hormones. Women who undergo bilateral oophorectomy before the age of 40 can reduce their risk by 50%. However, this risk reduction disappears if the woman takes hormone replacement.

Pregnancy

The number of pregnancies a woman has and the age at which she has her first full-term pregnancy can influence breast cancer risk as well. The protective effect comes from the full cellular differentiation in the breast that occurs during and after pregnancy (Chapter 1). Nulliparous women have a relative risk of about 1.5. Whether multiple pregnancies decrease that risk is unclear. Also somewhat confusing is the impact of the age of a woman at her first full-term pregnancy. As a general rule, women giving birth at older ages have a higher risk than their younger counterparts. However, it is not so simple. For example, women who give birth to their first child after the age of 30 appear to have a higher risk than nulliparous women. And women are at a higher risk of breast cancer in the years immediately after pregnancy, with the decrease in risk not coming until later in life (about 10 years after delivery).

This protection is conferred by full-term pregnancy, so this does not apply to disrupted pregnancies. Because abortion disrupts the pregnancy and the cellular differentiation of the breast, opponents to abortion have promoted the idea that abortion increases the risk of breast cancer. Population-based cohort studies, however, fail to support an association between abortion and breast cancer risk, and the National Cancer Institute accepted the conclusions of a workshop examining reproductive events and breast cancer that there is no evidence of a link between induced abortion and breast cancer risk.

Hormone Levels

The association between reproductive factors and breast cancer risk centers on exposure to hormones, primarily estrogen. This is supported by observational data, epidemiologic studies, animal models, and the clear evidence of risk reduction by decreasing estrogen levels. So it is reasonable to believe that measuring serum estrogen levels would identify high-risk individuals. However, the correlation between breast cancer risk and the levels of hormones in the blood have not been consistent. Part of this is due to difficulties with the assays. More responsible is the large variability between patients, and within individuals, of hormone concentrations. Estrogen levels fluctuate during the menstrual cycle, so studies of premenopausal women, particularly when only one blood sample is used, are difficult to interpret. The data are clearer for postmenopausal women, in whom multiple prospective epidemiologic studies have found a positive relationship between serum estradiol concentration and breast cancer risk. The association is strongest when looking at ER- and PR-positive tumors.

A surrogate for circulating estrogen levels is bone mineral density, in that bone contains estrogen receptors and is highly sensitive to estrogen levels. Women with high bone density appear to have a higher risk of breast cancer than those with low bone density.

Hormone Replacement Therapy

There is clear evidence of an association between the use of hormone replacement therapy (HRT) and breast cancer. Although this risk has received extensive media attention and is consistent across studies, it is a relatively modest risk, estimated to be about a 1.24-fold increase. However, the link between HRT and breast cancer is not so straightforward. Although the risk has been demonstrated for women taking combined estrogen/progesterone compared to placebo, the same risk has not been demonstrated for women taking unopposed estrogen, which may even be associated with a lower breast cancer risk. The length of time a woman uses HRT is also important. Long-term use of HRT is associated with the highest risk. Using HRT for a limited amount of time does not appear to increase the risk of breast cancer significantly.

Oral Contraceptives

The evidence is also fuzzy about whether oral contraceptives are linked to breast cancer. Multiple studies were unable to demonstrate an increased risk, although a large metaanalysis calculated a small but significant increase in the relative risk (RR 1.24). The risk appears to decrease after stopping use and by 10 years after stopping is back to normal. This metaanalysis has been criticized, however, for limited follow-up, and two subsequent studies found no evidence of increased risk, including among women with a family history of breast cancer.

Depot medroxyprogesterone acetate (DMPA) is a long-lasting, injectable contraceptive that suppresses ovulation for 90 days. It is approved for contraceptive use in the United States. It was thought that the serum estradiol-lowering effects of this drug might decrease breast cancer risk but there is no evidence for this in epidemiologic studies. In contrast, a case control study by the World Health Organization showed a slight increased breast cancer among current users, but not in past users.

Dietary Factors

Many of the factors discussed are beyond the control of the individual. Family history, age, race, genetic factors, and age of menarche or menopause are all factors that cannot be altered. Other factors, such as age at first pregnancy or the number of pregnancies, can be altered, but more important considerations tend to influence family planning decisions. The decision to breast-feed and for how long, and the decision to take hormone replacement therapy are controlled by the patient. Other areas within the control of the individual are factors related to diet and exercise.

Height and Weight

The height and weight of an individual has been associated with a higher risk of breast cancer in a number of studies. The reasons for this are complex. A woman's height and weight varies with her nutritional status in her developmental years, which is also related to the age of menarche. Young women who have significant nutritional deficiencies, such as those with anorexia nervosa, have a decreased incidence of breast cancer. In addition, a high body mass index (BMI) is associated with increased levels of estrogens. Obesity is strongly associated with an increased risk of breast cancer.

Physical Activity

Exercise has been linked to a decreased risk of breast cancer, but again, the reasons are complex. This does not need to be overly strenuous exercise, because a decreased risk of breast cancer can be seen in women who do brisk walking for 10 hours or more per week. The protective effect is seen in both premenopausal and postmenopausal women. Several mechanisms might explain this. The most obvious would be the link between exercise and reducing obesity, although a direct link between weight loss and risk reduction has not been demonstrated. Physical activity also appears to reduce serum estrogens, particularly in postmenopausal women, and this may also play a role in the decreased risk among women with increased physical activity.

Specific Foods

Epidemiologic studies of diet and cancer are extremely difficult for obvious reasons. They are often heavily dependent upon patient recall, which can often be inaccurate. The great variability of foods within a particular group makes categorization difficult. There are often confounding factors associated with diet that may bias the results. It is therefore difficult to make any solid recommendations on risk reduction based on dietary factors. However, many of the recommendations (decreased dietary fat, increased fruits and vegetables) have other health benefits.

Ecologic studies comparing breast cancer incidence and *dietary fat* intake have shown a strong positive correlation between the two, and for many years this was suspected to be the primary reason for the increased breast cancer risk seen in many Western countries. However, the results of prospective case control and cohort studies have been mixed. In the Nurses' Health Study, women who had the lowest fat intake had a decreased risk of breast cancer compared to those women with the highest fat intake. This was among premenopausal women. A pooled analysis of more than 300,000 women, mostly postmenopausal, failed to demonstrate any connection between dietary fat and breast cancer. It may be that the influence of dietary fat is more significant in younger women, particularly in the prepubertal years. This may have more impact on age of menarche and subsequent BMI. A prospective study, The Women's Health Study, which randomly assigns women to a low-fat or average American diet, is presently under way and may provide more answers on this topic.

There is presently no convincing evidence that taking vitamins or nutrients, such as vitamins A, C, E, or selenium, will alter the risk of breast cancer. Although caffeine is linked to fibrocystic disease of the breast, a number of studies have failed to show any increased risk of breast cancer with caffeine intake.

Alcohol is associated with an increased risk of breast cancer. This effect may be additive with HRT.

There has been considerable interest in the effects of *phytoestrogens* on breast cancer risk. Phytoestrogens are natural plant substances that have potential antioxidant activity. There are several types of phytoestrogens: isoflavones, coumestans, and lignans, which are found in a variety of fruits and vegetables. Overall, the data suggesting a protective effect of phytoestrogens in general have been weak. However, two phytoestrogens found in soy, the isoflavones genistein and daidzein, may function as weak estrogens in the body. In effect, these isoflavones may behave like tamoxifen, functioning as relative antiestrogens by displacing estradiol. Given the high soy intake in Asia and the low rates of breast cancer, many people believe that soy consumption decreases breast cancer risk.

Factors Related to the Breast

Previous History of Breast Cancer

One of the strongest risk factors for the development of breast cancer is a personal history of either in situ or invasive breast cancer. The risk of a second breast cancer in women with a history of breast cancer is approximately 1% per year among premenopausal women and 0.5% per year for postmenopausal women.

Breast Density

Dense breast tissue often hampers both physical examination of the breast as well as mammographic detection of breast cancers. There is some evidence now that the presence of dense breast tissue is also associated with an increased risk of developing breast cancer, with a relative risk between 1.8 and 6 times that of women with less dense tissue.

Breast-Feeding

Epidemiologic studies correlating breast-feeding with breast cancer have been quite variable, with no clear results. Studies in the United States have failed to demonstrate a connection, although studies from Asian countries have. It should be pointed out that women in these countries tend to breast-feed longer than American women. An analysis of 47 studies investigating this question concluded that the risk for breast cancer was decreased with breast-feeding, but this effect is quite small, perhaps a 4.3% decrease in risk for every 12 months of breast-feeding. This is in addition to a decrease of 7% for each birth. The exact mechanisms for this protective effect is unknown, although it is most likely due to a delay in the return of the ovulatory cycles and a decrease in estrogen production.

Proliferative Lesions without Atypia

Many women will present with complaints of breast masses or mammographic abnormalities that will ultimately turn out to have benign disease. While these lesions may not require immediate treatment, some may indicate an increased risk of breast cancer for the individual. Benign lesions can be categorized as proliferative or nonproliferative. Nonproliferative lesions are not associated with an increased risk for breast cancer, whereas proliferative lesions may be associated with an increased risk of either noninvasive or invasive disease. The risk associated with proliferative lesions depends upon the degree of atypia associated with the lesion.

Proliferative lesions without atypia include fibroadenoma, moderate or florid hyperplasia, sclerosing adenosis, radial scar, and intraductal papillomas. In these women, the relative risk of breast cancer is approximately 1.3 to 2 times that of other women. This varies with the specific lesion and the features of that lesion. For example, the presence of a fibroadenoma appears to be associated with an overall risk of breast cancer of 1.4 to 1.7 that of the general population. However, the risk is not uniform among all fibroadenomas. The majority of the elevated risk is among women with fibroadenomas exhibiting a complex histology or hyperplasia or those that occur in women with a first-degree relative with breast cancer (a risk above that of the family history alone). The remainder of women with a fibroadenoma (about 70%) are left without an apparent increased risk.

Proliferative Lesions with Atypia (Atypical Hyperplasia and Lobular Carcinoma in Situ)

When atypia is present in a proliferative lesion, the risk of breast cancer is significantly increased. The relative risk of developing breast cancer in a patient with atypical hyperplasia is increased 4.5 to 5 times. Atypical hyperplasia includes patients with atypical ductal hyperplasia and atypical lobular hyperplasia. Lobular carcinoma in situ is sometimes categorized as a proliferative atypical lesion and sometimes categorized as in situ disease. It is most appropriately discussed as a risk factor, associated with a 7 to 9 times increased risk and an absolute lifetime risk of breast cancer of 20%.

The atypical hyperplasias are proliferative lesions that possess some, but not all, of the features of carcinoma in situ. Atypical ductal hyperplasia (ADH) has some of the architectural and cytologic features of low-grade ductal carcinoma in situ (DCIS), and a distinction between the two is sometimes difficult. ADH is typically confined to a single lobular unit, seldom larger than about 3 mm overall. The hyperplastic cells may form tufts, micropapillae, or bridges within the involved space. The cells are relatively uniform with monomorphic round nuclei (Fig. 8–1). Atypical lobular hyperplasia (ALH) usually involves multiple lobular units with or without involvement of intervening ducts. The cells are monomorphic and evenly spaced with round or oval eccentric nuclei. The cytoplasm is pale with intracytoplasmic vacuoles. (Fig. 8–2).

Lobular carcinoma in situ (LCIS) is a noninvasive lesion that arises from the lobules and terminal ducts of the breast. LCIS is almost always an incidental finding in a breast biopsy in that it does not form a mass, does not have calcifications or other mammographic findings, and does not lead to nipple discharge or other breast symptoms. When LCIS is

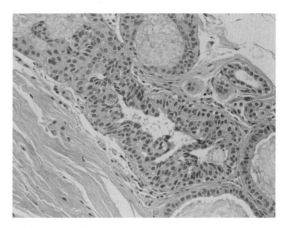

Figure 8–1. Histology of atypical ductal hyperplasia. There is a proliferation of relatively uniform cells with monomorphic round nuclei, in some but not all areas. In other areas the cells maintain their orientation to each other. Thus there are some of the features of low-grade DCIS. (Image courtesy of Maria Braman, MD, Department of Pathology, University of Michigan.)

discovered on a biopsy prompted by calcifications, the calcifications are often located in normal epithelial cells adjacent to the LCIS, rather than the involved lobules.

Histologically, LCIS is characterized by acini filled with a monomorphic population of small, round, polygonal, or cuboidal cells. The cells are often pale and slightly eosinophilic. These possess a thin rim of clear cytoplasm with a high nuclear-to-cytoplasm ratio. The nuclei are uniform. Many cells contain clear vacuoles.

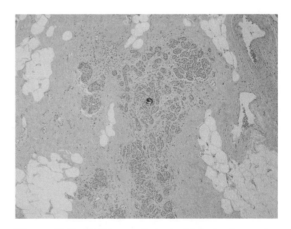

Figure 8–2. Histology of atypical lobular hyperplasia (ALH). Within the acini are small, uniform, evenly spaced cells. When less than half the acini are filled, distorted, or distended, a diagnosis of ALH is favored over lobular carcinoma in situ. (Image courtesy of Maria Braman, MD, Department of Pathology, University of Michigan.)

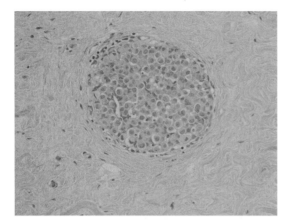

Figure 8–3. Histology of lobular carcinoma in situ. There is a solid proliferation of small, uniform round/cuboidal cells within the acini. (Image courtesy of Maria Braman, MD, Department of Pathology, University of Michigan.)

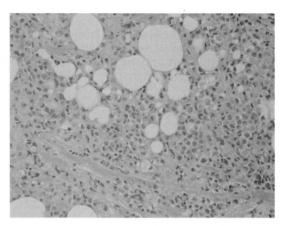

Figure 8–5. Pleomorphic lobular carcinoma in situ (PLCIS). The cells are larger, more pleomorphic, and eccentric. Some may have necrosis and dystrophic microcalcifications, making differentiation from DCIS difficult. (Image courtesy of Maria Braman, MD, Department of Pathology, University of Michigan.)

The cells are loosely cohesive and regularly spaced. Without disturbing the overall lobular architecture, the cells fill and distend the acini (Fig. 8–3). A characteristic of LCIS is *pagetoid spread*, wherein the neoplastic cells extend along adjacent ducts between intact overlying epithelium and underlying basement membrane (Fig. 8–4).

When the LCIS cells demonstrate marked pleomorphism and distinctly larger, eccentrically placed nuclei, this is a distinct entity known as *pleomorphic LCIS (PLCIS)*. Sometimes these cells have a signet ring cell appearance (Fig. 8–5). These cells are more discohesive than in classic LCIS, and central necrosis and calcifications, which are rarely seen with LCIS,

are more common with PLCIS. Recognition of the pleomorphic subtype is important for several reasons. The cellular features, necrosis, and calcifications can often make the differentiation from DCIS difficult. Frequently, PLCIS is associated with an infiltrating pleomorphic lobular carcinoma, which has a similar cytologic appearance. Whereas the treatment paradigm for typical LCIS is one of prevention (see later), the treatment of PLCIS is more akin to that of DCIS: complete excision of the lesion with tumor-free margins and no residual calcifications on mammography, either via lumpectomy or mastectomy. If a pleomorphic invasive component is present, axillary staging should also be performed. The exact role of radiation after lumpectomy is unclear because the natural history of PLCIS is unknown.

Overall, the diagnosis of atypical hyperplasia implies an increased risk of 3.5 to 5.0 times that of the general population. The risk appears to be greater for ALH (RR 5.0 to 6.0) than that of atypical ductal hyperplasia (RR 3.5 to 5.0). ALH involving both lobules and ducts appear to have a higher risk than ALH involving only the lobules. The risk is much higher when atypical hyperplasia is diagnosed in a patient with a family history of breast cancer.

The risk of subsequent cancer is significantly higher when LCIS is diagnosed. The risk of developing an invasive cancer ranges from 5% to more than 30%, depending on the population being studied and the length of time patients are followed. Overall, the risk of developing subsequent invasive breast cancer

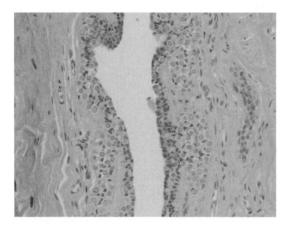

Figure 8–4. Pagetoid spread. The atypical cells are extending beneath the luminal epithelium of the extralobar ducts. This is characteristic of lobular carcinoma in situ. (Image courtesy of Maria Braman, MD, Department of Pathology, University of Michigan.)

is approximately 1% per year, a similar risk that is quoted for patients with a previous history of invasive breast cancer.

Surprisingly, the subsequent cancer is more likely to be ductal rather than lobular. Even so, the incidence of infiltrating lobular cancer is higher than that seen in the general population without LCIS (25% to 37% of cancers compared to 5% to 10% in the general population). The subsequent cancer is also possible in either breast. More than 50% of patients with LCIS show multiple foci, and about 30% of patients have further LCIS in the contralateral breast. This is one reason why LCIS has been considered to be only an indicator of risk rather than a direct precursor of invasive cancer, and management is based on risk reduction and not surgical excision of the LCIS.

Other Factors

Cigarette smoking has been implicated as increasing breast cancer risk, but the relationship is controversial and weak at best. *Silicone breast implants, electromagnetic fields, electric blankets, antiperspirants,* and *hair dyes* have all been implicated as causes of breast cancer, but have shown no increased risk in most studies.

An association between *antibiotic use* and breast cancer was suggested by a case control study and received significant media attention. When cases and controls were compared, increasing cumulative days of antibiotic use for any condition was associated with a significantly greater risk of breast cancer. However, there were several confounding factors including the fact that women with greater antibiotic use were older, had a younger age at menarche, were more likely to have a family history of breast cancer, and had a higher use of hormone replacement. There may also have been a detection bias at play. It is unclear biologically how antibiotic use (or infections) may be associated with breast cancer and the clinical significance of these data is uncertain. Clearly, antibiotics should not be withheld among high-risk women when indicated, although careful consideration should be given to prescribing antibiotics in the absence of a clear indication.

Viruses have been linked to other solid tumors (nasopharyngeal cancer, cervical cancer, hepatocellular carcinoma) and have been suggested as a possible cause of breast cancer. Fragments of the Epstein-Barr virus genome and sequences similar to the mouse mammary tumor virus (MMTV) have been identified in invasive breast cancers, although the significance of this finding is unclear. Further research is needed to determine whether viruses play a role in breast cancer etiology.

Exposure to *ionizing radiation* at a young age is associated with an increased risk of breast cancer. Women may have been exposed for therapeutic purposes (Hodgkin's lymphoma, thymic enlargement) or accidental exposure (nuclear fallout). Women are most vulnerable during the prepubertal years (10–14) but even women in their 40s who are exposed to radiation have an increased risk. The low radiation associated with diagnostic imaging and the older age at which imaging studies are usually obtained make it highly unlikely that diagnostic x-rays increase breast cancer risk. *Electromagnetic radiation exposure* has been suggested as a risk factor for breast cancer. Most women are exposed to electromagnetic radiation from power lines, transformer substations, or use of electrical appliances. Residential magnetic field exposure does not appear to increase breast cancer risk.

The link between *melatonin* and estrogen has been proposed as a risk factor for breast cancer, specifically women who are awake at night. Melatonin is produced by the pineal gland and exposure to light at night suppresses this nocturnal process. This might result in increased estrogen exposure. Three studies have shown an increased risk of breast cancer among women who work at night or who did not typically sleep between 1 AM and 2 AM (when melatonin levels are highest). Again, the exact association between nocturnal light exposure and breast cancer has not been elicited and the strength of the association is variable.

Statistical Models to Estimate the Risk of Breast Cancer

It is apparent that with so many different factors potentially related to an individual woman's risk of developing breast cancer, it may be difficult to counsel patients. Models of risk prediction have been created using the strongest risk factors. These were created before genetic testing for BRCA1 and BRCA2, but may still be useful for women who have not undergone genetic testing. Other models are available that may predict a woman's risk of harboring a BRCA mutation, such as the BRCAPRO model. Each model is based on slightly different data and study designs, so they may result in slightly different risk estimations.

Gail and Claus Models

Gail and colleagues, using data from more than 2800 patients and more than 3000 matched controls, created the Gail model for unaffected individuals with a limited family history. This model boils down to five variables: current age, age at first live birth, age at menarche, number of first-degree relatives with breast cancer, and number of prior breast biopsies. Tables and computer programs (including several on the Internet) are available to estimate the 5-year and lifetime risks of developing breast cancer. The Claus model is based on data from more than 4300 breast cancer cases and 4600 control cases and is based primarily on age and family history.

Even though these models are widely used, particularly the Gail model, they are not without limitations. They are not relevant for women with AH or LCIS. The Gail model does not include information on race, which can impact breast cancer risk (see Chapter 22) and so may overestimate the risk among African-Americans or Asian-Americans. It does not take into account the age at diagnosis of the relative's breast cancer, so the woman whose mother had breast cancer at age 70 has the same reported risk as the woman whose mother developed the disease at age 30. By not including second-degree relatives, it overlooks the possible contribution from the paternal side of the family. The Claus model does include second-degree relatives and the age of onset, but does not include nonfamilial risk factors such as hormonal factors. Neither model takes into account bilateral breast cancer or ovarian cancer.

The newest model is the Tyler-Cuzick model. This model not only takes into account many of the relevant details of family history and hormonal factors, but also includes BMI and the presence of LCIS. A computerized version of this model is not yet available.

What Can I Do to Decrease My Risk?

Many of the factors related to an increased risk of breast cancer cannot be altered. A woman cannot change her parents or genes.

TABLE 8–3 • *Factors That May Be Modified to Decrease the Risk of Breast Cancer*

Factor	Comments
Pregnancy before age 25 years or multiple pregnancies	20% to 30% decreased risk but family planning should be based on other factors
Breast-feeding	Small decrease in risk but multiple benefits to the baby
Stopping or avoiding oral contraceptives	Impact unclear
Stopping or avoiding hormone replacement therapy	Balanced against symptoms
Stopping or minimizing alcohol intake	
Exercise	
Maintaining a healthy body weight	
Maintaining a low-fat diet	
Consuming low-fat dairy products, calcium, and vitamin D	Impact unclear
Consuming fruits and vegetables	Impact unclear
Soy products	Impact unclear

While it is possible to delay the onset of menarche (through increasing physical activity, altering the diet, or using LH-releasing agonists), this seems a rather extreme approach to decreasing risk and offers little to most women who explore risk reduction strategies in their adult years. Likewise, having a child before the age of 25 years will decrease breast cancer risk, but the decision whether and when to have a child is influenced by many factors.

There are some changes that women can make to decrease their risk of developing breast cancer (Table 8–3). Their relative impact varies, and some are only theoretical.

Lifestyle Changes

Breast-feeding may decrease the risk of developing breast cancer, although supporting data are not definitive. Given the benefits of breast-feeding for the infant, however, there is little reason not to encourage breast-feeding.

Alcohol consumption has been clearly shown to increase the risk of breast cancer, and limiting alcohol intake is an effective way to reduce risk (in addition to other health benefits). For those who do drink, adding folic acid to the diet may counteract the effects of alcohol on breast cancer and mitigate this risk.

Even though a woman may not have control over when she goes into menopause, she does have a choice as to whether she takes postmenopausal estrogens. HRT is effective at reducing the symptoms associated with menopause, but it does increase the risk of breast cancer. Menopause symptoms can be managed using nonhormonal therapies, such as citalopram, fluoxetine, venlafaxine, or gabapentin.

Dietary changes, although difficult to implement for many women, can decrease breast cancer risk. A healthy body weight should be maintained through both diet and moderate exercise. These have been clearly associated with a decreased risk of breast cancer, although the mechanisms still need further investigation.

Data are less clear when one looks at specific foods or diets. Some epidemiologic studies have noted a lower risk of breast cancer among patients who eat a relatively large amount of fruits and vegetables, although a direct connection is difficult to show. Soy consumption has also been linked to a decreased risk of breast cancer, but this likely needs to be implemented at a young age. There is no strong evidence that supplementing the typical Western diet with soy-based products will impact risk. Low-fat diets have been suggested to not only decrease the risk of breast cancer but also decrease the risk of recurrence after treatment for breast cancer patients. However, this involves lowering fat levels far below that of the average American woman. Intake of low-fat dairy products may exert a protective effect, especially in premenopausal women. In the Nurses' Health Study, an inverse association between breast cancer risk and intake of low-fat dairy products, calcium, and vitamin D was suggested for premenopausal women. The exact impact that this may have on breast cancer risk is unclear, but again, it has other health benefits and should be encouraged.

Chemoprevention

Aspirin

Because nonsteroidal antiinflammatory drugs (NSAIDs), through their inhibition of COX-2, have been shown to inhibit polyp formation and the development of colon cancer, there was hope that a similar effect would be seen in breast cancer. Whereas a modest benefit has been suggested by population-based studies, the results are not clear and are difficult to interpret. In addition, data from the Nurses' Health study showed no protective effect of NSAIDs' use on breast cancer risk. At this time, there is no evidence to suggest that aspirin use will decrease breast cancer risk, although there are other health benefits associated with daily low-dose aspirin.

Tamoxifen

Tamoxifen was originally synthesized in the mid-1960s during a search for oral contraceptives and fertility agents. It failed at both, but it was found to bind to the estrogen receptor and halted the growth of malignant breast cancer cells in vitro. Further studies revealed that in both normal breast tissue and in breast cancer, tamoxifen could act as an estrogen antagonist, occupying the estrogen receptor and blocking the effects of estrogen. This results in a decrease in epithelial cellular proliferation (Box 8–1). Ultimately, randomized clinical trials established a role for tamoxifen in the treatment of metastatic disease and as an adjuvant treatment for breast cancer. (See Chapter 17, Hormonal Therapy). It was noted in these trials that the risk of a contralateral breast cancer was decreased by 40% to 50%, leading to the idea that tamoxifen might be used for breast cancer prevention. This led to four large trials of breast cancer chemoprevention using tamoxifen.

The *Royal Marsden Hospital Prevention Trial* randomized 2471 healthy women with a family history of breast cancer to receive tamoxifen or a placebo. After a median of 70 months, there was no difference in the incidence of breast cancer between the two groups (34 for tamoxifen and 36 for placebo).

BOX 8–1 MECHANISMS BY WHICH TAMOXIFEN DECREASES EPITHELIAL CELLULAR PROLIFERATION

- Reduces in transforming growth factor-alpha (TGF-α)
- Reduces insulin-like growth factor-I (ILGF-1)
- Stimulates transforming growth factor-beta (TGF-β)
- Binds to calmodulin
- Inhibits protein kinase activity

The *Italian Tamoxifen Prevention Study* randomized 5408 women to receive tamoxifen or placebo. These patients were at low to normal risk of breast cancer. Overall, there was no difference in the development of breast cancer between the two groups (45 and 34, respectively). One subset that did appear to benefit was the group of women who were taking hormone replacement therapy. There was a significant reduction in breast cancer cases among women taking HRT and tamoxifen compared with women taking HRT and placebo (6 vs. 17, $P = .02$).

The *International Breast Cancer Intervention study (IBIS-I)* randomized 7152 women with a family history of breast cancer (either one first-degree relative with bilateral breast cancer or onset before age 50, or two or more relatives with breast cancer) to receive tamoxifen or placebo.

With a median follow-up of 50 months, there were significantly less breast cancers among tamoxifen users than women receiving placebo (69 vs. 101, $P = .013$). Although this translated to a risk reduction of 32%, there was an excess of deaths in the tamoxifen group (25 vs. 11). The thromboembolic risk was increased 2.5-fold with tamoxifen.

The largest study of tamoxifen for chemoprevention is the *Breast Cancer Prevention Trial (NSABP P-01)* (Table 8–4.) Between June 1, 1992, and September 30, 1997, a total of 13,388 women were randomized to receive tamoxifen (20 mg/day) or placebo. High risk was defined as (1) age older than 60 years, (2) a Gail model 5-year estimated risk of at least 1.66%, or (3) 35 years of age or older with a history of LCIS. After a median follow-up of 48 months (the study was stopped early when

TABLE 8–4 • *Average Annual Rates for Outcomes in the NSABP Breast Cancer Prevention Trial by Patient Characteristic*

	Invasive Breast CA per 1000 Women		
	Tamoxifen	**Placebo**	**Risk Ratio (95% CI)**
Age			
<49	3.8	6.7	0.56 (0.37-0.85)
50 to 59	3.1	6.3	0.49 (0.29-0.81)
>60	3.3	7.3	0.45 (0.27-0.74)
LCIS	5.7	13.0	0.44 (0.16-1.06)
Atypical hyperplasia	1.4	10.1	0.14 (0.03-0.47)
# Relatives with breast CA			
0	3.0	6.4	0.46 (0.24-0.84)
1	3.0	6.0	0.51 (0.35-0.73)
2	4.8	8.7	0.55 (0.30-0.97)
3 or more	7.0	13.7	0.51 (0.15-1.55)
Gail model 5 year risk			
<2	2.1	5.5	0.37 (0.18-0.72)
2.01-3.0	3.5	5.2	0.68 (0.41-1.11)
3.01-5.0	3.9	5.9	0.66 (0.39-1.09)
>5.0	4.5	13.3	0.34 (0.19-0.58)
Complications per 1000 Women			
Invasive endometrial CA <49	1.3	1.1	1.21 (0.41-3.6)
Invasive endometrial CA >50	3.0	0.8	4.01 (1.7-10.90)
Fractures	4.3	5.3	0.81 (0.63-1.05)
Stroke	1.4	0.9	1.59 (0.93-2.77)
Transient ischemic attack	0.7	1.0	0.76 (0.40-1.44)
Pulmonary embolism	0.7	0.2	3.01 (1.15-9.27)
Deep vein thrombosis	1.3	0.8	1.60 (0.91-2.86)

Data from Fisher B, Constantino JP, Wickerham DL, et al. Tamoxifen for prevention of breast cancer: Report of the NSABP P-1 Study. J Natl Cancer Inst 1998;90:1371–1388.
CA, Cancer; LCIS, lobular carcinoma in situ.

an interim analysis found statistical significance), it was found that tamoxifen decreased the relative risk of breast cancer by 49%. The reduction was entirely in ER-positive tumors; there was no change in the occurrence of ER-negative tumors. The reduced risk was seen among all age groups in the trial (0.56 for women 49 years or younger; 0.49 for women 50 to 59; 0.45 for women 60 years or older).

Although not as dramatic as with the IBIS-I study, there were significant increases in adverse effects with tamoxifen. Most were in women older than 50 years of age. These included increases in endometrial cancer, stroke, pulmonary embolus (PE), and deep vein thrombosis (DVT).

When the data from all four trials are combined, the overall risk reduction associated with tamoxifen is approximately 32% to 38%. However, the differences in the studies make it difficult to compare them. The Royal Marsden and IBIS trials were limited to women with a strong family history, the P-01 trial had a broad range of what was defined as high-risk, and the Italian study was limited to low to normal risk. There are also variations in sample size and compliance. The P-01 trial was the largest and had more power to detect a small difference; however, it has been criticized for including patients who developed tumors shortly after initiation. Thus some of the benefit demonstrated may have been in treating occult primary tumors rather than preventing cancers.

Who Should Be Considered for Tamoxifen Chemoprevention?

Tamoxifen has been approved for the prevention of breast cancer for women at high risk. However, the potential benefits of tamoxifen must be weighed against the risks on an individual basis (Box 8–2). The two most worrisome adverse events are endometrial cancer and thromboembolic events. These occurred predominantly in women older than age 50. The relative risk of endometrial cancer in the P-01 trial was 2.53. All were localized (stage I) and no deaths from the disease occurred. In addition, several cases of uterine sarcoma have been seen with long-term follow-up among the tamoxifen uses (compared to no cases in the control group). The relative risk of thrombolic events was also increased in older women, with risk ratios of 1.59, 3.01, and 1.60 for stroke, pulmonary embolism, and DVT, respectively. Therefore the risks of

> **BOX 8–2** WOMEN FOR WHOM THE BENEFIT OF TAMOXIFEN APPEARS TO OUTWEIGH THE RISK
>
> - Women younger than age 50 who have a projected 5-year risk of invasive breast cancer of between 1.5% and 7%
> - Women ages 50 to 59 years who have a uterus and a projected 5-year risk of invasive breast cancer of $\geq 6.0\%$
> - Women age 50 to 59 years without a uterus who have a projected 5-year risk of invasive breast cancer of $\geq 3.0\%$
> - Women ages 60 to 69 years without a uterus who have a projected 5-year risk of invasive breast cancer of $\geq 5.5\%$

tamoxifen are going to be higher in older women, particularly those who have not had a hysterectomy. Women with a history of stroke, transient ischemic attack (TIA), DVT, or PE should not use tamoxifen. Tamoxifen also has other side effects to consider. There was an increase of approximately 14% in the rate of cataract development compared to placebo, so women with a history of cataracts or cataract surgery should also avoid tamoxifen use. Hot flashes and vaginal discharge also increased significantly with tamoxifen use.

Women with LCIS, ALH, or ADH

Women with LCIS have an annual risk of invasive breast cancer of more than 1% per year. In the P-01 trial, 6% of the participants had LCIS and 9% had atypical hyperplasia. A benefit was seen in both women with LCIS (RR 0.44, 95% CI 0.16 to 1.06) and atypical hyperplasia (RR ratio 0.14, 95% CI 0.03 to 0.47).

Women with a Family History of Breast Cancer

Women with a strong family history should be counseled by a medical geneticist or genetic counselor about the appropriateness of genetic testing. If they are found to harbor a BRCA1 or BRCA2 mutation, tamoxifen is one option for preventing breast cancer (see later). In women who do not choose to be tested or who do not possess a mutation, tamoxifen is an appropriate consideration for reducing risk. Data from the P-01 trial did demonstrate a risk reduction even in women with 3 or more immediate relatives with breast cancer.

Women with BRCA1 and BRCA2 Mutation

Women with a mutation in BRCA1 or BRCA2 genes are at the highest risk of developing breast cancer. Unfortunately, the data are not clear as to the benefit of tamoxifen in this population. A case control study looking at tamoxifen use in 593 breast cancer patients with either a BRCA1 or BRCA2 mutation showed a decreased risk of contralateral breast cancer with tamoxifen. However, data from the NSABP P-01 trial suggest that a preventive benefit might only be in women with a BRCA2 mutation. Whereas there was a 62% reduction in the incidence of breast cancer in women with BRCA2 mutations, there was no reduction in women with BRCA1 mutations. Although these are based on very small numbers, in that genetic testing was performed on only a small fraction of the patients, these findings may be due to the fact that only a small percentage of tumors in BRCA-1 carriers are ER positive (17% to 24%) compared to BRCA-2 carriers (76% to 78%).

Women with a High Risk of Breast Cancer Based on Their Gail Model

As described earlier, the Gail model takes into account several factors when assessing a woman's risk of breast cancer, including age, age at menarche, age at first live birth, number of first-degree relatives with breast cancer, and the number of breast biopsies. High risk is typically defined as at least a 1.66% chance of developing breast cancer in the next 5 years. However, the benefits of tamoxifen in this population must be weighed against the potential risks.

Raloxifene

Raloxifene (Evista) resulted from efforts to design selective estrogen receptor modulators (SERMs) that have estrogen activity in bone and cardiovascular tissue but not in the reproductive tissues, for the purpose of lowering the risk of osteoporotic fractures. The Multiple Outcomes of Raloxifene Evaluation (MORE) trial randomized 7705 postmenopausal women with osteoporosis (and no history of breast or endometrial cancer) to either receive one of two doses of raloxifene or placebo. Although the trial was designed to look at osteoporosis, it was found that with 4 years of follow-up, there was an 84% relative reduction in the incidence of ER-positive breast cancer. There was no effect on ER-negative breast cancer. As with tamoxifen, raloxifene was associated with an increased risk of venous thromboembolic disease, but it was not associated with an increased risk of endometrial cancer.

These data prompted the Study of Tamoxifen and Raloxifene (STAR) trial, which randomized postmenopausal women who are high-risk for the development of breast cancer to receive either tamoxifen or raloxifene. One of the largest breast cancer prevention studies ever, STAR took place at more than 500 centers across the United States, Canada, and Puerto Rico. Initial results of STAR show that the drug raloxifene is as effective as tamoxifen in reducing the breast cancer risk of the women in the trial. In STAR, both drugs reduced the risk of developing invasive breast cancer by about 50%. In addition, within the study, women who were assigned to take raloxifene daily had 36% fewer uterine cancers and 29% fewer blood clots than the women who were assigned to take tamoxifen.

Aromatase Inhibitors

Aromatase inhibitors reduce circulating estrogen by approximately 90% in postmenopausal women and have been shown to be beneficial in the adjuvant therapy of breast cancer (see Chapter 17). The ATAC trial (anastrazole, tamoxifen, alone and in combination) randomized postmenopausal women with early-stage breast cancer to tamoxifen, anastrazole, or the combination. Anastrozole was superior to tamoxifen in prolonging disease-free survival. It also reduced the incidence of contralateral primary invasive breast cancers. However, additional data from trials looking specifically at aromatase inhibitors as chemoprevention are needed before this class of drugs can be used in this manner.

Surgery

Prophylactic Mastectomy

Bilateral prophylactic mastectomy is the most logical preventive measure, although it is also the most extreme. Prophylactic mastectomy should be a simple mastectomy, incorporating the nipple-areola complex and the breast tissue extending into the axilla, but not the axillary lymph nodes. Subcutaneous mastectomy is generally not thought to be appropriate as cancer can form in the nipple-areolar complex, but studies are examining the potential of nipple and areolar sparing mastectomies. Immediate reconstruction is appropriate and may reduce the psychological stress associated with the procedure. It must be stressed that mastectomy does not remove all mammary tissue. Residual mammary tissue can be found in the axilla and pectoralis fascia. Therefore it does not provide 100% protection against breast cancer. Studies of both high-risk women and breast cancer patients have shown that bilateral mastectomy reduces the risk by 90% to 95%.

While there is a clear reduction in the risk of developing breast cancer (possibly for a second time), the fact that even among high-risk women, most will not develop cancer and the cancers they do develop are usually curable, bilateral prophylactic mastectomy may not improve overall survival. This varies with the age and health of the patient, the risk of cancer, and the risk of systemic disease among patients already diagnosed with breast cancer. Thus a careful discussion needs to be held with the patient regarding what she can expect, and not expect, from bilateral mastectomy. The benefits of bilateral prophylactic mastectomy must be balanced against the physical and psychological consequences.

Prophylactic Oophorectomy

Observational studies have suggested that bilateral oophorectomy among premenopausal women reduces their risk of breast cancer. Even though this is probably not a reasonable intervention for the typical high-risk woman, it is a reasonable consideration for women with a heritable predisposition to breast cancer. Women with a BRCA1 and BRCA2 mutation are at an increased risk of not only breast cancer but also ovarian cancer. One study suggests that bilateral oophorectomy in women with a BRCA mutation will significantly reduce the risk of developing a breast or gynecologic cancer. This should be strongly considered for premenopausal women known to have a BRCA mutation and who have completed child bearing. It should also be considered in postmenopausal women with a BRCA mutation for the ovarian cancer benefit, but it is unclear what impact this might have on their subsequent breast cancer risk.

Management of the Patient with Lobular Carcinoma In Situ

The true incidence of LCIS in the population is unknown but it is discovered incidentally on approximately 0.5% to 3.8% of benign breast biopsies. Management is based on the fact that LCIS is not considered a malignant or premalignant lesion, but rather an indicator lesion for the risk of subsequent invasive carcinoma. The presence of LCIS in a breast biopsy specimen is one of the strongest risks currently known for the subsequent development of invasive carcinoma. Efforts to identify features of LCIS that are associated with a higher likelihood of invasive disease have been unsuccessful. Therefore all women with LCIS must be considered high risk.

The management of atypical hyperplasia or LCIS is twofold. The first step is to rule out the presence of an invasive cancer. When ADH, ALH, or LCIS is diagnosed by a core-needle biopsy, a wire-localized excisional biopsy is recommended to establish definitive histologic results. Often the diagnosis is upgraded to DCIS or invasive cancer (7% to 17% of cases). If an excisional biopsy demonstrates LCIS extending to the margins, however, reexcision is not necessary to obtain negative margins. Bilateral mammograms should be reviewed with increased suspicion, and biopsy of any additional suspicious lesions should be undertaken.

Once it is confirmed that the patient does not have DCIS or invasive cancer, a discussion must be held with the patient regarding her individual risk and prevention strategies. It often takes some time to explain the nuances of LCIS. It is important to explain why unilateral mastectomy or wide surgical excision with histologically negative margins and radiation therapy are not needed. Patients often come to the office having been told they have cancer, and they are confused when informed otherwise. Some surgeons and pathologists prefer the term "lobular neoplasia" to "LCIS" to decrease anxiety of patients and help avoid confusion, but LCIS remains the most commonly used name.

Patients diagnosed with LCIS have the following choices (Box 8–3):

1. Observation. As one might do for any woman known to have an increased risk of developing breast cancer, observation is a reasonable option. Women should be counseled that they have an approximately 1% per year risk of developing cancer. Attempts to further stratify this risk, such as by the extent of LCIS in the biopsy specimen, have been unsuccessful, although women with LCIS and a first-degree relative with breast cancer may have an even higher risk. In the

BOX 8–3 OPTIONS FOR WOMEN DIAGNOSED WITH ATYPICAL HYPERPLASIA OR LOBULAR CARCINOMA IN SITU

- Careful clinical follow-up is appropriate for most women with LCIS; the risk of invasive breast cancer is approximately 1% per year.
- Tamoxifen reduces the risk of invasive breast cancer by 55% and should be considered. Raloxifene may also be considered for postmenopausal women.
- Bilateral prophylactic mastectomy, usually with reconstruction, is an alternative approach for women unwilling to undergo careful observation or tamoxifen therapy.
- Excision to negative margins, radiation therapy, and chemotherapy have no role in treatment of women with LCIS.

absence of intervention, it is important for these women to undergo appropriate screening for breast cancer. At a minimum, this should include monthly self breast examinations, clinical examinations at 6-month intervals, and annual mammograms. There is no evidence that more frequent mammography is of benefit. Are there other more intensive options for screening for the woman with LCIS? MRI has recently been shown to increase the detection of cancer in women at high risk based on known genetic defects or strong family history (see Chapter 2). However, it has not been studied in the setting of LCIS, and it is important to note that MRI will detect many benign lesions. MRI-guided biopsy is still not available at many institutions, so a woman who has LCIS and an MRI-detected abnormality could find herself in a difficult situation. For now, MRI as a screening examination in women with LCIS cannot be routinely recommended. Another surveillance examination being touted for high-risk women is ductal lavage. Ductal lavage detects epithelial atypia among ductal cells collected from microcatheter lavage. Although this may someday be a promising tool for women at risk for invasive breast cancer, the role of ductal lavage in the surveillance of women with LCIS is uncertain.

2. Bilateral prophylactic mastectomy. A second and more drastic option for women with LCIS is bilateral simple mastectomy, usually with immediate reconstruction. Treatment strategies addressing one breast are not recommended because the risk of cancer in the contralateral breast is roughly the same as the risk in the biopsied breast. With the significant reduction in invasive breast cancer with tamoxifen treatment, recent trends of fewer women undergoing mastectomy to treat LCIS seem appropriate. However, some women may opt for prophylactic surgery.

3. Tamoxifen or Raloxifene. Before the advent of tamoxifen as chemoprevention, women with LCIS had only two options: continued observation or bilateral mastectomy. Today, the use of tamoxifen in women with LCIS is worthy of serious consideration. In the NSABP P1 Breast Cancer Prevention Trial, the rate of development of invasive breast cancer in women with LCIS was significantly less in the tamoxifen-treated group compared to the controls (5.69 versus 12.99 per 1000 women). The 56% risk reduction was slightly higher than that seen in women at risk for breast cancer based on other factors. Raloxifene is also an option for postmenopausal women. This is not to say that tamoxifen or raloxifene is ideal for all women with LCIS. Many women choose not to take tamoxifen because of the adverse effects, which can include hot flashes (an estrogen antagonist effect), endometrial hyperplasia, fibroids, and an increased risk of endometrial cancer and venous thromboembolism. Furthermore, women who receive tamoxifen need to be seen for ongoing follow-up every 3 months, with regular screening blood work to evaluate for the possibility of adverse effects; this is not necessary in women who undergo observation alone.

Management of the Patient with a BRCA Mutation

Recent estimates of breast cancer risk would suggest that a woman with a BRCA1 mutation has a 90% risk of breast cancer and a 24% risk of ovarian cancer by age 80. A woman with a BRCA2 mutation has a 40% risk of breast cancer and an 8% risk of ovarian cancer.

The rates of survival for these cancers are roughly similar to those of cancers in non-BRCA mutation carriers.

Management of these patients is difficult because several issues must be considered and the exact risk of breast cancer or ovarian cancer for any individual BRCA mutation carrier is difficult to assess. Counseling is of the utmost importance, taking into account the family history, personal medical history of the patient, ethnic group, and specific mutation. Family members must also be counseled regarding recommendations for testing and screening. A thorough discussion of the risks and benefits of increased surveillance, chemoprevention, and prophylactic surgery is necessary. It is quite unlikely that a breast surgeon has the time or expertise to discuss all of these issues with the patient, which is why genetic counseling is so important at this juncture. The surgeon must work with not only the genetic counselor, but also the medical oncologist (if chemoprevention is an option), the plastic surgeon (if bilateral mastectomy is considered), and the gynecologist (if bilateral salpingo-oophorectomy is considered) to determine the best strategy for each individual patient.

Increased Surveillance

Breast Examination

There are minimal data either supporting or refuting the importance of self breast examination for women with a hereditary risk of breast cancer. For women at average risk, self breast examinations do not appear to be associated with a decrease in breast cancer mortality but are associated with an increase in breast biopsies. Clinical breast examination will detect additional cancer beyond mammographic screening, although the numbers are small; roughly 3% to 8% of cancers were detected solely by clinical examination. Even among women with a hereditary risk, clinical examination detects only a small number of cancers above and beyond imaging. However, there are benefits to both self breast examination and clinical breast examination beyond cancer detection and most cancer societies continue to recommend their use for all women, not just women with a hereditary predisposition. There is minimal evidence to support high-risk women undergoing a clinical breast examination more often than every 6 months.

Mammogram

As opposed to breast examination, screening mammograms have been clearly shown to increase breast cancer detection and decrease breast cancer mortality (see Chapter 2). However, mammographic screening among BRCA carriers has several limitations compared to the screening in the general population. Patients are generally younger than 40 years of age, in whom mammographic screening is less sensitive due to breast density, and it is common for these patients to have interval cancers (cancers that become clinically apparent between yearly mammograms). Specialized mammogram screening programs among women with a familial risk have failed to demonstrate either an improved survival or a decreased stage at presentation, and the sensitivity of mammograms specifically among BRCA mutation carriers has been questioned.

Even so, yearly mammography is recommended for any woman with a known BRCA mutation who has not opted for bilateral mastectomy, beginning between the ages of 25 and 30. Digital mammography is recommended because studies have suggested a higher accuracy among women with dense breast tissue. At this time, there is no evidence to suggest that mammography more frequently than once a year is of added benefit.

Ultrasonography

Ultrasound is typically thought of as a complement to mammography; a tool to further scrutinize a palpable mass or abnormality seen on screening mammogram. Whole-breast screening ultrasonography does not yield a high enough rate of breast cancer detection to recommend its routine use. Even among high-risk patients, it is of questionable worth. It will detect some mammographically occult cancers, and for women who do not have access to MRI, may be worth adding to yearly mammography. However, in women undergoing screening MRI (see later), the addition of ultrasonography is of minimal value.

Magnetic Resonance Imaging

The use of MRI in the management of breast disease is controversial and still evolving, but one area where MRI has documented superiority is in the screening of the high-risk woman. Prospective studies of high-risk patients, including many women with BRCA mutations, have shown that MRI more than doubles the number of cancers detected using routine physical examination, mammography, and ultrasonography. Rates of interval cancers are less than 10% when MRI is included in the screening.

Despite the high sensitivity of MRI, it is not perfect, and both in situ and invasive cancers may be missed. Thus MRI should be performed with mammograms and should not be considered a substitute. Another problem with MRI has been the specificity. MRI will lead to the further evaluation and biopsy of a number of benign lesions that would not have been picked up on mammography and ultrasound. Specificity has varied in these studies, but has ranged from 81% to 97%. This variable specificity will affect the positive predictive value (PPV). However, PPV is dependent upon the frequency of the disease in question among the population being studied. Therefore the PPV is acceptable for high-risk women but significantly lower and less likely to be cost-effective among average risk women. Thus MRI screening should be limited to patients at high risk, especially those with BRCA mutations. At this time, yearly MRI as an adjunct to physical examination and mammography is recommended, although further research is necessary to define the most appropriate intervals, and the ideal population for MRI screening including what age to begin and what age to stop MRI screening.

The National Comprehensive Cancer Network (NCCN) has recommended that women with a genetic high risk of breast cancer be counseled to perform self breast examination on a monthly basis starting at age 18. Clinical breast examination should be performed every 6 months starting at age 25. Mammography and MRI should be performed yearly starting at age 25 (Box 8–4).

Other

BRCA mutations predispose patients to non–breast malignancies as well. Screening for other BRCA-associated cancers (ovarian, prostate, pancreas) is recommended, although there are little data to suggest a survival benefit or the ideal screening protocols (beyond those recommended for the general population). Although popular, screening BRCA mutation carriers for ovarian cancer through serum CA-125 measurements and transvaginal ultrasounds has not been shown to downstage ovarian tumors or improve survival. Likewise there are no data to support serum CA19-9

BOX 8–4 INCREASED SCREENING STRATEGY FOR WOMEN WITH A KNOWN BRCA1/BRCA2 MUTATION WHO DO NOT DESIRE RISK-REDUCING SURGERY

- Monthly breast self-examination beginning at age 18.
- Clinical breast examination every 3 to 6 months beginning at age 25.
- Annual mammography and magnetic resonance imaging study beginning at age 25.
- Twice yearly ovarian cancer screening with ultrasound and serum CA-125 levels beginning at age 35.

measurements or abdominal CT scans to screen for pancreatic cancer outside of a clinical trial. The benefit of mammography for male BRCA2 carriers is also unknown and not recommended, although these patients should be examined regularly by their internists for signs of breast cancer. Male carriers should also be monitored for signs of prostate cancer.

Risk Reduction Strategies

Tamoxifen

Five years of tamoxifen clearly decreases the risk of breast cancer, decreasing the incidence by 43% in the Breast Cancer Prevention Trial. Raloxifene will provide a similar risk reduction, with a lower risk of uterine cancer or venous thromboembolism among postmenopausal women. It is unclear, however, if this same degree of benefit can be expected among BRCA mutation carriers. A subgroup analysis of the Breast Cancer Prevention Trial failed to demonstrate a benefit, but the numbers were too small to exclude this possibility. Tamoxifen does appear to decrease the risk of contralateral cancers among BRCA patients treated for breast cancer.

Bilateral Prophylactic Mastectomy

Bilateral prophylactic mastectomy (BPM) reduces the risk of breast cancer by at least 90% among carriers of a BRCA mutation, and it should be presented and discussed with any affected patient. The exact benefits of bilateral mastectomy on survival are unclear. Even though mathematical models would suggest a survival benefit of bilateral mastectomy to routine surveillance, the degree of that benefit compared with oophorectomy and/or surveillance with MRI is not clear. Immediate reconstruction is strongly recommended to minimize the psychological trauma associated with bilateral mastectomy. Patients still need close follow-up because this prophylactic measure does not completely eradicate the risk of breast cancer.

Risk-Reducing Salpingo-Oophorectomy

Bilateral salpingo-oophorectomy (BSO) has not been evaluated in randomized trials, but both retrospective and prospective data strongly support its use. BSO can result in an 80% to 96% reduction in the risk of a BRCA-associated gynecologic cancer. In addition, it can reduce the risk of breast cancer by almost 50%. Certainly there are drawbacks; it will prematurely put young women into menopause with the associated symptoms and diminished quality of life. In addition, it should be delayed until after the woman has completed child bearing, although this can be a difficult compromise in a younger woman, particularly one who is not married. Women who undergo BSO are still at a small risk of primary peritoneal carcinoma, estimated at about 0.2% annually.

Suggested Readings

1. Ahlgren M, Melbye M, Wohlfahrt J, Sorensen TIA. Growth patterns and the risk of breast cancer in women. N Engl J Med 2004;351:1619–1626.
2. American Society of Clinical Oncology Policy Statement Update: Genetic Testing for Cancer Susceptibility. J Clin Oncol 2003;21:2397.
3. Antoniou A, Pharoah PDP, Narod S, et al. Average risks of breast and ovarian cancer associated with mutations in BRCA1 or BRCA2 detected in case series unselected for family history: A combined analysis of 22 studies. Am J Hum Genet 2003; 72(5):1117–1130.
4. Beral V, Bull D, Doll R, et al. Breast cancer and abortion: Collaborative re-analysis of data from 53 epidemiological studies, including 83,000 women with breast cancer from 16 countries. Lancet 2004;363:1007.
5. Berry DA, Iversen ES Jr, Gudbjartsson DF, et al. BRCAPRO validation, sensitivity of genetic testing of BRCA1/BRCA2, and prevalence of other breast cancer susceptibility genes. J Clin Oncol 2002; 20(11):2701–2712.
6. Bodian CA, Perzin KH, Lattes R. Lobular neoplasia: Long term risk of breast cancer and relation to other factors. Cancer 1996;78:1024.
7. Breast cancer and breastfeeding: Collaborative reanalysis of individual data from 47 epidemiological studies in 30 countries, including 50302 women with breast cancer and 96973 women without the disease. Lancet 2002;360:187.
8. Breast cancer and hormonal contraceptives: Collaborative reanalysis of individual data on 53, 297 women with breast cancer and 100,239 women without breast cancer from 54 epidemiological studies. Collaborative Group on Hormonal Factors in Breast Cancer. Lancet 1996;347:1713.
9. Calle EE, Rodriguez C, Walker-Thurmond K, Thun, MJ. Overweight, obesity, and mortality from cancer in a prospectively studied cohort of U.S. adults. N Engl J Med 2003;348:1625.
10. Cauley JA, Norton L, Lippman ME, et al. Continued breast cancer risk reduction in postmenopausal women treated with raloxifene: 4-year results from the MORE trial. Multiple Outcomes of Raloxifene Evaluation. Breast Cancer Res Treat 2001;65:125.
11. Chemoprevention of breast cancer: Recommendations and rationale. Ann Intern Med 2002;137:56.
12. Chlebowski RT, Collyar DE, Somerfield MR, Pfister DG. American Society of Clinical Oncology technology assessment on breast cancer risk reduction strategies: Tamoxifen and raloxifene. JCO 1999;17:1939.
13. Chlebowski RT, Col N, Winer EP, et al. American Society of Clinical Oncology technology assessment of pharmacologic interventions for breast cancer risk reduction including tamoxifen, raloxifene, and aromatase inhibition. J Clin Oncol 2002;20:3328.
14. Chlebowski RT, Hendrix SL, Langer RD, et al. Influence of Estrogen Plus Progestin on Breast Cancer and Mammography in Healthy Postmenopausal Women: The Women's Health Initiative Randomized Trial. JAMA 2003;289:3243.
15. Clemons M, Goss P. Estrogen and the risk of breast cancer. N Engl J Med 2001;344:276.
16. Cuzick J, Powles T, Veronesi U, et al. Overview of the main outcomes in breast-cancer prevention trials. Lancet 2003;361:296.
17. Fisher B, Constantino JP, Wickerham DL, et al. Tamoxifen for prevention of breast cancer: Report of the National Surgical Adjuvant Breast and Bowel Project P-1 Study. J Natl Cancer Inst 1998;90:1371.
18. Fisher B, Costantino JP, Wickerhan L, et al. Tamoxifen for prevention of breast cancer: Report of the National Surgical Adjuvant Breast and Bowel Project P-1 study. J Natl Cancer Inst 1998;90:1371.
19. Fisher B, Costantino JP, Wickerham DL, et al. Tamoxifen for the prevention of breast cancer: Report of the National Surgical Adjuvant Breast and Bowel Project P-1 study. J Natl Cancer Inst 1998;90:1371.
20. Foote FW, Steward FW. Lobular carcinoma in situ: A rare form of mammary carcinoma. Am J Surg Pathol 1941;19:74.
21. Ford D, Easton DF, Bishop DT, Narod SA, Goldgar DE, and the Breast Cancer Linkage Consortium. Risk of cancer in BRCA-1 mutation carriers. Lancet 1994;343:692–695.
22. Ford D, Easton DF, Stratton M, et al. The Breast Cancer Linkage Consortium: Genetic heterogeneity and penetrance analysis of the BRCA1 and BRCA2 genes in breast cancer families. Am J Hum Genet 1998;62:676–689.
23. Foster MC, Helvie MA, Gregory NE, et al. Lobular carcinoma in situ or atypical lobular hyperplasia at core-needle biopsy: Is excisional biopsy necessary? Radiology 2004;231:813–819.
24. Frank TS, Deffenbaugh AM, Reid JE, et al. Clinical characteristics of individuals with germline mutations in BRCA1 and BRCA2: Analysis of 10,000 individuals. JCO 2002;20:1480–1490.

25. Gail MH, Brinton LA, Byer DP, et al. Projecting individualized probabilities of developing breast cancer for white females who are being examined annually. J Natl Cancer Inst 1989;81:1879.

26. Goldberg JI, Borgen PI. Breast cancer susceptibility testing: Past, present and future. Exp Rev Anticancer Ther 2006;6(8):1205–1214.

27. Gump FE. Lobular carcinoma in situ: Pathology and treatment. Surg Clin N Am 1990;70: 873.

28. Hartmann LC, Schaid DJ, Woods JE, et al. Efficacy of bilateral prophylactic mastectomy in women with a family history of breast cancer. N Engl J Med 1999;340:77–84.

29. Hartmann LC, Sellers TA, Schaid DJ, et al. Efficacy of bilateral prophylactic mastectomy in BRCA1 and BRCA2 gene mutation carriers. J Natl Cancer Inst 2001;93:1633–1637.

30. IBIS investigators. First results from the International Breast Cancer Intervention Study (IBIS-I): A randomised prevention trial. Lancet 2002;360: 817–824.

31. Lippman ME, Krueger KA, Eckert S, et al. Indicators of lifetime estrogen exposure: Effect on breast cancer incidence and interaction with raloxifene therapy in the multiple outcomes of raloxifene evaluation study participants. J Clin Oncol 2001;19:3111.

32. Martino S, Cauley JA, Barrett-Connor E, et al. Continuing outcomes relevant to Evista: Breast cancer incidence in postmenopausal osteoporotic women in a randomized trial of raloxifene. J Natl Cancer Inst 2004;96:1751.

33. Meijers-Heijboer EJ, van Geel B, van Putten WLJ, et al. Breast cancer after prophylactic bilateral mastectomy in women with a BRCA1 or BRCA2 mutation. N Engl J Med 2001;345:159–164.

34. Metcalfe K, Lynch HT, Ghadirian P, et al. Contralateral breast cancer in BRCA1 and BRCA2 mutation carriers. J Clin Oncol 2004;22:2328.

35. Narod SA, Brunet JS, and the Hereditary Breast Cancer Clinical Study Group. Tamoxifen and risk of contralateral breast cancer in BRCA1 and BRCA2 carriers: A case control study. Lancet 2000;356:1876–1881.

36. Narod SA, Brunet JS, Ghadirian P, et al. Tamoxifen and risk of contralateral breast cancer in BRCA1 and BRCA2 mutation carriers: A case-control study. Hereditary Breast Cancer Clinical Study Group. Lancet 2000;356:1876.

37. NCCN Guidelines on Genetic/Familial High-Risk Assessment: Breast and ovarian. Available at www.nccn.com/physician_gls/f_guidelines.html.

38. Page DL, Kidd TE, Depont WD, et al. Lobular neoplasia of the breast: Higher risk for subsequent invasive cancer predicted by more extensive disease. Hum Pathol 1991;22:1232.

39. Page DL, Schuyler PA, Dupont WD, et al. Atypical lobular hyperplasia as a unilateral predictor of breast cancer risk: A retrospective cohort study. Lancet 2003;361:125.

40. Rebbeck TR, Lynch HT, Neuhausen SL, et al. Reduction in cancer risk after bilateral prophylactic oophorectomy in BRCA1 and BRCA2 mutation carriers. N Engl J Med 2002;346:1616–1622.

41. Risks and benefits of estrogen and progestin in healthy postmenopausal women: Principal results from the Women's Health Initiative randomized controlled trial. JAMA 2002;288:321.

42. Rivers A, Newman LA. Ductal lavage for breast cancer risk assessment. Surg Oncol Clin North Am 2005;14:45–68.

43. Robson M, Offit K. Management of an inherited predisposition to breast cancer. N Engl J Med 2007;357:154.

44. Rosen PP, Lieberman PH, Braun DW, et al. Lobular carcinoma in situ of the breast: Detailed analysis of 99 patients with average follow-up of 24 years. Am J Surg Pathol 1978;2:225.

45. Russo J, Moral R, Balogh GA, et al. The protective role of pregnancy in breast cancer. Br Canc Res 2005;7(3): 131–142.

46. Sasco AJ, Kaaks R, Little RE. Breast cancer: Occurrence, risk factors and hormone metabolism. Exp Rev Anticancer The 2003;3(4):546–562.

47. Singletary KW, Gapstur SM. Alcohol and breast cancer: Review of epidemiologic and experimental evidence and potential mechanisms. JAMA 2001; 286:2143.

48. Struewing J, et al. The risk of breast cancer associated with specific mutations of BRCA1 and BRCA2 among Ashkenazi Jews. N Engl J Med 1997; 336:1401–1407.

49. Wysowski DK, Honig SF, Beitz J. Uterine sarcoma associated with tamoxifen use. N Engl J Med 2002; 346:1832.

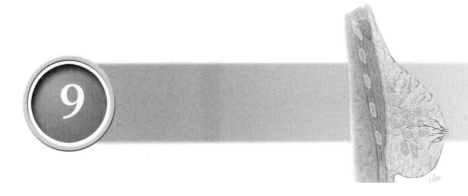

Reading the Pathology Report

Reading the Pathology Report: Key Points

Be familiar with the different subtypes of invasive breast cancer and the implications on surgical management.

Know how margins are assessed and the need for reexcision for either a close or positive margin.

Understand how tumor size, grade and other histologic features may impact surgical or adjuvant therapy.

Although there are many important relationships among the various members of the breast cancer multidisciplinary team, the relationship between the surgeon and the pathologist is a unique one. The two are closely tied because the success of surgical therapy is dependent upon the accuracy of the pathology report, and the accuracy of the pathology report depends upon a firm grasp of the surgical procedure performed. To succeed, this relationship requires excellent communication, including the accurate labeling of specimens, the proper orientation of specimens, and possibly the presence of the surgeon in the pathology laboratory to help facilitate the process.

Histology

The first question when one receives a pathology report back after a biopsy is what type of cancer is this? Specifically is this in situ or invasive disease and what type of invasive cancer is it? The pathology of in situ disease is discussed in Chapter 11. For invasive cancers, the two most common histologic types are invasive ductal and invasive lobular. However, there are many other subtypes that may have different implications in terms of surgical or adjuvant therapy (Box 9–1).

Invasive Ductal Carcinoma

Invasive ductal carcinoma is the most common type of invasive breast cancer. Tumors can be either pure invasive ductal carcinoma, or mixed, which consists of combinations of ductal carcinoma and other types. Grossly, invasive ductal tumors are hard in consistency, with a gray-white color. This is secondary to an often present stromal desmoplasia. The tumors can either be well circumscribed or be spiculated with irregular margins. Histologically, the tumor cells are arranged as glandular structures, either as nests, cords, trabeculae, or solid sheets (Fig. 9–1). Depending on the differentiation, the cells can look similar to normal breast epithelial cells or show marked cellular and nuclear pleomorphism.

Overall, invasive ductal carcinoma has the worst prognosis of the invasive histologies; however, ductal cancers can be quite heterogeneous,

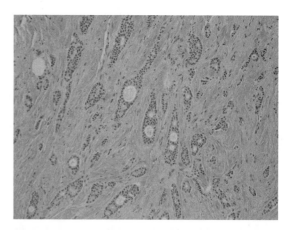

Figure 9–1. Histology of invasive ductal carcinoma. The cancer cells form glandular structures with cellular and nuclear pleomorphism. These nests infiltrate the surrounding breast tissue in a haphazard fashion. (Image courtesy of Maria Braman, MD, Department of Pathology, University of Michigan.)

and within this group, subsets can be identified with more favorable prognoses.

Invasive Lobular Carcinoma

The second most frequent type of invasive breast cancer, invasive lobular carcinomas, account for approximately 10% to 15% of breast cancers. Even though invasive lobular tumors can be hard and discrete like ductal carcinomas, they are often much more subtle. There may not be a hard palpable mass, but rather a vague thickening with indiscrete margins. The same goes for imaging studies, wherein invasive lobular carcinomas may be mammographically occult or may be poorly defined areas of asymmetry. Often, the tumor is larger than expected based on physical examination or imaging studies.

Histologically, classic invasive lobular carcinoma is composed of a uniform population of cells that infiltrate the breast parenchyma in a so-called "single file" (Fig. 9–2). The cells follow each other in a linear fashion to surround both benign ductal or lobular structures. Cytologically, the cells are relatively small with minimal cytoplasm, large nonpleomorphic nuclei, and few if any mitoses. There are several variants of lobular carcinoma based on cytology (pleomorphic, histiocytoid, signet-ring cell) or pattern (alveolar, solid, tubulolobular). Sometimes the diagnosis is made not only by pathology, but also by taking into account the clinical and radiologic presentation.

BOX 9–1 TYPES OF BREAST CANCER

In situ cancer
  Ductal carcinoma in situ
  Lobular carcinoma in situ
  Paget disease
Invasive cancer
  Invasive lobular
  Invasive ductal
  Tubular
  Cribriform
  Papillary
  Secretory
  Cystic hypersecretory
  Mucinous
  Medullary
  Apocrine
  Acinic cell
  Adenoid cystic
  Sarcomatoid

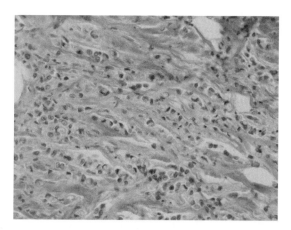

Figure 9–2. Histology of invasive lobular carcinoma. The cancer cells infiltrate the parenchyma in a linear, "single-file" pattern. The cells themselves are small with minimal cytoplasm and large nuclei. (Image courtesy of Maria Braman, MD, Department of Pathology, University of Michigan.)

Overall, lobular carcinoma is prognostically similar to ductal carcinoma, although some studies have shown better survival rates for lobular carcinoma. However, studies that include both classic lobular carcinoma and its variants are difficult to interpret (Box 9–2). Pure, classic invasive lobular carcinoma appears to have a slightly better prognosis compared with solid or alveolar patterns. Pleomorphic lobular carcinoma and the signet ring cell variant appear to have a worse prognosis.

There are two misconceptions regarding invasive lobular carcinoma. The first is that breast conservation therapy is inappropriate for invasive lobular carcinoma, because the tumors are often larger than what is found on physical examination or on mammography. Even though this is true and reexcision may be necessary to ultimately achieve negative margins, if an adequate lumpectomy can be performed, breast conservation is perfectly appropriate. The second assumption is that because lobular carcinoma in situ (LCIS) is associated with an increased risk of bilateral breast cancer, patients with invasive

lobular carcinoma are at an increased risk of contralateral breast cancer compared to other histologies. Thus some clinicians recommend bilateral mastectomies more often for lobular carcinomas. However, long-term follow-up of patients with invasive lobular carcinoma shows a similar rate of contralateral breast cancer to invasive ductal carcinoma.

Tubular Carcinoma

Tubular carcinoma is an extremely well-differentiated form of breast cancer. Tubular carcinoma is rare, representing only 2% of breast cancers. Histologically, tubular carcinoma is composed of small, single-layered, angulated tubules that are surrounded by a dense cellular stroma, rich in hyaline and elastotic tissue (Fig. 9–3). In this way, it is similar to benign conditions such as sclerosing adenosis and radial scar.

Compared with invasive ductal carcinoma, tubular carcinoma tends to be more common in older patients. It is more commonly multicentric and bilateral. They appear to be very slow growing, with most (80% to 90%) being less than 1 cm. Because they rarely get large enough to cause a palpable mass and they are often associated with microcalcifications (50% of cases), they are almost always detected by mammography. Thus the incidence of tubular carcinoma is rising with increased mammographic screening.

The prognosis is quite good. The tumors are usually small, rarely larger than 2 cm with

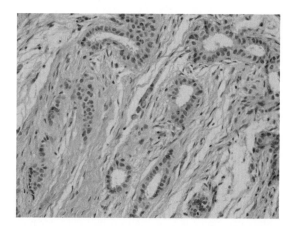

Figure 9–3. Histology of tubular carcinoma. Tubular carcinoma is characterized by small, single-layered angulated tubules. They are surrounded by a dense cellular stroma. (Image courtesy of Maria Braman, MD, Department of Pathology, University of Michigan.)

BOX 9–2 VARIANTS OF LOBULAR CARCINOMA

Classic
Solid variant
Loose alveolar variant
Tubuloalveolar
Pleomorphic lobular

a median size of 0.8 cm. Axillary node metastases are less common than other invasive subtypes, but not unheard of, so lymphatic mapping is still recommended. Axillary node involvement is more common when multicentric disease is present, but even when nodes are involved, the prognosis is favorable.

Cribriform Carcinoma

Another well-differentiated form of invasive cancer is cribriform carcinoma. It is also rare, with an incidence of 0.3% to 4%. A cribriform pattern of growth is characterized by nests of tumor cells containing round to oval arched glandular spaces. This gives it a fenestrated pattern with sharp "cookie-cutter" spaces within a desmoplastic stroma. The cells in these nests have low-grade nuclei and low mitotic rates.

There are very few studies specifically addressing cribriform carcinoma. Axillary node metastases are again less common than other subtypes, but can occur, so lymphatic mapping is worthwhile. Cribriform carcinoma appears to be a low-grade malignancy, with a better prognosis than other forms of breast cancer.

Medullary Carcinoma

Medullary carcinomas are nicely circumscribed tumors with a good prognosis despite a poorly differentiated appearance. The pathologist

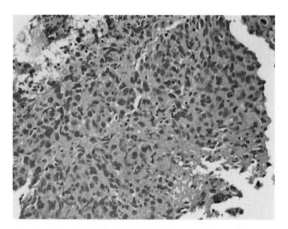

Figure 9–4. Histology of medullary carcinoma. Medullary carcinoma is characterized by broad irregular sheets of cells devoid of glandular differentiation. The borders between the cells are indiscriminate and the cells are poorly differentiated, with high-grade nuclei and frequent mitoses. (Image courtesy of Maria Braman, MD, Department of Pathology, University of Michigan.)

> **BOX 9–3** CRITERIA FOR DIAGNOSING MEDULLARY CARCINOMA
>
> - Microscopically circumscribed, characterized by a smooth pushing border
> - A lymphoplastic reaction present within and at the periphery of the tumor
> - Germinal centers may be present, mimicking an intramammary lymph node
> - A syncytial growth pattern is present, characterized by broad irregular sheets or islands of cells devoid of glandular differentiation
> - Poorly differentiated cells
> - High nuclear grade
> - Mitotic activity

must be certain that they are dealing with a pure medullary carcinoma, and not an invasive ductal carcinoma with medullary features, because the latter has a prognosis similar to invasive ductal cancer (Fig. 9–4). Medullary carcinoma is often overdiagnosed. There are strict criteria that must be met to call a cancer medullary (Box 9–3).

Medullary carcinomas are more common in younger women, as well as in both Japanese and African-American women in the United States. Because they are so well circumscribed, they are often confused for fibroadenomas. Prognosis is good, even when lymph node involvement is present. Not uncommonly, medullary carcinomas are associated with a reactive lymphadenopathy that may be confused for clinical nodal involvement. fine-needle aspiration should be performed to confirm metastatic disease, and if negative, sentinel node biopsy should be performed in the presence of palpable adenopathy to avoid unnecessary node dissection.

Mucinous Carcinoma

These tumors comprise less than 2% of invasive breast cancers and, as their name implies, are composed of large amounts of extracellular mucin. Mucinous carcinomas are also known as *colloid* or *gelatinous carcinoma*. They are more common in older women and present as a softer mass. Sometimes crepitance, known as a "swish sign," can be heard on palpation. Most are mammographically occult; others appear benign on imaging. Even follow-up mammograms may not increase suspicion

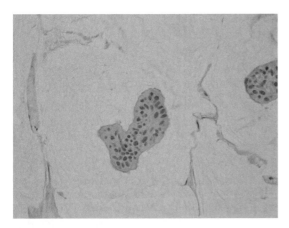

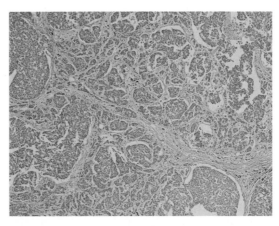

Figure 9–5. Histology of mucinous carcinoma. Well-defined cells floating in a sea of extracellular mucin separated by fibrous septa. (Image courtesy of Maria Braman, MD, Department of Pathology, University of Michigan.)

Figure 9–6. Histology of papillary carcinoma. Within the network of thin fibrovascular cores are layers of cuboidal or columnar epithelial cells. (Image courtesy of Maria Braman, MD, Department of Pathology, University of Michigan.)

because they are relatively slow growing. Grossly, they are well-circumscribed with a soft, currant-jelly gelatinous cut surface. Histologically, they are defined by the presence of well-differentiated cells floating in a sea of extracellular mucin separated by fibrous septa (Fig. 9–5). The mucin is composed of neutral and acidic mucopolysaccharides expressing MUC-5 and MUC-2. It is possible that the MUC-2 contributes to the favorable prognosis of mucinous carcinomas, by not only conferring tumor suppressor activity but also hindering the spread of cells. Mucinous carcinomas have a lower rate of axillary node metastases and an improved survival compared to other subtypes. It is reasonable to treat small, node-negative mucinous carcinomas without the need for systemic adjuvant therapy. Recurrence can be quite late after initial treatment, as long as 25 to 30 years after therapy.

Papillary Carcinoma

Another rare form of breast cancer that is more common in elderly women is papillary carcinoma. As with papillomas, papillary carcinomas are more common in the subareolar region and can be associated with nipple discharge. However, papillary carcinomas are not limited to this area and can occur anywhere in the breast. Papillary carcinomas can be difficult in that on mammography they are well circumscribed, suggesting a benign pathology. If part of the peripheral contour lacks circumscription, invasion should be suspected.

Under the microscope, papillary carcinoma consists of a complex network of papillae: thin fibrovascular cores covered by layers of cuboidal or columnar epithelial cells (Fig. 9–6). The cells have high nuclear-to-cytoplasm ratio and hyperchromatic nuclei. It is not only difficult to differentiate benign from malignant on mammography and ultrasound, but it is also difficult on pathology. For these reasons, core biopsies of a papillary lesion usually need to be followed up by an excisional biopsy to completely rule out a carcinoma. Papillary-like lesions on mammography are therefore often best removed by wire-localized biopsy to make the diagnosis.

There are several variants of papillary carcinoma. *Intracystic papillary carcinoma* describes a papillary carcinoma that is entirely contained within a large cystic duct. Alone, it is an in situ papillary carcinoma with an excellent prognosis and an extremely low rate of axillary metastases. However, in many cases, nonpapillary invasive ductal carcinoma is seen in association with intracystic papillary carcinoma. *Papillary transitional cell carcinoma* is a variant that has both intraductal and intracystic papillary growth and bears similarities to papillary urothelial neoplasms. *Invasive micropapillary carcinoma* is a much more aggressive form of breast cancer, and compared with other forms of papillary carcinoma, occurs in relatively younger women. Often mammographically occult, it more commonly presents with advanced disease and axillary metastases. Chest wall recurrences are common and 50% of patients succumb to widespread disease within 2 years. Histologically invasive micropapillary carcinoma has a distinct pattern of neoplastic cells in small micropapillae and ring-shaped nests. These are immersed in a hyaline stroma giving a "spongy" appearance. There is often extensive lymphatic invasion, and the disease is often hormone receptor-positive and HER-2/neu-positive.

Secretory Carcinoma

Secretory carcinoma, also known as juvenile carcinoma, is a rare form of breast cancer that can occur in children and teenagers as well as in adults. It occurs over a wide age range (3 to 73 years) but most patients are younger than 30. A well-circumscribed mass, it has several histologic growth patterns that can include cribriform, microcystic, solid, and papillary areas. The cells have abundant pale and finely granular cytoplasm, round nuclei, and prominent nucleoli. These can be confused with apocrine or acinic carcinoma.

A low-grade neoplasm, the carcinoma appears to have a good prognosis in children and is slightly more aggressive in adults. Tumor size less than 2 cm and an absence of stromal invasion at the periphery also portend a good prognosis. Wide excision is the treatment of choice, with special attention being paid to preserving the breast bud in prepubertal girls. Recurrences do occur after lumpectomy alone, as late as 20 years after therapy. However, the benefit of radiation or chemotherapy is difficult to assess given the rarity of secretory carcinoma. Sentinel node biopsy should be done because there may be axillary metastases in up to 30% of cases.

Metaplastic Carcinoma

Metaplastic breast cancers are rapidly growing tumors, often presenting as a well-circumscribed, firm mass larger than the average invasive ductal carcinoma. The mean size is 3 to 4 cm with more than half being more than 5 cm and some are larger than 20 cm. The tumors may be necrotic, and the largest tumors can have associated skin and nipple changes. These cancers are thought to be invasive ductal cancers transforming to nonglandular components, and they consist of a combination of mammary carcinoma with spindle, squamous, chondroid, or osseous elements (metaplasia is defined as a change from one cell type to

another). Despite the unusual appearance, the prognosis is roughly equal to that of invasive ductal carcinoma.

Metaplastic carcinomas are subdivided into two categories: squamous and heterologous. *Squamous metaplasia* has histologic features similar to squamous cell carcinoma: intercellular bridges, dyskeratotic cells, and keratin pearl formation. Focal squamous metaplasia can be seen in a small percentage of cases of invasive ductal carcinoma, but squamous metaplastic carcinoma consists predominantly of squamous-type changes. *Heterologous metaplastic carcinomas* have two components, an epithelial one and a heterologous one, which can be quite bland or can contain spindle cells, bone, cartilage, muscle, adipose tissue, and vascular differentiation. When bone or cartilage is present, the carcinoma is known as a *matrix-producing carcinoma*. When these components are poorly differentiated, it is called *carcinosarcoma*.

Other Forms of Breast Cancer

Apocrine carcinomas are characterized by apocrine differentiation of ductal cells. There are two types of normal apocrine cells within the mammary gland. Type A apocrine cells have eosinophilic granular cytoplasm while type B apocrine cells have abundant foamy cytoplasm filled by small vacuoles. These apocrine cells can proliferate into atypical or malignant lesions. Apocrine features can be seen with in situ disease, invasive ductal carcinoma, and invasive lobular carcinomas. Pure apocrine carcinomas are rare, constituting 1% to 2% of breast carcinomas. They possess similar growth patterns to invasive ductal carcinoma and similar clinical features. What makes apocrine carcinoma different is the appearance of the cells, which have abundant granular eosinophilia or cytoplasm with fine empty vacuoles.

Adenoid cystic carcinomas are low-grade tumors that usually arise in the salivary gland but can occur in the breast, albeit quite rarely. They often present as painful or tender masses in the subperiareolar region. They have a good prognosis with few cases of axillary or distant metastases. Distant metastases occur in about 10% of patients, usually to the lungs.

Neuroendocrine carcinomas are defined by an endocrine growth pattern and the expression of neuroendocrine markers. They are more common in older women and may occasionally present with symptoms related to ectopic hormone production such as adrenocorticotropic hormone (ACTH), parathyroid hormone (PTH), calcitonin, and epinephrine.

Tumor Size

Besides the presence of regional metastases, the size of the invasive component of the tumor is, to date, the most important factor used in therapy decisions. The size of a breast cancer is generally determined by the measurement of the largest contiguous area of invasive cancer. Pathologic size does not necessarily correspond with imaging size (although ultrasound is slightly more accurate than mammogram) or clinical estimations. This may be due to a lack of discrimination on the imaging studies, the presence of benign components, as well as decreased tumor size secondary to multiple core-needle biopsies.

Multifocal tumors may extend over a larger area, but the tumor size is reported as the largest microscopic area of contiguous invasive tumor. For staging and adjuvant therapy decisions, this is most accurate, but it may not reflect the true area needed to be resected surgically. This is particularly true for lobular carcinoma and after neoadjuvant chemotherapy. Tumor size is also difficult to reconstruct in situations in which a portion of the tumor was removed by an excisional biopsy with residual tissue on the reexcision lumpectomy. For example, if 6 mm of tumor is reported in the biopsy and 8 mm of tumor is reported in the reexcision lumpectomy, is the tumor 8 mm (the size of the largest component) or 14 mm (the combined size), which would upstage it from T1b to T1c? It is not reasonable to assume the two portions add together (Fig. 9–7), so this is generally discouraged, with the tumor size being reported as the larger of the two components.

Margin Status

One of the most important aspects of the pathology report to the surgeon is the margin status. In theory, tumors are generally unicentric and pathologic assessment of negative margins should mean complete excision. Even when ductal carcinoma in situ (DCIS) is present, it is usually a contiguous spread through the ductolobular tree rather than multiple foci.

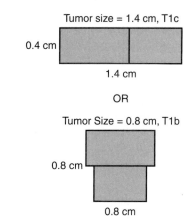

Figure 9–7. Difficulty in accurately determining the true tumor size when there is residual tissue on the reexcision. Depending on how the two sections combine, the tumor may have a maximal dimension of 1.4 cm (and be staged as T1c) or 0.8 cm (and be staged as T1b).

However, theory does not match practice in that there is tissue artifact and it is impossible to completely examine the entire periphery of a tumor. Negative margins do not preclude the possibility of residual disease just as positive margins do not necessarily mean that tumor was left behind. However, there is an inverse relationship between the likelihood of a complete excision and the proximity of the tumor to the margins (as well as the amount of tumor near the margin).

It is clear that positive margins are not acceptable for breast conservation and require reexcision. In an older study of lumpectomy alone (no radiation), early local recurrence rates were 45% for positive margins and 9% for negative margins. In the modern era of breast conservation (lumpectomy and radiation), even though radiation improves local recurrence, it does not compensate for positive margins. Local recurrence rates range from 0% to 9% for negative margin lumpectomies followed by radiation therapy (XRT) compared with 10% to 20% when margins are positive.

The more controversial question regarding margin status is the "close margin." This is variably defined as margins that are negative but within 0.1 and 3 mm. Some authors say a margin less than 1 mm is close, whereas other authors say a margin within 3 mm is close. Studies have shown inconsistent results as to the local recurrence risk associated with close margins. In general, however, studies show an increasing risk of recurrence with the distance between the tumor and the margin, and several studies have shown a significant risk of finding residual disease when reexcisions are performed for close margins. This should prompt an aggressive use of reexcision when margins are within 2 to 3 mm although this needs to be balanced against the size of the close margin (broad vs. focal), the age of the patient, the impact of re-excision and whether a boost is planned by radiation oncology.

Grade

The grade of a tumor is primarily used for invasive ductal carcinomas, recognizing the fact that these can be quite heterogeneous. This allows clinicians to stratify those invasive ductal cancers with a better prognosis from those with a worse outcome. The grade of the tumor is based on the degree of differentiation of the cells, comparing the nuclear and structural features with those of normal mammary cells. This can be based on the nuclear features, the architecture, or a combination of features. The most commonly used grading system in breast cancer is based on three features: nuclear grade, tubular formation, and mitotic rate. Originally known as the Bloom-Richardson grade, it was modified by Elston and Ellis to remove some of the subjective qualities and make the grading of breast cancer more reproducible. Thus a semiquantitative evaluation of the three variables is given (Box 9–4). Along with tumor size and lymph node status, the grade of the tumor is the only other prognostic factor that repeatedly and significantly correlates with recurrence and survival. Although grade is not included in the staging system, it is used in adjuvant therapy decisions.

Hormone Receptor and Her-2/neu Expression

Several factors have been identified that can help select which patients are most likely to benefit from adjuvant therapy. Most are controversial or of limited benefit (Ki-67, p53, S-phase, ploidy), although two are extremely

---

BOX 9–4 ELSTON AND ELLIS MODIFICATION OF BLOOM-RICHARDSON GRADE

Tubules	
>75% of tumor composed of tubules	1 point
10 to 75% of tumor	2 points
<10% of tumor	3 points
Nuclear Grade	
Nuclei small and uniform	1 point
Moderate variation in nuclear size and shape	2 points
Marked nuclear proliferation	3 points
Mitotic Rate (Dependent on Microscopic Field)	
Low	1 point
Intermediate	2 points
High	3 points
Point Total	**Histologic Grade**
3 to 5	1 (well-differentiated)
6 to 7	2 (moderately differentiated)
7 to 9	3 (poorly differentiated)

---

important and should be considered standard of care in the histopathologic assessment of breast cancer. These include staining for hormone receptors (estrogen and progesterone) and for Her-2/neu. These not only help select appropriate therapies (hormonal therapy is only effective in patients who express the hormone receptors, and trastuzumab [Herceptin] is only effective in patients who overexpress Her-2/neu), but also provide prognostic information because their expression correlates with outcome. Both of these are most commonly evaluated by direct immunohistochemistry, which allows the pathologist to not only visually evaluate the number of cells involved and the intensity of the reaction, but also confirm that the expression is truly on the invasive component. If the immunohistochemical staining for Her-2/neu is equivocal, fluorescence in situ hybridization (FISH) is recommended. These are discussed in more detail in Chapters 16 and 17.

Lymphovascular Invasion

Angiolymphatic invasion, lymphovascular invasion, lymphatic invasion, and vascular invasion

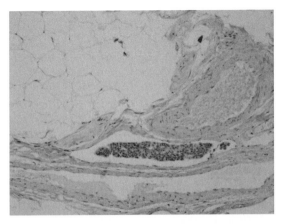

Figure 9–8. Angiolymphatic invasion. Tumor cells are seen within the dilated endothelial lined space. The cells conform to the shape of the lymphatic space, but appear to float in it. (Image courtesy of Maria Braman, MD, Department of Pathology, University of Michigan.)

are terms often used interchangeably among pathologists to describe the histologic finding of tumor cells within a vessel (Fig. 9–8). The term "vascular invasion" should be restricted to cases in which tumor cells are seen within a vessel containing a muscular wall (with or without red blood cells) and the term "lymphatic invasion" should be limited to evidence of intraluminal groups of tumor cells conforming to the shape of the endothelial-lined space. Whereas the former is relatively rare, the latter is much more common. The term "lymphovascular invasion" should be limited to cases in which both are seen, but this is rarely the case in practice. In addition, the reproducibility of this finding is in question because it is often hard to tell the difference between lymphatic invasion and artifact. Immunohistochemical stains are emerging that will help differentiate true lymphatic invasion; this is important because this finding implies a higher chance of finding nodal metastases. Likewise, the finding of lymphatic or vascular invasion correlates with prognosis in node-negative patients, including decreased disease-free survival and increased local recurrence after breast conservation therapy (BCT). Even though lymphovascular invasion is not a contraindication to BCT, its presence may influence adjuvant chemotherapy and radiation therapy decisions.

Extensive Intraductal Component

Extensive intraductal component (EIC) refers to cases in which at least 25% of the mass of an invasive tumor is intraductal carcinoma, and the intraductal component is present both within and outside of the tumor mass. EIC is important because EIC-positive patients have a higher risk of residual DCIS in reexcision lumpectomy specimens. In some series, EIC has been associated with an increased local recurrence rate, whereas other studies found no difference, that is if negative margins around both the invasive and intraductal component are obtained. This emphasizes the importance of attaining negative margins for both invasive and in situ disease when performing a lumpectomy, but does not preclude breast conservation in EIC-positive patients. However, EIC may be a contraindication to newer, experimental approaches to breast cancer including in situ ablation and partial breast irradiation.

Suggested Readings

1. Colleoni M, Rotmensz N, Maisonneuve P, et al. Prognostic role of the extent of peritumoral vascular invasion in operable breast cancer. Ann Oncol 2007;18(10):1632–1640.
2. Harris L, Fritsche H, Mennel R, et al. American Society of Clinical Oncology. American Society of Clinical Oncology 2007 update of recommendations for the use of tumor markers in breast cancer. J Clin Oncol 2007;25(33):5287–5312.
3. Hayes DF. Prognostic and predictive factors revisited. Breast. 2005;14(6):493–499.
4. Kapoor A, Vogel VG. Prognostic factors for breast cancer and their use in the clinical setting. Expert Review in Anticancer Therapy 2005;5(2):269–281.
5. Mirza AN, Mirza NQ, Vlastos G, Singletary SE. Prognostic factors in node-negative breast cancer: A review of studies with sample size more than 200 and follow-up more than 5 years. Ann Surgery 2002;235(1):10–26.
6. Wong SL, Chao C, Edwards MJ, et al. University of Louisville Breast Cancer Study Group. Frequency of sentinel lymph node metastases in patients with favorable breast cancer histologic subtypes. Am J Surg 2002;184(6):492–498.
7. Yoder BJ, Wilkinson EJ, Massoll NA. Molecular and morphologic distinctions between infiltrating ductal and lobular carcinoma of the breast. Breast J 2007; 13(2):172–179.

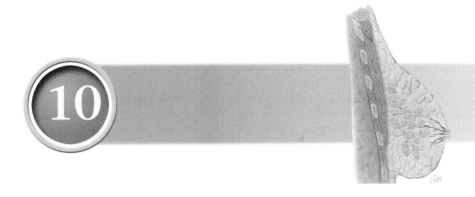

10

Workup and Staging of the Breast Cancer Patient

Workup and Staging of the Breast Cancer Patient: Key Points

Know the TNM staging system for breast cancer.

Describe the preoperative assessment of the woman diagnosed with breast cancer.

Appreciate the potential benefits and drawbacks to obtaining an MRI to stage breast cancer.

Develop an algorithm for evaluating the lymph nodes (N stage) in the clinically node-negative and clinically node-positive patient.

Understand which patients need a more thorough staging (CT, bone scan) before proceeding with surgery.

Appreciate which patients might benefit from meeting with a genetic counselor before proceeding with therapy.

Understand the advantages of discussing the patient's case and formulating a treatment plan in a multidisciplinary setting.

Breast Cancer Staging

The purpose of staging breast cancer patients, or all cancer patients for that matter, is to classify groups of patients with similar outcomes. Even though patients are often extremely concerned with their stage, the information is of limited use to them and to us, because even with our current methods of stratifying patients there is still considerable heterogeneity within each stage. A primary reason for staging patients is to provide consistency for both clinical and basic science research. By staging patients appropriately, outcomes across different populations can be effectively compared. In this manner, the efficacy of specific treatments can be better assessed.

Staging patients is also important in delineating a treatment plan, but in breast cancer treatment, decisions are based on factors well beyond simple TNM staging. Therefore it is important not to focus only on garnering information to provide the TNM staging, but rather on information that will impact how the patient is treated. Conversely, it is often a waste of time and money to order a battery of tests that are unlikely to influence treatment, either because they are of low yield or because treatment would not change pending the results of the test. It is therefore necessary to use clinical acumen when deciding what staging tests to order before proceeding with therapy.

Staging systems for breast cancer began in 1940 with the Manchester classification, a clinical four-stage system based on the local extent of the primary tumor and the involvement of axillary lymph nodes. This gave way to the Columbia staging system, which had more clinical utility in predicting which patients were appropriate for surgery. The Columbia classification served as a precursor to the TNM classification system, introduced in 1958 by the International Union against Cancer (UICC). Whereas the Manchester and Columbia systems were entirely clinical, the TNM system was based on histopathology. Independent of the UICC, the American Joint Committee on Cancer (AJCC) developed a series of site-specific staging systems in the late 1960s and early 1970s, including breast cancer. Ultimately, in the late 1980s, the two bodies agreed on a single staging system, which is in use today.

It is important to remember that the staging systems are fabricated, based on our knowledge of important prognostic factors in breast cancer. As our understanding of the biology of breast cancer changes and as new prognostic tests emerge, the staging system is updated. The AJCC updates the staging system every few years, incorporating new data, so that the staging system better stratifies patients into homogenous groups. This, however, makes staging more complicated and more difficult to commit to memory. In addition, as we understand more about the molecular biology

of breast cancer, TNM staging may become more archaic, replaced by a more sophisticated stratification based on the presence, absence, overexpression, or mutation of particular genes within the tumor.

TNM staging of breast cancer patients is typically done at two points. The first is the clinical staging, which is based on physical examination and imaging studies. The patient is usually restaged after surgery using pathologic information. Even though the pathologic TNM stage is generally more important and better stratifies patients, clinical staging is often used to base treatment decisions on, particularly surgery and the use of neoadjuvant chemotherapy. After neoadjuvant chemotherapy, the pathologic stage may change (hopefully the patient will be downstaged), and the pretreatment pathologic stage may never be truly known. It is important to clarify whether one is referring to clinical or pathologic staging when discussing an individual patient, as well as knowing when additional clinical staging information may be necessary to make treatment decisions.

T Stage

The first component of the TNM staging system is the size of the tumor (T). Table 10–1 outlines the present T-staging system. The T stage is based solely on the invasive component of the tumor, thus a 3-cm area of ductal carcinoma in situ (DCIS) with a 4-mm invasive component is staged as T1a based on the 4 mm of invasive breast cancer. This can only be determined after surgery and evaluation of the resected specimen. The T stage is based on the maximum diameter of the primary tumor. Even after surgery, however, the T stage is not always clear. For patients with more than one tumor within the breast, the T stage is based on the largest of the two lesions and *not* the sum of the greatest diameter. Thus a patient with a 1.3-cm tumor and a 1.0-cm tumor is a T1b tumor (based on the 1.3 cm) and *not* a T2 tumor based on the sum of 1.3 and 1.0. For patients with bilateral cancers, each cancer is staged separately. However, when a patient has multifocality within a tumor, the T stage is less clear. Whether it should be based on the size of the largest single focus or based on the entire extent of the multifocality is less clear and varies among tumors and among pathologists. Either way, it is important to document the presence of multifocality.

TABLE 10-1 • *Primary Tumor Staging*

TX	Primary tumor cannot be assessed	
T0	No evidence of primary tumor	
Tis	Carcinoma in situ	
	Tis (DCIS)	Ductal carcinoma in situ
	Tis (LCIS)	Lobular carcinoma in situ
	Tis (Paget's)	Paget disease of the nipple with no tumor
T1	Tumor 2 cm or less in greatest dimension	
	T1mic	Microinvasion 0.1 cm or less
	T1a	0.1 to 0.5 cm
	T1b	>0.5 to 1.0 cm
	T1c	>1.0 to 2.0 cm
T2	Tumor >2 to 5 cm in greatest dimension	
T3	Tumor >5 cm in greatest dimension	
T4	Tumor of any size with direct extension to chest wall or skin	
	T4a	Extension to chest wall not including pectoralis muscle
	T4b	Skin involvement, including edema, peau d'orange, ulceration, or ipsilateral satellite skin nodules
	T4c	T4a and T4b
	T4d	Inflammatory carcinoma

The maximum dimension of the invasive component strongly correlates with the risk of regional and distant disease and hence prognosis. Thus it is crucial information upon which to base adjuvant therapy decisions. However, for the surgeon, the most important question in planning surgical therapy is the size of the tumor relative to the size of the breast and specifically whether a lumpectomy is possible. In our patient with 3 cm of DCIS and 4 mm of invasive cancer, the 3 cm becomes the more important variable. Accurate clinical T staging helps determine the patient's surgical options.

Clinical T staging is done by physical examination, mammography, ultrasonography, and possibly magnetic resonance imaging (MRI). Bilateral mammography is essential, not only for estimating the size of the tumor but also for looking for synchronous lesions or diffuse microcalcifications. These may preclude breast conservation or mandate biopsies of other lesions before proceeding with surgery. Ultrasound is not mandatory, but can often provide additional information about the primary tumor. In addition, ultrasound of the regional nodes can provide crucial staging information and potentially alter surgical therapy (see later).

A more controversial topic is the routine role of MRI in the staging of the primary tumor. Several studies have suggested that MRI is the preferred method for detecting the extent of disease within the breast before surgical decision making. This appears particularly true for younger women with dense breasts, women with an extensive intraductal component, and women with invasive lobular carcinoma. MRI also has been shown to increase the detection of contralateral breast cancers over mammography alone.

MRI is not without its drawbacks, however. The primary concern is the specificity, in that MRI has been associated with a high false-positive rate. This partly depends upon the technique and expertise of whoever is reading the MRI, but even in the best hands, MRI can be associated with false-positive findings. The decision to perform a mastectomy based on an MRI finding without tissue diagnosis will lead to unnecessary mastectomies. Therefore any abnormality discovered on MRI that might alter the surgical management must be biopsied; however, not all of the institutions performing MRI have the capability of performing MRI-guided biopsy. Patients should be guided to only undergo breast MRI at an institution where subsequent biopsy can be performed if necessary, because it is very difficult and not always possible (given the differences in machines, protocols, and interpretations between institutions) to have a lesion seen at one hospital biopsied at another.

A more important, and unanswered question, is what impact MRI might have on recurrence rates. Proponents of MRI would point out the frequency at which MRI detects lesions that alter surgical management, leading to either a wider excision or a mastectomy. However, this appears to be occurring at a frequency higher than local recurrence rates, suggesting that much of the disease seen on MRI but missed on mammography is eradicated by radiation or systemic therapy. This has raised a significant concern that MRI in this setting may lead to considerable surgical overtreatment and a sharp increase in the mastectomy rate.

Until more data are available, the routine use of MRI as a preoperative staging test cannot be recommended. It may be considered in cases wherein mammography is limited by breast density or in cases of invasive lobular carcinoma, but even in these situations the exact benefit of MRI has yet to be established. It may also be used after lumpectomy if there is a concern that bulky residual disease may be present at the margins or elsewhere in the breast, which may preclude an attempt at reexcision (although MRI cannot detect microscopic disease and cannot be used to decide whether a positive or close margin should be reexcised). Patients should be counseled to both the potential benefits of MRI and the risks, and if an MRI is to be performed, patients should be steered only to centers that have the ability to perform MRI-guided biopsies.

N Stage

The absence or presence of disease in the regional lymph nodes represents the N stage and has undergone dramatic changes in recent years (Table 10–2). This is secondary not only to changes in our understanding of biology, but also to changes in how the regional lymph nodes are approached surgically. Sentinel lymph node (SLN) biopsy has essentially replaced axillary lymph node dissection (ALND) as the method for surgically staging the regional lymph nodes. This has not only reduced the morbidity of breast cancer surgery, but also allowed for more detailed histologic evaluation of the regional nodes. Extremely small foci of disease within the lymph nodes can now be detected that would have been missed on routine ALND. The clinical implications of these findings are a source of confusion and controversy, so care must be taken not to overestimate or underestimate the importance of these micrometastases.

As with T stage, the N stage is first approached clinically, with the pathologic N stage determined after surgery. In contrast to the T stage, there are two different N-staging systems, depending on whether the patient was assessed clinically or pathologically. Table 10–2 demonstrates the clinical N staging. The stage is based on not only the absence or presence of adenopathy, but also the location of disease (axillary, internal mammary, supraclavicular) and physical examination findings (movable versus fixed or matted). Thus a careful physical examination of the axilla and neck is a crucial part of the clinical N stage. It is important to point out that not all palpable adenopathy identified on clinical examination of the breast cancer patient represents regional disease; in some cases reactive lymph nodes may be present. Fine-needle aspiration (FNA) biopsy of palpable nodes in this setting is highly accurate and should be routinely obtained to confirm the presence of regional metastases.

Clinical staging of the regional nodes has primarily been based on physical examination. Imaging studies were rarely indicated to look at the regional nodes, and the identification of regional disease was usually an incidental finding on a computed tomography (CT) scan obtained to look for distal disease. However, the use of axillary ultrasound is expanding and should be considered either a selective (based on tumor size) or routine part of the staging workup in any patient with invasive breast cancer. (See Chapter 13.) The identification of axillary metastases by ultrasound and ultrasound-guided FNA biopsy can spare patients from undergoing an unnecessary sentinel node biopsy, instead proceeding directly to axillary node dissection. This not only decreases the number of operations performed but also decreases the costs of breast cancer care. In addition, the identification of disease in the regional nodes before neoadjuvant chemotherapy not only accurately stages the patient, but also allows for the assessment of response after chemotherapy.

Pathologic staging has become more complex with the introduction of the SLN biopsy. With the staging ALND, the pathologist bisected each identified node in search of metastases. With only one to three nodes to examine, SLN allows the pathologist to analyze multiple sections and allows more time to identify metastases. The use of immunohistochemical (IHC) staining and molecular detection of disease by polymerase chain reaction (PCR) have also become possible, although the clinical significance is still in question. The new staging guidelines for breast cancer incorporate these changes into the staging system, including designations for the identification of small metastases of unknown significance under N0. Disease not visible on hematoxylin and eosin (H&E) but visible on IHC and less than 0.2 mm is designated N0(i+) and usually referred to as "isolated tumor cells." These are still categorized as N0, and until more information is available, should be treated as such. Likewise, disease detected by reverse transcriptase PCR (RT-PCR) but not by H&E or IHC is designated as N0(mol+) and likewise should still be treated as N0 disease (RT-PCR of SLN should only be done as research).

TABLE 10–2 • *Regional Nodal Staging: Clinical and Pathologic*

Clinical

NX	Regional lymph nodes cannot be assessed
N0	No regional lymph node metastases
N1	Metastasis in movable ipsilateral axillary lymph nodes
N2	Metastasis in ipsilateral axillary lymph nodes fixed or matted, or in clinically apparent ipsilateral internal mammary nodes in the absence of clinically evident axillary lymph node metastasis
N2a	Metastasis in ipsilateral axillary lymph nodes fixed to one another (matted) or to other structures
N2b	Metastasis only in clinically apparent ipsilateral internal mammary nodes in the absence of clinically evident axillary lymph node metastasis
N3	Metastasis in ipsilateral infraclavicular lymph node(s) with or without axillary lymph node involvement, or in clinically apparent ipsilateral internal mammary lymph node(s) and in the presence of clinically evident axillary lymph node metastasis; or metastasis in ipsilateral supraclavicular lymph node(s) with or without axillary or internal mammary lymph node involvement
N3a	Metastasis in ipsilateral infraclavicular lymph node(s)
N3b	Metastasis in ipsilateral internal mammary lymph node(s) and axillary lymph node(s)
N3c	Metastasis in ipsilateral supraclavicular lymph node(s)

Pathologic (pN)

pNX	Regional lymph nodes cannot be assessed (e.g., previously removed or not removed for pathologic study)
pN0	No regional lymph node metastasis histologically, no additional examination for isolated tumor cells
pN0(i-)	No regional lymph node metastasis histologically, negative IHC
pN0(i+)	No regional lymph node metastasis histologically, positive IHC but no IHC cluster greater than 0.2 mm
pN0(mol-)	No regional lymph node metastasis histologically, negative molecular findings (RT-PCR)
pN0(mol+)	No regional lymph node metastasis histologically, positive molecular findings (RT-PCR)
pN1	Metastasis in 1 to 3 axillary lymph nodes and/or in internal mammary nodes with microscopic disease detected by SLN biopsy but not clinically apparent
pN1mic	Micrometastasis (greater than 0.2 mm, none greater than 2.0 mm)
pN1a	Metastasis in 1 to 3 axillary lymph nodes
pN1b	Metastasis in internal mammary nodes with microscopic disease detected by SLN biopsy but not clinically apparent
pN1c	Metastasis in 1 to 3 axillary lymph nodes and in internal mammary nodes with microscopic disease detected by SLN biopsy but not clinically apparent
pN2	Metastasis in 4 to 9 axillary lymph nodes, or in clinically apparent internal mammary lymph nodes in the absence of axillary lymph node metastasis
pN2a	Metastasis in 4 to 9 axillary lymph nodes (at least one tumor deposit >2 mm)
pN2b	Metastasis in clinically apparent internal mammary lymph nodes in the absence of axillary lymph node metastasis
pN3	Metastasis in 10 or more axillary lymph nodes, or in infraclavicular lymph nodes, or in clinically apparent ipsilateral internal mammary lymph nodes in the presence of 1 or more positive axillary lymph nodes; or in more than 3 axillary lymph nodes with clinically negative microscopic metastasis in internal mammary lymph nodes; or in ipsilateral supraclavicular lymph nodes
pN3a	Metastasis in 10 or more axillary lymph nodes or metastasis to the infraclavicular lymph nodes
pN3b	Metastasis in clinically apparent ipsilateral internal mammary lymph nodes in the presence of 1 or more positive axillary lymph nodes; or in more than 3 axillary lymph nodes with microscopic metastasis in internal mammary lymph nodes detected by SLN biopsy
pN3c	Metastasis in ipsilateral supraclavicular lymph nodes

IHC, Immunohistochemistry; SLN sentinel lymph node.

TABLE 10–3 • *Distant Metastatic Staging*

MX	Distant metastasis cannot be assessed
M0	No distant metastasis
M1	Distant metastasis

TABLE 10–4 • *Stage Grouping*

Stage	T	N	M
Stage 0	Tis	N0	M0
Stage 1	T1	N0	M0
Stage 2A	T0-1	N1	M0
	T2	N0	M0
Stage 2B	T2	N1	M0
	T3	N0	M0
Stage 3A	T0-3	N2	M0
	T3	N1	M0
Stage 3B	T4	N0-2	M0
Stage 3C	Any T	N3	M0
Stage 4	Any T	Any N	M1

Metastases greater than 0.2 mm in size but less than 2.0 mm in size are referred to as *micrometastases* and are staged as N1mi. The term *micrometastases* is often used inappropriately, both to describe lesions less than 0.2 mm or greater than 2.0 mm. As N1 disease, micrometastases should be treated as such, prompting a completion node dissection (see Chapter 13) and considered when contemplating adjuvant systemic therapy. The nodal staging goes up with the number of nodes involved, as well as with the location of metastases, as outlined in Table 10–2.

Metastases to the internal mammary and supraclavicular nodes must also be considered in the N stage. Previously, supraclavicular nodes were considered metastatic disease, and patients with documented disease in the supraclavicular nodes were considered stage IV. However, outcomes of patients with locally advanced breast cancer with supraclavicular involvement are similar to those of patients with locally advanced breast cancer without supraclavicular disease, and both are significantly better than those with metastatic disease, prompting reclassification of these metastases as pN3c disease.

The internal mammary nodes were not a significant issue before sentinel node biopsy came into use because they were only rarely discovered incidentally on a staging CT study. However, lymphatic mapping often demonstrates drainage to the internal mammary nodes and some surgeons routinely or selectively excise these nodes (see Chapter 13). Whether the disease is clinically discovered or discovered on SLN biopsy and whether there are internal mammary (IM) metastases in conjunction with axillary metastases or not are factored into the staging system.

M Stage

Finally, the M stage documents the presence of distant metastases (see Table 10–3). The staging system is simple: MX if the patient cannot be clinically assessed, M0 if there are no distant metastases, and M1 if there are. The TNM staging can then be used to determine the AJCC stage (Table 10–4).

Whether a patient is M0 or M1 will in some part depend on how hard one looks. All patients should have a thorough history (including complete review of systems) and physical as part of their staging workup (as well as their diagnostic workup), and any symptoms consistent with possible metastases should be fully evaluated. Bone is the most common site of distant spread (Box 10–1). Up to 70% of women who die of breast cancer will have bone metastases. However, very few women will have identifiable bone metastases at presentation. Patients with bone pain, recent fractures, lower extremity weakness, or bowel or bladder dysfunction (signs of spinal cord involvement) should have a thorough workup including bone scan, and CT scans or x-ray studies as indicated. Lung metastases are the next most common site of distant spread, representing about 25% of patients with stage IV breast cancer, although again only a small percentage have identifiable disease at presentation. Whereas lung metastases often cause no symptoms initially, the presence of dyspnea, a dry cough, chest pain, or heaviness or pain on deep inspiration should prompt a chest CT and further studies as indicated. Liver is the third most common site

BOX 10–1 BONES MOST COMMONLY AFFECTED BY METASTASES

Spine
Ribs
Pelvis
Skull
Long bones of the extremities

BOX 10–2 SYMPTOMS OF CENTRAL NERVOUS SYSTEM INVOLVEMENT BY BREAST CANCER METASTASES

Motor deficit or gain disturbance
Seizures
Headaches
Cognitive dysfunction
Nausea and vomiting
Visual changes
Cranial nerve dysfunction
Cerebellar symptoms
Speech disturbances

of spread. It is exceedingly uncommon for patients to have any symptoms suggestive of liver disease. Finally, the central nervous system (brain, cranial nerves, spinal cord, leptomeninges) is involved in 20% of patients with stage IV disease (Box 10–2). Symptoms of brain or spinal cord involvement should prompt an MRI of the brain.

Even though the indications for imaging studies in symptomatic patients are clear, the majority of breast cancer patients are asymptomatic and the question arises as to which, if any, of these patients should have a workup for distant metastases. Clearly, not all patients need to undergo a complete workup. The prevalence of detectable metastases is extremely low in the early stage of breast cancer, and while their presence might alter therapy, a complete workup in all patients is not only exceedingly costly, but also leads to unnecessary stress, repeat studies, and biopsies prompted by false-positive results or indeterminate lesions often detected on these studies. The evidence is clear that bone, CT, MRI , and positron emitting tomography (PET) scans are not indicated in asymptomatic patients with early-stage disease. They have an extremely low detection rate and poor sensitivity.

Chest x-ray studies are a common preoperative staging examination. However, they have a very low yield, detecting disease in only approximately 0.3% of breast cancer patients. Several studies have shown that their routine use is neither cost-effective nor clinically useful. However, many surgeons obtain a chest x-ray study not so much to look for distant disease but rather to look for cardiopulmonary disease before administering general anesthesia. Although the use of chest x-ray studies in asymptomatic patients without known underlying pulmonary disease is debatable, it is a well-established practice. If a chest x-ray study was obtained and demonstrates an abnormal finding, a follow-up CT scan is usually indicated.

Serum blood tests are often part of the routine preoperative search for distant disease and include a complete blood count (CBC) comprehensive metabolic panel including alkaline phosphatase and liver function tests. Some physicians also order tumor markers such as CA15-3 or CEA. A further metastatic workup would then be initiated in patients with anemia or abnormalities in any of these laboratory values. As with radiographic studies, however, the yield of detecting metastases based on serum laboratory abnormalities is extremely low, and this approach does not appear to be cost-effective.

For the symptomatic patient, the patient with a more advanced cancer, and even the asymptomatic patient with newly diagnosed breast cancer, PET scanning is being examined as an alternative to CT and bone scan. The Center for Medicare and Medicaid Services approved the use of PET scanning in breast cancer patients in 2002, although how PET scanning should be used is not yet clear. Even though it is being used more often, the yield of PET scanning in asymptomatic patients with small primary tumors and clinically negative nodes is very low (<1%) and not recommended. For the symptomatic patient, or the patient with more advanced disease, PET scanning may be complementary to CT of the chest/abdomen/pelvis and bone scan. As an alternative, however, because infection and inflammation will lead to increased uptake of fluorodeoxyglucose, false-positive findings are not uncommon, and treatment decisions should not be based on PET scan results alone. PET scan may play a bigger role in the workup of the patient suspected to have recurrent disease (see Chapter 21).

Other Information Not Included in Staging

Although the TNM staging system does a reasonable job at stratifying the risk of recurrence, and hence the benefit of therapy, there is additional information that goes into the decision-making process, particularly with regard to adjuvant systemic therapy (see Chapter 16). As our knowledge of breast cancer genetics advances and genetic analysis of breast cancer specimens become commercially available, the TNM staging system becomes less relevant. For years, factors beyond TNM have been examined as methods to stratify risk.

Bone marrow micrometastases can be detected through the use of monoclonal antibodies against cytokeratins found specifically on epithelial cells. The detection of micrometastases in the bone marrow of breast cancer patients may help predict prognosis and guide adjuvant therapies. Approximately 2 mL of marrow is drawn from each anterosuperior iliac crest and then studied using an anticytokeratin monoclonal antibody immunocytochemical technique, PCR, or flow cytometry. The relatively simple procedure can be done at the time of surgical resection with intravenous sedation and local anesthesia. Numerous studies have shown that bone marrow micrometastases not only correlate with the size and grade of the primary tumor, but also with distant recurrence and survival, and can stratify patients with similar TNM staging. More importantly, bone marrow micrometastases may be present in patients with negative SLN nodes, identifying a subset of patients with unrecognized micrometastases. Risk can be further stratified by the quantity of breast cancer cells in the marrow.

Ongoing prospective studies will further quantify the risk associated with the presence of bone marrow micrometastases, but there are, at present, no data on the outcome of bone marrow micrometastases–negative patients who avoid chemotherapy. Therefore, while the finding of bone marrow micrometastases may argue for the addition of systemic therapy in the patient who was otherwise not a strong candidate (node-negative, small primary tumor), the absence of bone marrow micrometastases cannot be used to withhold chemotherapy from an otherwise reasonable candidate. It is also not clear how much bone marrow micrometastases adds in the era of Oncotype DX and genetic analysis of the primary tumor (see Chapter 16). For now, bone marrow aspiration should only be performed as part of an investigational trial.

Markers of tumor cell proliferation have also been examined for their prognostic and predictive value. *S-phase fraction, DNA ploidy,* and an elevated *thymidine labeling index (TLI)* are signs of increased proliferation and have been correlated with tumor size, grade, and stage. Positive IHC staining for *Ki-67* (a cell-cycle–specific nuclear antigen present only in proliferating cells) has also been correlated with advanced grade and stage and worse outcome. However, none of these tests has been shown to impact management of the breast cancer patient and their routine use is not recommended.

Genetic Counseling

As stated, there is information that, although not considered "standard" staging information, greatly impacts the workup, treatment, and surveillance of the breast cancer patients. One example of this is the family history of the patient and the implications regarding their risk of a second breast cancer. It has been known for some time that families with a disproportionate amount of breast and/or ovarian cancer exist. Careful analysis of these families suggested that the malignancy was transmitted as an autosomal dominant trait. This ultimately led to the discovery of mutations in the genes BRCA1 and BRCA2. It is estimated that these genes account for approximately 5% and 10%, respectively, of all breast and ovarian cancer. Chapter 8 discusses the risk of cancer among BRCA carriers in more detail. However, patients with breast cancer, especially young patients, must be concerned with their risk of developing a second cancer. Thus a discussion of that risk and options to minimize it, including surgical, must be part of the preoperative assessment.

The question will arise as to whether to pursue genetic testing before proceeding with surgery. The ultimate question is whether this patient would benefit from bilateral mastectomy, not only to treat the known cancer but also to prevent the development of a second breast cancer. However, obtaining genetic testing is not as simple a decision as that of obtaining a staging chest x-ray study or CT scan. There are implications not only for the patient but also the patient's family. Interpreting the results is not always straightforward. Most importantly, genetic testing may not impact surgical decision making. Patients with a strong family history of breast cancer may have decided to proceed with bilateral mastectomy regardless of their BRCA results. In contrast, candidates for breast conservation may not be willing to undergo prophylactic mastectomies regardless of risk. The benefit of prophylaxis must also be weighed against the risk of recurrence and death resulting from the primary tumor. Thus genetic testing should almost never be ordered by the surgeon, but rather by a genetic counselor after an adequate assessment of the likelihood of

BOX 10–3 PATIENTS WITH INVASIVE BREAST CANCER FOR WHOM GENETIC COUNSELING/TESTING SHOULD BE CONSIDERED

- Diagnosed at a young age (<40)
- Patients with bilateral cancers or both breast and ovarian cancer
- Patients with two or more close relatives with breast or ovarian cancer
- Patients with a family member who developed breast or ovarian cancer before age 50, had both breast and ovarian cancer, or bilateral breast cancer
- Patients with a male relative who had breast cancer
- A positive BRCA1 or BRCA2 genetic test in a relative
- Ashkenazi (Eastern European) Jewish ancestry

BOX 10–4 PARTICIPANTS IN A BREAST CANCER TUMOR BOARD

- Genetic counselors
- Medical oncologists
- Nurse coordinators
- Pathologists
- Psychologists/psychiatrists
- Radiation oncologists
- Radiologists
- Research nurses
- Social workers
- Surgeons

harboring disease and discussion of the interpretation and potential benefits of testing.

Who should be referred to a genetic counselor? Genetic counseling is appropriate for any patient who believes that she or her family is at increased risk of developing breast or ovarian cancer. Not all of these patients do carry an increased risk, and counseling may help alleviate fears and stop patients from choosing extensive surgery that may not be in their best interest. In addition, patients determined to have an increased risk of possessing a genetic predisposition to breast or ovarian cancer, based on a thorough history, should be referred for genetic counseling (Box 10–3). It is also important not to overlook syndromes other than BRCA1 or BRCA2 that may be associated with breast cancer. Li-Fraumeni syndrome (p53 mutation) should be suspected in a young woman with breast cancer who has a personal or family history that includes soft tissue sarcomas, osteosarcomas, brain tumors, or leukemias. Histories that include breast cancer, benign breast disease, thyroid, renal, and endometrial cancer may suggest Cowden syndrome (PTEN).

Presentation at a Multidisciplinary Tumor Board

Finally, before proceeding with treatment, it is prudent to present patient cases at a breast cancer multidisciplinary tumor board (Box 10–4). The treatment of breast cancer is multimodal and increasingly complex. The old scenario in which the surgeon evaluates the patient, proceeds with surgery, and then refers the patient to medical and radiation oncologists is becoming less appropriate as the management of breast cancer changes. There are several advantages to the multidisciplinary approach.

One significant advantage is that it allows for review of the pathology and radiology in a group setting. This is particularly important if the patient had x-ray studies or biopsies at an outside institution because it allows for a second and potentially an expert review of the findings. In many cases, this review may change the recommended surgery. Review of the mammogram may reveal a second area of suspicion that requires biopsy before proceeding with lumpectomy or calcifications that preclude breast conservation. Review of the pathology may change the margin status, affecting the need for reexcision, or it may find or question the presence of an invasive component in predominantly in situ disease, changing recommendations for axillary staging. The tumor board setting also facilitates direct communication between the surgeon, radiologist, and pathologist in planning surgery.

Given that radiation is a crucial component of breast conservation therapy, it is prudent to have the radiation oncologist and the surgeon review the history, physical, and imaging findings together before deciding upon breast conservation. Concerns of the radiation oncologist, based on comorbidities, underlying medical conditions, body habitus, or mammographic findings, may prevent a scenario wherein the surgeon feels lumpectomy is appropriate, only to have the patient return for a mastectomy after a consultation with a radiation oncologist. For patients who require a mastectomy, the need for postmastectomy radiation might influence the type and timing of reconstruction, and in some cases this may prompt an SLN biopsy before mastectomy to determine whether immediate reconstruction is appropriate.

One of the most important angles of the multidisciplinary tumor board is the dialogue between the medical oncologist and surgeon on the use of neoadjuvant chemotherapy. Chemotherapy before surgery is increasingly used to downstage operable tumors, and it has other advantages as well (see Chapter 18). Many patients may be better served by completing chemotherapy before surgery, assuming the patients are deemed appropriate candidates for chemotherapy. The tumor board setting allows for a discussion of not only when neoadjuvant chemotherapy might be appropriate, but also how to handle regional staging (SLN before or after chemotherapy), whether BCT would be appropriate even if the primary tumor is downstaged, and whether neoadjuvant hormonal therapy may be preferred to chemotherapy. Even when neoadjuvant chemotherapy is not necessary, having medical oncologists review the case in the beginning can change surgical management, especially in cases of recurrent disease.

Beyond the oncologists, surgeons, and radiation oncologists, there are other aspects to the tumor board setting that are advantageous to both the clinicians and the patients. Reviewing the family history with the genetic counselor present helps determine who should be referred for genetic counseling and facilitates this process. Likewise, the early intervention of social workers and psychologists may help patients having a difficult time with their diagnosis or other obstacles to receiving appropriate care.

Also important is the presence of research nurses who can help identify patients appropriate for open research protocols.

Patients are often concerned that the time it takes to get a second opinion from a multidisciplinary team may be detrimental. They feel that the cancer needs to be removed as soon as possible and any delay may lead to the development of metastatic disease. Patients should be assured that they have time to get all the necessary information and make the right decision without jeopardizing their chance of cure. Another question is whether all patients need to be reviewed or if just the "complex cases" should be. It may not be feasible to present all new patients in this manner; however, it is often in the "straightforward" cases that a change in the radiology or pathology report alters surgical management. Thus it seems most prudent to review most cases with the tumor board, although the reality of this depends upon the resources available.

Suggested Readings

1. Green FL, Page DL, Fleming ID, Fritz A, eds. AJCC Cancer Staging Manual, 6th ed. Chicago: American Joint Committee on Cancer, 2002.
2. National Comprehensive Cancer Network (NCCN) Clinical Practice Guidelines in Oncology. Available at http://www.nccn.org/professionals/physician_gls/default.asp.
3. Newman EA, Guest AB, Helvie MA, et al. Changes in surgical management resulting from case review at a breast cancer multidisciplinary tumor board. Cancer 2006;107(10):2346–2351.
4. Singletary SE, Allred C, Ashley P, et al. Revision of the American Joint Committee on Cancer staging system for breast cancer. JCO 2002;20(17):3628–3636.
5. Singletary SE, Connolly JL. Breast cancer staging: Working with the 6th edition of the AJCC Cancer Staging Manual. CA Cancer J Clin 2006;56:37–47.

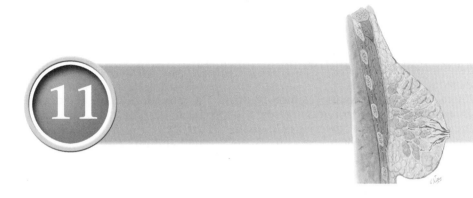

Management of Ductal Carcinoma In Situ and Paget Disease

Management of Ductal Carcinoma In Situ and Paget Disease: Key Points

Appreciate the presentation of DCIS and the changes in incidence since the introduction of screening mammograms.

Understand the natural history of DCIS and the implications for treatment.

Know the advantages and disadvantages of breast conservation therapy versus mastectomy for patients with DCIS.

Be familiar with the NSABP and EORTC trials of radiation after lumpectomy for DCIS.

Understand the role of tamoxifen after surgery for DCIS.

Describe the clinical presentation and appearance of Paget disease.

Know the treatment options for patients with Paget disease and the implications of the mammographic findings.

Ductal carcinoma in situ (DCIS) is a non-invasive form of ductal carcinoma, limited to the confines of the basement membrane of the duct (also referred to as intraductal carcinoma). It represents an intermediate stage in the histologic progression of normal breast tissue to invasive ductal carcinoma. Most invasive ductal carcinomas appear to originate from DCIS, as evidenced by similar genetic changes in invasive cancers adjacent to in situ disease, although the exact mechanisms and pathways of tumorigenesis are not well understood.

Before the era of screening mammography, DCIS was a relatively uncommon presentation of breast cancer. Today, however, DCIS makes up about 15% to 30% of breast cancer cases. DCIS typically starts in the small to medium-sized ducts with exaggerated ductal cellular proliferation and is generally thought to be a precursor to invasive ductal carcinoma. Although DCIS is stage 0 breast cancer and thought of as an innocuous lesion, the term DCIS encompasses a variable group of lesions with a wide spectrum of histologic and pathologic features, diverse malignant potential, and multiple treatment options. The treatment of DCIS within the breast is extremely similar to that of invasive ductal carcinoma, while the concern for regional or distant disease is much less.

Incidence

The detection of noninvasive breast cancer increased dramatically with screening mammography. Before this, DCIS was a very different disease entity, often presenting as either a palpable mass, nipple discharge, or Paget disease (see later). It represented only a small fraction of breast cancer cases (approximately 1% to 3%). Unsure exactly how to treat it, recommendations ranged from simple observation to modified radical mastectomy. Between 1983 and 1992, as screening mammography became widespread, incidence rates increased dramatically. This increase in the incidence of DCIS has been most pronounced among women between the ages of 40 and 69.

The incidence of DCIS continues to increase, with more than 62,000 cases in 2007. Today, DCIS accounts for more than 20% of all new cancer diagnoses and approximately 42% of all mammographically detected malignancies. How much of the increase is due to increased screening and how much may be a true increased incidence of DCIS is unknown. The risk factors for DCIS and invasive cancer are identical and include a personal history of breast cancer, family history, nulliparity, or older age at first birth.

Although the concept of a localized preinvasive form of breast cancer dates back to 1906, the actual term *in situ* was not coined until 1932. Basically, DCIS is thought to be an exaggerated multiplication of cells in the ductal system with a propensity toward longitudinal rather than radial growth; these cells remain within the confines of the basement membranes. A constellation of subtypes have been recognized, each with their individual architectural characteristics, invasive potential, and prognostic significance (Box 11–1).

BOX 11–1 Terms Used to Describe DCIS

- *Multifocal DCIS* is an entity wherein multiple, apparently separate foci of disease occur within the same quadrant of the breast. Upon closer evaluation by three-dimensional reconstructions of the cross-sectional segments, 99% of these seemingly disconnected areas are in essence *unifocal*, harboring disease arising from convolutions of the same duct system.

- *Multicentric DCIS* on the other hand refers to foci of disease present in different quadrants of the breast arising simultaneously in different disconnected duct systems. On average, 30% of cases of DCIS are believed to be multicentric.

- *Microinvasive DCIS* has been defined by the American Joint Committee on Cancer (AJCC) as the extension of cancer cells beyond the basement membrane into adjacent tissues with no focus more than 1 mm in greatest dimension. Lesions fulfilling this criterion are staged as T1*mic*, a subset of T1 breast cancer. It is important to remember that with multiple foci of microinvasion, only the focus with the largest dimension is used to classify the lesion and the sizes of individual foci are not added together.

- *Extensive intraductal component* (EIC) is a term used to describe a particular morphology of invasive carcinoma with associated DCIS comprising more than 25% of the tumor volume along with an additional extra-tumoral focus of DCIS.

- *Paget disease* of the breast is defined clinically by the finding of eczematous, scaly skin at the nipple-areolar complex. It is associated with underlying breast cancer (invasive and/or in situ) in 97% of cases. A less common presentation of breast cancer, it is important to consider Paget disease in any patient presenting with a persistent nipple-areolar complex abnormality.

TABLE 11-1 • *Traditional Architectural Classification for DCIS*

Architectural Pattern	Cytologic Features	Calcifications	Cell Necrosis
Micropapillary	Intraluminal projection of cells, club shaped, lack fibrovascular	Minimal, small	Limited to single cells
Papillary	Intraluminal projection of tumor cells, fibrovascular cores	Minimal, small	Variable
Cribriform	Small cells, small hypochromatic nuclei, back-to-back glands	Minimal, small	Limited to single cells
Solid	Not as well defined, tumor cells fill and distend involved space	Variable	Not significant
Comedo	Large cells, nuclear pleomorphism, mitotic activity, often associated with microinvasion	Linear, branching	Prominent

Historically DCIS has been classified into five subtypes (postulated to represent steps in evolution and worsening malignant potential) based on architectural pattern: micropapillary, papillary, cribriform, solid, and comedo (Table 11-1) (Figs. 11-1 through 11-3). More recently the emphasis has been on the presence of necrosis and nuclear grade (Fig. 11-4). This is based on the fact that these factors have the most significant association with microinvasive disease and the propensity for recurrence. DCIS is not associated with a high risk of regional or distant recurrence, so the focus centers on local control, particularly on preventing an invasive recurrence. This is particularly true as more women opt for breast conservation. Hence the current recommendation is for each histopathologic report to individually comment upon morphology, nuclear

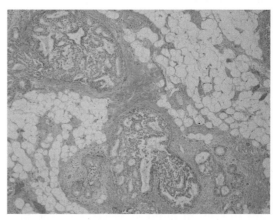

Figure 11-2. Cribriform growth pattern of ductal carcinoma in situ. These cells entirely fill the ducts and the cells form secondary glandular lumina. (Image courtesy of Maria Braman, MD, Department of Pathology, University of Michigan.)

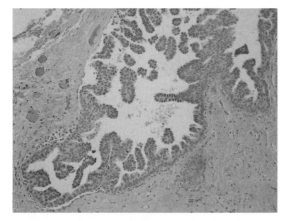

Figure 11-1. Micropapillary growth pattern of ductal carcinoma in situ. A proliferation of neoplastic cells replace the epithelium lining and form small projections. These can coalesce, forming curvilineous structures. (Image courtesy of Maria Braman, MD, Department of Pathology, University of Michigan.)

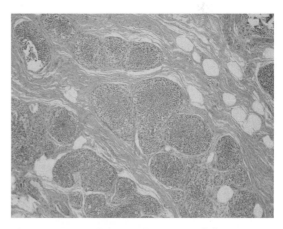

Figure 11-3. Solid growth pattern of ductal carcinoma in situ. The cells completely fill the duct without necrosis. (Image courtesy of Maria Braman, MD, Department of Pathology, University of Michigan.)

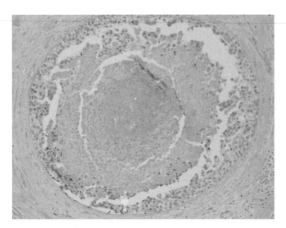

Figure 11–4. Comedonecrosis. The cells completely fill the duct, but the central core becomes necrotic. (Image courtesy of Maria Braman, MD, Department of Pathology, University of Michigan.)

grade, and necrosis. Several systems exist for classifying DCIS by these features (Table 11–2).

Natural History

Ductal carcinoma in situ is generally thought to be a precursor lesion to invasive carcinoma; a step in the transition from normal cells of the duct to frankly invasive cancer. It is important to keep in mind, however, that the progression from cellular proliferation, to atypical hyperplasia, to noninvasive cancer, and ultimately to invasive cancer has been hypothesized yet never proven. Some have suggested that a good portion of mammographically detected DCIS is clinically indolent and would never lead to invasive cancer. If this is the case, we may be overtreating DCIS, extending surgery and radiation therapy to patients unlikely to benefit. This argument is supported in part by autopsy studies showing DCIS occurring in 1% to 18% of women.

Past studies of patients with DCIS left untreated due to missed diagnoses provide valuable insights; there is convincing evidence that most DCIS would proceed to invasive cancer. After 30 years of follow-up, approximately two thirds of these patients progressed to invasive disease. This clearly demonstrates that most DCIS lesions will evolve into invasive cancers, yet a significant proportion do not. The disease-free subset most likely represents low-grade disease with small residual tumor burden or even lesions that were incidentally completely excised upon biopsy. The fact that the same risk factors exist for DCIS and invasive ductal carcinoma is additional proof. However, better definition of the molecular factors required for DCIS to progress to invasive disease is needed to better differentiate between the cases of DCIS that could in the future be safely observed versus those cases that may need treatment.

Studies suggest that DCIS most commonly originates from a single site with longitudinal extension along the ductal systems. Cross-sectional proliferation and progression to invasion occurs concurrently, so the larger the area of DCIS, the more likely it is that there are microinvasive foci. There is a much higher prevalence of invasive disease in cases of diffuse DCIS.

By definition, unless microinvasive disease is present, DCIS does not invade through the basement membrane and therefore cannot spread to the regional lymph nodes or distally. Review of modified radical mastectomy specimens performed for DCIS more than two decades ago shows concurrent axillary disease in only 2% to 3% of patients. Similar proportions were seen to develop distant metastasis despite adequate local treatment. This most likely represents missed foci of microinvasion, although the possibility of an inherently aggressive form of DCIS cannot be ruled out.

Classification

Although DCIS has classically been classified by morphology, for clinical purposes, many authors have simply characterized DCIS as comedo and noncomedo. The cells of comedo DCIS have a more malignant appearance; this is reflected biologically because comedo DCIS is more likely to be associated with invasive cancer than noncomedo DCIS. Even this simple classification system is complicated by the fact that larger lesions may have more than one pattern and there is significant interobserver

TABLE 11–2 • *Histopathologic Classifications for DCIS*		
European	**Van Nuys**	**Lagios**
Well differentiated	Non–high grade No necrosis	Low grade
Moderately differentiated	Non–high grade with necrosis	Intermediate grade
Poorly differentiated	High grade	High grade

variation in labeling DCIS as comedo or noncomedo. Two other important pathologic features are nuclear grade and the presence of necrosis. Silverstein and colleagues have proposed dividing DCIS into three groups: (1) high-grade, (2) non–high-grade with comedonecrosis, and (3) non–high grade without comedonecrosis. Again, however, it is difficult to find concordance among pathologists using this system and more importantly, none have been able to accurately stratify DCIS by risk of local recurrence or development of invasive breast cancer.

Presentation

Although today most patients present with an abnormality on routine screening mammogram, approximately 9% of patients still present with a palpable mass, nipple discharge, or as Paget disease of the breast (a chronic eczematous, scaly rash at the nipple-areolar complex) (Fig. 11–5). Any patient presenting with these findings should undergo mammographic imaging.

Because more than 90% of DCIS lesions diagnosed today are clinically occult, dependence on imaging modalities has become obligatory. Mammography has emerged as the primary imaging tool for the detection and diagnosis of DCIS. Microcalcifications are the most common mammographic characteristic of DCIS and are observed in more than 90% of cases (Fig. 11–6). Less frequently mammographic findings may include prominent ducts, mass, or architectural changes.

There is evidence to suggest correlation between the histopathologic subtype of DCIS and features of associated mammographic calcifications. The most characteristic feature of comedo DCIS is casting-type calcifications— linear branching patterns depicting alignment in a ductal distribution. Conversely noncomedo DCIS is more often associated with fine punctuate calcifications, usually presenting as a cluster or a noncalcific mass. Up to 94% of comedo DCIS have mammographic calcifications, 87% of which are linear. On the other hand, only 53% of noncomedo DCIS had calcifications. In addition, the mammographic estimation of lesion size for comedo DCIS was more accurate than for the other subtypes.

Other available imaging techniques, including ultrasonography, magnetic resonance imaging, scintimammography, and computerized thermography, are relatively insensitive in the absence of invasion. Sonographic features of DCIS include a higher proportion of oval- or lobulated-shaped areas with uniform isoechoic texture and bilateral edge shadowing. Calcifications may be detected by a high frequency probe in up to 60% of lesions, usually the comedo subtype. Ultrasound's sensitivity is estimated as 62% for comedo DCIS versus only 30% for noncomedo lesions. Breast magnetic resonance imaging (MRI) is the most recent adjunct to breast imaging. The use of MRI in evaluating invasive breast cancer is still evolving, and recent data suggest a possible role in accurately assessing the extent of disease as well as detecting multicentricity or residual disease after resection. While estimating the extent of disease in DCIS is equally as important, the ability of MRI to do this accurately is still under investigation, and the role of MRI for DCIS remains experimental.

An abnormality detected on mammography obligates histopathologic evaluation. The various available options include fine-needle aspiration (FNA), percutaneous core-needle biopsy under stereotactic, sonographic, or tactile guidance (when palpable), and surgical biopsy with or without wire localization. The absolute sensitivity of FNA in the diagnosis of DCIS is only in the range of 51% to 55% with more than 35% of indeterminate cytology lesions later confirmed as DCIS. Cytology cannot differentiate in situ versus invasive cancer and therefore FNA is inadequate for the diagnosis of DCIS. On the other hand, stereotactically guided core biopsy with specimen imaging to confirm retrieval of microcalcifications has a sensitivity up to 91% to 94%. Ultrasound-guided biopsy techniques have similar results. Wire localization of microcalcifications with surgical excision is used for

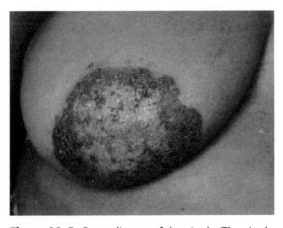

Figure 11–5. Paget disease of the nipple. The nipple areolar complex is scaly and eczematous. (Image courtesy of Celina Kleer, MD, Department of Pathology, University of Michigan.)

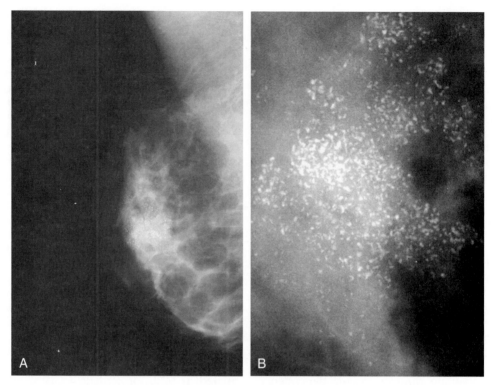

Figure 11–6. Mediolateral oblique and magnification views demonstrate regionally distributed pleomorphic calcifications. Pathology demonstrated ductal carcinoma in situ. (Images courtesy of Dr. Alexis Nees, Department of Radiology, University of Michigan.)

diagnosis if the aforementioned procedures cannot be performed due to technical or patient-related factors, a situation that is becoming increasingly rare.

It is important to remember that image-guided core biopsy techniques may understage malignant microcalcifications. Studies indicate that approximately 10% to 15% of 14-gauge core biopsy specimens revealing atypical ductal hyperplasia (ADH), a benign condition, get histopathologically upgraded to DCIS, microinvasive carcinoma, or frankly invasive carcinoma after complete excision. Similarly, DCIS diagnosed by core biopsy may get upgraded correspondingly. This rate of upstaging may be reduced by using larger 11-gauge or 8-gauge core samples. It is recommended that ADH diagnosed on core biopsy be completely excised via wire localization excision to rule out any residual DCIS or invasive cancer.

Treatment

With the evolution of our knowledge of the disease process and its pattern of behavior, the treatment options have evolved accordingly.

Today, a variety of treatment options, ranging from excision alone (lumpectomy or breast-conserving therapy) to mastectomy, with or without radiation therapy (XRT), have been proposed for DCIS. When treating invasive breast cancer, local control efforts may be tempered by the likelihood of distant recurrences and overall survival. For noninvasive breast cancer, there is an extremely low likelihood of distant disease and the overall survival should approach 99% to 100%. Therefore the goal of therapy centers squarely on local control. Approximately one half of all recurrences will be invasive, carrying the associated risks of metastases and decreased survival.

Once DCIS has been established with tissue biopsy, the treatment is directed at complete resection of all disease and the prevention of recurrence. Treatment must be individualized to each patient to accomplish these goals. The extent of disease, the size of the lesion, any prior history of breast cancer and/or XRT, occult invasive cancer coexisting with the in situ lesion, and multicentricity are important factors in determining the best treatment for disease control. Patients should be counseled and involved in the decision-making process.

Mastectomy

Historically, mastectomy was the treatment of choice for DCIS, with cure rates approaching 98% to 99%. Reported failure rates after mastectomy are in the range of 1% to 3%, and almost all of these are invasive carcinomas, presenting as chest wall, axillary or distant recurrence. This may be explained by the fact that high-grade comedo DCIS may contain areas of invasion or microinvasion that remain undiagnosed with standard histopathologic evaluation protocols, or these are new primary cancers in residual breast tissue.

Although mastectomy has the lowest reported failure rate and is considered the gold standard for the management of DCIS, it may be more aggressive than is necessary for most women with DCIS. With the advent of breast conservation therapy (BCT) options for invasive cancer, its application was successfully extended to DCIS. However, mastectomy is still the treatment of choice in several specific situations (Box 11–2). Multicentric DCIS is one indication for mastectomy. Some patients will have diffuse microcalcifications throughout the breast on mammography. This often represents diffuse disease and even in those cases where these calcifications are associated with benign disease, they hamper the ability to detect recurrence on surveillance mammography. When DCIS is not multicentric but limited to one area within the breast, the size of this region relative to the size of the breast is an important consideration for whether mastectomy is indicated. This is obviously relative and must be individually considered for each patient, but a large area of disease that cannot be excised with a cosmetically acceptable result should be a relative indication for mastectomy. Likewise, the inability to obtain histologically negative margins after multiple attempts is another indication to proceed with mastectomy. Contraindications to radiation, which plays a significant role in breast conservation, must be considered. These include women in the first or second trimester of pregnancy, women with connective tissue disorders such as scleroderma who have unusually high complications from radiation, and women who have had previous radiation to the area.

Breast Conservation Therapy

During the mid 1980s to 1990s, there were various authors who reported their experiences with BCT for DCIS, employing lumpectomy as the primary treatment modality with or without local XRT (Table 11–3). These indicated compelling evidence in favor of BCT. A strong argument for the use of adjuvant radiation came unintentionally from the National Surgical Adjuvant Breast and Bowel Project (NSABP) protocol B-06. Designed to evaluate invasive breast cancers, the protocol recruited a small group of women (78 patients) who were confirmed to have DCIS upon histopathologic reevaluation. Recurrence rates were in the range of 43% for lumpectomy alone, but only 9% for the lumpectomy plus XRT arm.

This prompted the NSABP to launch protocol B-17, a prospective randomized trial comparing lumpectomy alone to lumpectomy plus XRT (50 Gy) for the treatment of DCIS. More than 800 patients were recruited in total

BOX 11–2 INDICATIONS FOR MASTECTOMY IN DUCTAL CARCINOMA IN SITU

- Multicentric disease
- Diffuse microcalcifications on mammography
- Large tumor size with predictably bad cosmetic outcome
- Contraindication to radiation
  - Pregnancy
  - Connective tissue disorder (scleroderma)
  - Previous radiation therapy
  - Patient preference

TABLE 11–3 • Trials of Lumpectomy With and Without Radiation for DCIS

	NSABP B-17	EORTC 10853	UK DCIS
Number of patients	813	1002	1030
Follow-up (yr)	12	4	4.4
RR Excision alone	32%	16%	14%
% Invasive	50%	50%	40%
RR Excision + XRT	12%	9%	6%
% Invasive	30%	40%	50%

RR, Recurrence rate; XRT, radiation therapy.

BOX 11-3 RADIATION THERAPY AFTER LUMPECTOMY FOR DUCTAL CARCINOMA IN SITU

- Radiation therapy (XRT) reduces ipsilateral breast tumor recurrence by 50% to 60%.
- XRT reduces ipsilateral invasive breast tumor recurrence by 50% to 60%.
- After XRT, the annual rate of an invasive recurrence is 0.5% to 1% per year.
- XRT does not improve necessarily survival.

for both arms of the study with a mean follow-up of 90 months. Local failure rate for the group treated with lumpectomy alone was approximately twice that of the lumpectomy plus XRT group: 26.8% vs. 12.1%, with half the recurrent tumors being invasive in the former and one third in the latter. Pathologic findings from protocol B-17 showed that the two biggest predictors of ipsilateral recurrence were comedo necrosis and the presence of involved specimen margins (Box 11–3).

A similar trial was simultaneously launched in Europe by the European Organization for Research and Treatment (EORTC). After a median follow-up time of 51 months, a recurrence rate of 16% was observed in the group treated with lumpectomy alone, and 50% of these were invasive cancers. Patients treated with lumpectomy with subsequent XRT revealed a recurrence rate of 9%, of which 40% were invasive cancers.

Although there have been no prospective randomized trials comparing mastectomy to BCT in the treatment of DCIS, the large treatment registries have suggested that, while local recurrence rates may be lower after mastectomy than after BCT, there is no difference in overall survival. The reported cause-specific mortality from DCIS treated with either mastectomy or lumpectomy plus XRT is similar (in the range of 1% to 2%). For DCIS, there is little risk of metastasis, yet the potential of an invasive recurrence remains. It is imperative that the basis of all treatment options for DCIS be the minimization of the potential risk of an invasive recurrence. At the present time, most patients are candidates for BCT. The initial attempt should be to widely excise the entire area with acceptable margins. Careful preoperative planning is paramount, because the initial operation is the best chance to achieve complete excision and offer good cosmetic results.

As with all breast biopsies, the surgical specimen should be accurately oriented and, if appropriate, imaged to confirm complete excision of the radiographic abnormality. If the lesion is seen to abut a specific margin, an additional adequate surgical margin should be obtained in the corresponding quadrant. Orienting the specimen correctly and inking it with a six-color system allows the pathologist to inform the surgeon whether a specific margin is either involved or close, allowing for a more directed reexcision. This provides a better cosmetic outcome compared to having to reexcise the entire lumpectomy cavity. Surgical clips left along all six biopsy cavity boundaries are instrumental in delineating the site for accurate planning of adjuvant radiation therapy boost dose or partial breast irradiation.

Accurate pathologic assessment of margin status is imperative. There is no consensus to date on what comprises the ideal negative margin for DCIS. Most institutions strive for at least 2 to 3 mm of circumferential disease-free tissue. Inadequate margins necessitate reexcision, hence the importance of orienting and labeling the specimen at the time of lumpectomy to guide subsequent surgery. Noninvasive cancers presenting with calcifications require postoperative mammography to ascertain complete excision. Residual suspicious calcifications require localization and reexcision even in the presence of negative margins.

Lumpectomy Alone for DCIS

It is clear that postoperative radiation as a component of BCT offers excellent local control. However, radiation is not without its side effects and cost. Whole breast irradiation is time consuming and can cause cardiac or pulmonary side effects. There is also the risk of second malignancies. Given the fact that many cases of DCIS treated by excision alone do not recur, it seems likely that there is a subset of patients who may be treated by lumpectomy alone. With careful attention to grade, size, and margin width, there should be a subset of patients who could consider treatment by lumpectomy alone. This may be appropriate treatment for patients with extremely low-risk mammographically detected DCIS exhibiting favorable histopathologic features (low grade, no necrosis) when resected with an adequate negative margin. Silverstein and colleagues have proposed that patients who have undergone excision with a minimal margin of 1 cm do not benefit from radiation therapy.

However, in an attempt to confirm this, a prospective study of patients with grade 1 or 2 DCIS underwent excision with margins of greater than 1 cm. There was a 12% local recurrence rate after 5 years, with 31% of these being invasive, and the trial needed to be stopped early due to the high rate of local failure. Other attempts to confirm that an adequate excision of a low-grade lesion may not require radiation have been hampered by the fact that the definition of "adequate margins of excision" varies amongst institutions and has not been clearly defined. Ongoing prospective studies in both Europe and the United States are attempting to answer these questions. To date, though, no subgroup has been identified that does not benefit from radiation therapy. Until then, for most patients qualifying for BCT, lumpectomy plus postsurgical XRT is the treatment of choice to minimize the risk of local recurrence, although the relative risks and benefits of radiation vary and should be discussed in detail with the patient.

Management of the Axilla (Box 11–4)

Because DCIS is noninvasive, theoretically there should be no possibility of finding disease within the regional lymph nodes. However, studies of modified radical mastectomy for the treatment of DCIS revealed axillary metastases in approximately 2% of cases. When patients with DCIS are found to have disease in the lymph nodes, the assumption is that there are possible foci of invasive disease somewhere in the breast that may have eluded discovery on pathologic tissue examination. This low risk of finding disease, however, prompted most surgeons to abandon the routine practice of performing a level I and II axillary lymph node dissection (ALND) in patients being treated for DCIS. Some surgeons, because of the possibility of invasive disease being present when there was diffuse DCIS throughout the breast,

BOX 11–4 INDICATIONS FOR SENTINEL LYMPH NODE BIOPSY IN DUCTAL CARCINOMA IN SITU

- Patients with microinvasion
- Patients undergoing mastectomy for diffuse disease
- Patients with a high suspicion of harboring invasive disease
  - Extensive high-grade disease or necrosis on core biopsy
  - Imaging studies suggesting invasion

continued to advocate a level I ALND when a mastectomy was performed.

When lymphatic mapping and sentinel lymph node (SLN) biopsy became routine in the management of breast cancer, this prompted a rethinking of whether the regional nodes should be looked at when treating DCIS. Because the pathologist may serial-section just one or two nodes, rather than bisecting 10 to 30 nodes as with an ALND specimen, SLN biopsy is more sensitive for finding micrometastatic disease. When SLN biopsy is used in DCIS, the results have shown wide variability, with some series describing 3% to 10% of patients with DCIS having a positive sentinel lymph node (SLN). This has prompted a handful of surgeons to recommend the routine use of SLN biopsy for DCIS; however, most surgeons question the prognostic significance of these findings. Most of the disease detected was found by immunohistochemistry, for which we do not know the prognostic implications. In addition, it is hard to reconcile long-term survivals of 99% for pure DCIS with a nodal positivity rate of 5% to 10%.

Therefore neither lymph node dissection nor lymphatic mapping and SLN biopsy should play a role in the routine management of pure DCIS, with two notable exceptions. The first is when there is a high likelihood of finding invasive disease. These would include cases in which the DCIS presents as a mass or there is a high suspicion of invasion on either the imaging studies or the biopsy specimen. In these cases it is reasonable to perform a sentinel node biopsy in conjunction with lumpectomy, although for patients being treated by BCT, axillary staging can just as reasonably be deferred until the diagnosis of invasion is confirmed. Any patients with documented microinvasion should have axillary evaluation by SLN biopsy. The second indication for lymphatic mapping in the management of DCIS is in the patient undergoing mastectomy for diffuse DCIS, particularly if it is high grade. In this case, if microinvasive disease is discovered on pathologic examination, it is not possible to then stage the patient by SLN biopsy and an ALND might be necessary. Immunohistochemistry should not be routinely performed for these cases.

Occasionally, patients undergo a mastectomy with SLN biopsy for DCIS and have metastatic disease identified in the sentinel node but no invasive disease identified in the breast. The first step should be to perform a more extensive pathologic examination of the breast for invasive disease that may have been over-looked. This may be facilitated by obtaining x-rays of the specimen so that more detailed examination can be performed on areas with suspicious calcifications. However, even if it cannot be identified, if there are true metas-tases in the sentinel nodes, it must be assumed that the patient does have an undetected focus of invasion and the patient should be consid-ered for completion ALND and systemic therapy.

Hormonal Therapy

Because systemic metastases are not a concern with in situ disease, there is no role for cytotoxic chemotherapy in the treatment of DCIS. DCIS does, however, express the estrogen receptor (ER), although not universally, prompting the investigation of tamoxifen as an adjuvant to surgical therapy. The NSABP B-24 protocol stud-ied the use of tamoxifen in women with DCIS undergoing BCT. More than 1800 women with DCIS were randomized to 5 years of tamoxifen versus placebo. At a median follow-up of 74 months, there was an overall risk reduction of 37% for patients receiving tamoxifen, regard-less of resection margin, tumor size, or grade. There was also a decreased risk of contralateral invasive and noninvasive cancer by 52% (Table 11–4). On the other hand, a trial from the United Kingdom, Australia, and New Zeal-and failed to demonstrate a significant benefit to tamoxifen in preventing either ipsilateral or contralateral events. The UK/ANZ trial was a smaller study, with a design that allowed for some patient choice, so the results must be interpreted with care.

These results suggest that a selective approach must be used when deciding which women with DCIS should receive adjuvant tamoxifen. The potential benefits of tamoxifen both on reducing recurrence and second breast malignancies must be weighed against the potential side effects, including venous throm-boembolism and uterine cancer. The baseline

risk of recurrence, the age of the patient, and the relative risk of side effects must be considered.

In addition, the ER status should be consid-ered. As stated, ER expression is not 100% among DCIS patients. In a study derived from the NSABP-B24 drug arm comparing the response of ER-positive versus ER-negative patients to tamoxifen, recurrence rates were 10% for the ER-positive group compared to 23% for the ER-negative group. Therefore many institutions have begun routinely evalu-ating DCIS for ER status by immunohisto-chemistry and limiting the use of tamoxifen for patients with ER-positive DCIS.

Recently, the aromatase inhibitor anastra-zole has received growing attention. Results of the ATAC (Anastrazole and Tamoxifen: Alone or in Combination) trial, which rando-mized 9000 patients with early-stage breast cancer to receive anastrozole versus tamoxifen versus the combination, revealed a statistically significant risk reduction of new breast cancers in the anastrozole arm ($P = .007$). However, there are no data on the use of aromatase inhi-bitors in patients with DCIS. There are pres-ently two trials ongoing to address this issue (NSABP B-35 in the United States and IBIS-II in Great Britain).

Paget Disease

In 1874, Sir James Paget described 15 women with chronic nipple ulceration who ultimately developed cancer of the involved breast within 2 years. He described an eruption on the nip-ple and areola, similar to acute eczema, with a copious clear yellowish exudation. Ulti-mately this would be known as Paget disease of the breast and is defined clinically as a scal-ing eczematous lesion of the nipple-areolar complex. Paget believed that the nipple changes were themselves benign, but later it was discovered that the cells of Paget disease were malignant and that Paget disease was

TABLE 11–4 • *Results of NSABP Protocol B24: Tamoxifen versus Placebo after Lumpectomy Plus Radiation Therapy*				
Study Arms	**Patients**	**Local Recurrence**	**Invasive Recurrence**	**Survival**
Lumpectomy + XRT + placebo	902	87 (9.6%)	40/87 (46%)	97%
Lumpectomy + XRT + tamoxifen	902	63 (7%)	23/63 (37%)	97%

XRT, Radiation therapy.

TABLE 11–5 • *Theories of Pathogenesis of Paget Disease*

Theory	Idea	Support
Epidermotropic	Neoplastic cells migrate from underlying malignancy to the epidermis of the nipple-areolar complex (NAC).	Paget is almost always associated with underlying ductal carcinoma. Immunohistochemical staining of Paget is usually identical to the underlying cancer. Molecular markers are also usually concordant.
Transformation	Epidermal keratinocytes in the nipple transform into Paget cells and then spread to the breast.	Not all cases of Paget have underlying parenchymal cancer. Tumors may be distal from the NAC. The "Toker cell" with an appearance between a keratinocyte and Paget cell is thought to be a precursor to Paget.

carcinoma arising from an intraductal carcinoma in the subareolar ducts.

Paget disease is associated with either in situ or invasive cancer in almost all cases. Paget disease is considerably less common than other presentations of breast cancer, accounting for only 1% to 3% of breast cancer cases diagnosed each year in the United States. Paget disease also can occur in men, although given the low incidence of male breast cancer overall, this is extremely rare. Paget disease must be a strong consideration in the differential diagnosis of any persistent nipple abnormality in either men or women.

Although the clinical definition of Paget disease is relatively straightforward, there is controversy as to its pathogenesis (Table 11–5). Two main theories have been put forward to explain the presence of Paget disease. The more commonly accepted theory is the *epidermotropic* theory, which suggests that the cells migrate from an underlying breast malignancy into the epidermis of the nipple. The second is the *transformation* theory, which suggests that Paget disease arises from malignant transformation of the cells within the epithelium of the nipple itself. Although there may be different underlying mechanisms, most evidence points to the epidermotropic theory.

Clinical Presentation

As stated, the hallmark of Paget disease is a scaly, raw, ulcerated lesion on the nipple and/or areola. Usually this starts with the nipple and then spreads to the areola. There may be ulceration or discharge (usually serous but possibly bloody). Associated nipple retraction suggests more advanced disease. The disease is almost always unilateral, although bilateral cases have been described (Box 11–5). All patients with nipple complaints should have a complete breast exam and bilateral mammography.

The lesion is typically present for several months before being accurately diagnosed. At first patients may have pain, burning, or pruritus without any obvious lesion. Patients with these symptoms should be followed, and further investigation initiated if the symptoms do not resolve. Many times the lesion is thought to be a benign dermatologic condition and is treated topically. Often the inflammatory component resolves, suggesting improvement. In some cases, these lesions may improve spontaneously. It is important not to completely rule out Paget disease even if there was some improvement with or without therapy. The differential diagnosis (Box 11–6) includes both

BOX 11–5 ASSOCIATED BREAST ABNORMALITIES IN PAGET DISEASE

- Palpable breast mass—50%
- Mammographic abnormality with no palpable mass—20%
- No underlying mass or mammographic abnormality—30%

BOX 11–6 DIFFERENTIAL DIAGNOSIS OF PAGET DISEASE

Benign
 Eczema
 Erosive dermatitis
 Pemphigus vulgaris
 Syphilitic lesion
 Herpes zoster
Malignant
 Bowen's disease
 Basal cell carcinoma
 Malignant melanoma

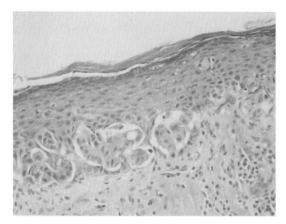

Figure 11–7. Pathology of Paget disease. The Paget cells are seen within the keratinizing epithelium of the nipple epidermis. The Paget cells are large, round cells with pale cytoplasm and pleomorphic nuclei. (Image courtesy of Maria Braman, MD, Department of Pathology, University of Michigan.)

benign (eczema, dermatitis) and malignant etiologies (Bowen's disease, basal cell carcinoma).

If benign disease is suspected, a short course of topical steroids is reasonable. If the lesion improves but fails to completely resolve, Paget should be considered. The next step in the workup should be biopsy. The diagnosis can be made by punch or wedge biopsy of the nipple. Shave biopsy or scrape cytology can be diagnostic, but a negative finding does not rule out Paget disease. In addition, core-needle biopsy of any mass or mammographic abnormality should be performed.

The pathologic hallmark of Paget disease is the presence of malignant, intraepithelial Paget cells, either singly or in small groups, within the epidermis of the nipple (Fig. 11–7). They are large in size with pale cytoplasm and have high-grade nuclei with prominent nucleoli. Retraction from the surrounding keratinocytes can give the appearance of a vacuole. Occasionally these cells can incorporate melanin, making them difficult to differentiate from melanoma. It is also sometimes difficult to differentiate Paget disease from squamous carcinoma of the epidermis (Bowen's disease) on routine histology. Immunohistochemical staining can usually make the diagnosis.

Treatment

Until recently, the standard treatment of Paget disease has been a simple mastectomy. More recent data suggest that BCT is feasible, but the nipple-areolar complex needs to be removed.

A thorough workup with particular attention paid to any associated palpable mass or mammographic abnormality is crucial to selecting the proper patients for BCT (Fig. 11–8).

Paget Disease with Palpable Mass or Mammographic Abnormality

When Paget disease is associated with a palpable mass, it is more frequently associated with invasive disease, axillary metastases, and multifocal underlying disease. Most of these patients will require mastectomy. However, if it is feasible to perform a lumpectomy that incorporates both the nipple-areolar complex and the palpable mass with adequate margins, and if this would result in acceptable cosmetic results after whole breast irradiation, then BCT is reasonable. The same can be said for a focal nonpalpable mammographic abnormality that can be resected in continuity with the nipple-areolar complex.

Many times the palpable mass or mammographic abnormality is a considerable distance from the nipple, and even when it is close, resection of both results in a poor cosmetic result. These patients may be better served by simple mastectomy with breast reconstruction. Patients with large breasts may allow for adequate resection while still allowing for acceptable breast contour and symmetry, often with contralateral breast reduction and nipple reconstruction. If the patient has a proven invasive component and clinically negative nodes, sentinel lymph node biopsy should be performed at the time of lumpectomy or mastectomy.

Patients with multicentric lesions or diffuse microcalcifications should be treated by simple mastectomy. Sentinel lymph node biopsy for staging the axilla is recommended in this situation because of the possibility of discovering invasive disease within the mastectomy specimen.

Paget Disease with No Mass or Mammographic Findings

Approximately one third of patients with Paget disease will not have an associated mass or mammographic abnormality, but the majority of these women will have an underlying carcinoma. Simple mastectomy (with or without reconstruction) has been the standard of care, but breast conservation is very reasonable. Breast conservation consists of resection of the nipple-areolar complex followed by whole breast irradiation. Although there are

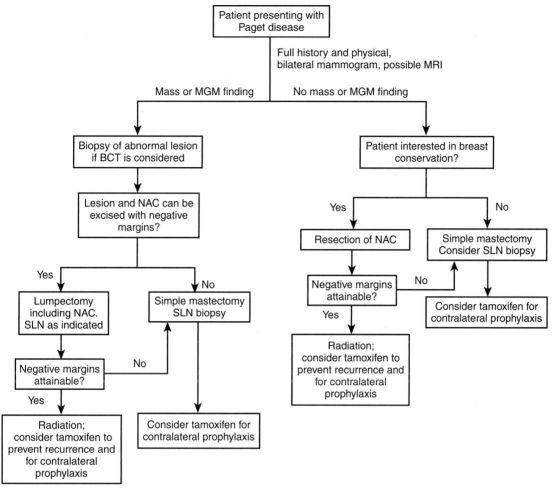

Figure 11–8. Management of Paget disease. In addition to a biopsy of the Paget to confirm the diagnosis, the workup should include a breast examination, bilateral mammogram, and possibly MRI to identify an associated mass or abnormality. Biopsy of this mass may help in planning treatment if breast conservation therapy (BCT) is a consideration. If the nipple-areolar complex (NAC) and any associated lesion can be resected with negative margins, a lumpectomy is an option, with subsequent radiation and possible NAC reconstruction in the future. If not, a simple mastectomy is indicated. Sentinel lymph node biopsy at the time of mastectomy is reasonable given the possibility of an unrecognized invasive component. The benefits of hormonal therapy can be extrapolated from the ductal carcinoma in situ data.

small series describing excision alone without radiation, local recurrence rates are concerning. Likewise, radiation alone has been described (after only tissue biopsy) but this approach has also been associated with high local recurrence rates.

The idea of excision and radiation for Paget disease is obviously based on the success of BCT for both invasive cancer and DCIS. Breast conservation should consist of complete nipple-areolar resection, because partial resection may lead to higher local recurrence rates. The largest series of BCT for Paget disease comes from a prospective study by the EORTC. After nipple-areolar resection with negative margins

followed by whole breast irradiation, the local recurrence rate was only 6.5% after a median follow-up of 6.4 years.

Negative margins are mandatory, and positive or close margins (<3 mm) should prompt reexcision. SLN biopsy is not essential at the time of nipple-areolar resection, because in the absence of a palpable mass, the underlying malignancy is typically intraductal and axillary node involvement is rare. However, it is not an unreasonable option. After completion of therapy, there are several techniques that can be used to reconstruct the nipple-areolar complex with excellent cosmetic outcomes. After surgery and radiation, patients should be considered for adjuvant hormonal therapy. Although there is no specific evidence supporting the use of tamoxifen or Arimidex after BCT for Paget disease, data can be extrapolated from the DCIS literature. Tamoxifen can also be considered after mastectomy for prophylaxis of the contralateral breast.

Suggested Readings

1. Bijker N, Rutgers EJ, Duchateau L, et al. Breast-conserving therapy for Paget disease of the nipple. A prospective European Organization for Research and Treatment of Cancer study of 61 patients. Cancer 2001:91:472.

2. Dupont W, Parl F, Hartmann W, et al. Breast cancer risk associated with proliferative breast disease and atypical hyperplasia. Cancer 1993;71:1258.

3. Fisher B, Dignam J, Wolmark N, et al. Lumpectomy and radiation therapy for the treatment of intraductal breast cancer: Findings from the National Surgical Adjuvant Breast and Bowel Project B-17. J Clin Oncol 1998;16:441–452.

4. Fisher B, Dignam J, Wolmark N, et al. National Surgical Adjuvant Breast and Bowel Project B24 randomized controlled trial. Lancet 1999;353:1993.

5. Fisher B, Dignam J, Wolmark N, et al. Tamoxifen in treatment of intraductal breast cancer: National Surgical Adjuvant Breast and Bowel Project B-24 randomised controlled trial. Lancet 1999;353:1993–2000.

6. Fisher ER, Contantino J, Fisher B, et al. Pathological findings from the National Surgical Adjuvant Breast and Bowel Project Protocol B-17. Cancer 1995; 75:1310.

7. Hutter RVP. The management of patients with lobular carcinoma in situ of the breast. Cancer 1984; 53:798.

8. Irvine T, Fentiman IS. Biology and treatment of ductal carcinoma in situ. Exp Rev Anticancer Ther 2007;7(2):135–145.

9. Julien, J-P, Bijker N, Fentiman IS, et al. Radiotherapy in breast-conserving treatment for ductal carcinoma in situ: first results of the EORTC randomized phase III trial 10853. EORTC Breast Cancer Cooperative Group and EORTC Radiotherapy Group. Lancet 2000;355;528–533.

10. Kawase K, Dimaio DJ, Tucker SL, et al. Paget's disease of the breast: There is a role for breast-conserving therapy. Ann Surg Oncol 2005;12:391–397.

11. Kollmorgen DR, Varanasi, JS, Edge SB, Carson WE 3rd. Paget's disease of the breast: A 33-year experience. J Am Coll Surg 1998;187:171.

12. Lagios MD, Margolin FR, Westdahl PR, et al. Mammographically detected ductal carcinoma in situ. Cancer 1989;63:618.

13. Marcus E. The management of Paget's disease of the breast. Curr Treat Options Oncol 2004;5:153–160.

14. Marshall JK, Griffith KA, Haffty BG, et al. Conservative management of Paget disease of the breast with radiotherapy: 10- and 15-year results. Cancer 2003;97:2142.

15. Mizra NQ, Vlastos G, Meric F, et al. Ductal carcinoma in situ: Long term results of breast conserving therapy. Ann Surg Oncol 2000;7:656.

16. Morrow M, Schnitt SJ. Treatment selection in ductal carcinoma in situ. JAMA 2000;283(4):453–455.

17. Orel SG, Mendonca MH, Reynolds C, et al. MR imaging of ductal carcinoma in situ. Radiology 1997;202:413.

18. Page DL, Dupont WD, Rogers LW, et al. Continued local recurrence of carcinoma 15-25 years after a diagnosis of low grade ductal carcinoma in situ of the breast treated only by biopsy. Cancer 1995; 76:1197.

19. Romero L, Klein L, Ye W, et al. Outcome after invasive recurrence in patients with ductal carcinoma in situ of the breast. Am J Surg 2004;188:371.

20. Silverstein MJ, et al. A prognostic index for ductal carcinoma in situ of the breast. Cancer 1996; 77:2267–2274.

21. Solin LJ, Kurtz J, Fourquet A, et al. Fifteen year results of breast-conserving surgery and definitive breast irradiation for the treatment of ductal carcinoma in situ of the breast. J Clin Oncol 1996; 14:754.

22. UK Coordinating Committee on Cancer Research (UKCCCR). Radiotherapy and tamoxifen in women with completely excised ductal carcinoma in situ of the breast in the UK, Australia and New Zealand: Randomized controlled trial. Lancet 2003;362 (9378):95–102.

23. Winchester DP, Jeske JM, Goldschmidt RA. The diagnosis and management of ductal carcinoma in-situ of the breast. CA J Clin 2000;50:184–200.

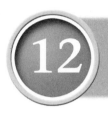

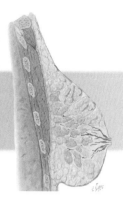

Surgical Management
of Primary Breast Cancer

Surgical Management of Primary Invasive Breast Cancer: Key Points

Understand the evolution of the surgical management of breast cancer.

Know the absolute and relative contraindications to breast conserving surgery.

Develop an algorithm for selecting the appropriate patients for breast conserving therapy.

Describe the surgical techniques for a lumpectomy, a wire-localized lumpectomy, and a simple or modified radical mastectomy.

Be familiar with the complications of breast surgery and their management.

Changes in Surgical Management of Breast Cancer

Going back to the late 1800s, the treatment of breast cancer was characterized by either wide excision or simple mastectomy. These resulted in extremely high rates of local recurrence and poor survival (Table 12–1). In 1894, William Halsted proposed that breast cancer was a local disease that spread by contiguous

TABLE 12-1 • *Local Recurrences after Mastectomy*

Surgeon	Dates	Number	Local Recurrence Rate (%)
Bergmann	1882-1887	114	51-60
Billroth	1867-1876	170	82
Czerny	1877-1886	102	62
Fischer	1871-1878	147	75
Gussenbauer	1878-1886	151	64
König	1875-1885	152	58-62
Küster	1871-1885	228	60
Lücke	1881-1890	110	66
Volkmann	1874-1878	131	60
Halsted	1889-1894	50	6

Hasted WS. The results of operations for the cure of cancer for the breast performed at the Johns Hopkins Hospital from June 1889 to January 1894. The Johns Hopkins Hospital Reports 1894-1895;4:297-350.

extension, and that more extensive resection would provide a better chance of disease control (Halsted's Theory). That year, he had performed 50 "complete" mastectomies and reported his experience. Halsted's radical mastectomy consisted of en bloc removal of the breast, the overlying skin, both the pectoralis major and minor muscles, and the entire axillary contents (level I, II, and III nodes) (Fig. 12-1).

The radical mastectomy resulted in a significant drop in local recurrence rates, and it quickly became the standard of care for the treatment of breast cancer. However, despite the improvement in local control, the curative potential of this operation remained limited. In one series of more than 1400 women over a course of 30 years, only 13% remained free of disease, and nearly 60% died of breast cancer. At first this was believed to be because the mastectomy was not extensive enough, and so the extended radical mastectomy, which included resection of the internal mammary nodes (IMNs) and/or supraclavicular nodes, was proposed. The Dahl-Iversen extended mastectomy included dissection of both the IMN and supraclavicular nodes with the radical mastectomy. An even more radical mastectomy was the "super-radical" mastectomy that included four parts (Box 12-1). However, these failed to improve survival. In a randomized comparison of the Dahl-Iversen extended radical mastectomy to simple mastectomy with radiation to the regional lymph nodes, with approximately 330 patients per arm, there was no difference in disease-free or overall survival. In a European randomized trial between radical mastectomy and extended radical mastectomy (including IMNs), there was again no improvement in survival. A much smaller randomized trial from the University of Chicago also showed no improvement to removing the IMNs.

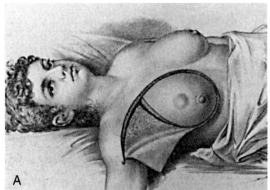 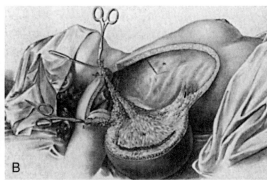

Figure 12-1. The Halsted radical mastectomy involved removing the breast with the overlying skin, the pectoralis major and minor muscles, and the level I, II, and III axillary lymph nodes. (From Bland KI, Copeland EM III. The Breast, 3rd ed. Philadelphia: WB Saunders, 2004.)

BOX 12-1 THE "SUPER RADICAL" MASTECTOMY

- Breast and axillary contents
- Internal mammary artery and vein with internal mammary lymph node chain
- Upper mediastinal nodes
- Low supraclavicular nodes

Disappointed by the failure of radical mastectomy to cure women with breast cancer despite significant morbidity, many surgeons proposed that a less extensive operation, the modified radical mastectomy (MRM), could be performed without compromising survival. The MRM involves complete removal of the breast tissue and the underlying fascia of the pectoralis major muscle, and removal of some but not all of the axillary lymph nodes (levels I and II). The overlying skin and underlying pectoralis muscles are not removed. Several prospective randomized trials documented equivalent survival rates with MRM as compared to radical mastectomy, with less morbidity. As a result of these data, the radical mastectomy has become an historical footnote in the treatment of breast cancer, and there are no absolute indications for radical as opposed to modified radical mastectomy in women with invasive breast cancer.

The fact that less radical surgery did not affect survival made people question whether Halsted's theory was correct; that breast cancer was not a local disease that spread contiguously, but instead, systemic disease was ultimately the main determinant of survival. The question arose as to whether the breast needed to be removed or could be preserved without compromising survival. There had

been several reports of breast cancer being treated by radiation alone (see Chapter 15), and there was evidence that radiation could eliminate subclinical foci of disease. This allowed for the combination of limited surgery and radiation therapy as a method of adequately treating breast cancer while avoiding mastectomy.

Although initially controversial, breast conserving therapy (BCT) has become a standard of care in the management of breast cancer. BCT refers to the surgical removal of the tumor (lumpectomy, wide excision, quadrantectomy) followed by moderate-dose radiation therapy to eradicate any residual disease. This chapter focuses on the surgical aspects of BCT and mastectomy. Chapter 15 focuses on radiation therapy.

Breast Conserving Therapy

The goals of BCT are to provide the survival equivalent of mastectomy, a cosmetically acceptable breast, and a low rate of recurrence in the treated breast. Although there was great resistance when it was first introduced, six randomized trials involving more than 4000 patients over 3 decades established that BCT was as effective as mastectomy for suitable patients with breast cancer (Table 12–2). It is difficult to compare one trial to another because they were quite different in design. Some required lumpectomy, whereas others required the more extensive quadrantectomy. Some required that the final margins be negative, whereas others allowed for positive resection margins. In the European Organization for Research and Treatment trial, surgical margins were microscopically positive in nearly half the patients. The size of the tumors included were also quite variable. Despite these

TABLE 12–2 • *Prospective, Randomized Trials of BCT vs. Mastectomy*							
Trial	Patients	Max Tumor Size	Median Follow-up	Overall Survival		Local Recurrence	
				BCT	Mastectomy	BCT	Mast.
NSABP B-06	1851	4	20	47%	47%	14.3%	10.2%
Milan I	701	2	20	58.3%	58.8%	8.8%	2.3%
NCI	237	5	18.4	54%	58%	22%	0%
EORTC	868	5	13.4	65%	66%	20%	12%
Institut Gustav Roussy	179	2	10	78%	79%	4%	NR
Danish	905	5	9.8	79%	82%	NR	NR

differences, none of the six trials demonstrated a difference in overall survival for BCT compared with mastectomy. The trials also demonstrated several points worth mentioning.

When discussing treatment options with patients, many lean toward mastectomy to avoid any chance of local recurrence. It is important to note that mastectomy does not guarantee freedom from local recurrence. This is true for all stages of breast cancer. Recurrence rates after mastectomy range from 3% to 20%, depending on the size of the tumor, the presence of regional metastases, and the use of systemic therapy. Overall the risk of a local recurrence is about the same for BCT and mastectomy. Chest wall recurrences after mastectomy tend to occur later than in-breast recurrences after breast conservation, although most will occur within the first 3 years after surgery for both groups.

Radiation eradicates microscopic residual foci that are present in the breast after surgery. The effects of radiation have no effect on the future risk of breast cancer. Therefore the risk of a second primary cancer in the treated breast is the same as in the contralateral breast.

The six randomized trials all demonstrated that even when local recurrence was higher (as with lumpectomy without radiation), overall survival was the same. This has been interpreted as meaning that local therapy has minimal if any effect on the risk of developing distant disease. Based on this interpretation, surgeons have been increasingly willing to accept therapies that have higher rates of local recurrence, arguing that even if an increased number of those patients ultimately require completion mastectomy, overall survival would not be affected. But these trials were all individually too small to detect a small impact on overall survival.

Even if there was no difference in overall survival when comparing BCT to mastectomy, patients who had BCT and developed a local recurrence do have a worse outcome. In one matched-pair analysis, BCT patients who had a local recurrence had an overall survival of 71% compared to 81% for those who did not have a local recurrence. This in itself did not prove that prospectively preventing a local recurrence would have improved survival by this degree. It could be that the local recurrence is a marker reflecting the propensity of the tumor to metastasize distantly. So rather than metastases developing from the recurrence, the patients with more aggressive tumors are more likely to develop both.

So does the prevention of a local recurrence improve overall survival? Yes, as demonstrated by the Early Breast Cancer Trialists Collaborative Group (ECGTCG) metaanalysis. Several of the randomized trials that established the efficacy of breast conservation included arms in which women underwent lumpectomy alone, without radiation, and most demonstrated that despite a significant increase in local recurrence, there was no impact on overall survival. However, these trials did not have the power to detect a small survival advantage from the improved local control provided by radiation therapy. In addition, the morbidity and mortality associated with radiation therapy negated some survival advantage, particularly with older methods for delivering radiation. The most recent update of the ECGTCG metaanalysis demonstrates that the 15-year breast cancer mortality risks were significantly lower in the patients who received radiation therapy (30.5 versus 35.9, $P = .002$). A pooled analysis of mortality data from 13 randomized trials also showed a worse survival in women who did not receive radiation therapy, with an 8.6% excess mortality. These data clearly demonstrate that improved local control does impact survival, and women with an exceedingly high risk of in-breast recurrence with BCT compared to mastectomy may be better served by the latter. It also establishes that radiation is a critical component of BCT.

Patient Selection

Although the surgeon plays many roles in the management of breast cancer, one of the most important is deciding whether the patient is a good candidate for BCT or whether the patient will require a mastectomy (Box 12–2).

BOX 12–2 WORKUP TO DETERMINE SUITABILITY FOR BREAST CONSERVATION

- Complete history and physical
  - Past medical history
  - Medications
  - Complete family history
  - Thorough bilateral breast examination
- Bilateral mammogram with diagnostic imaging of the cancer
- Review of the histology
- ? Ultrasound of the primary tumor
- ? Magnetic resonance imaging

There are several absolute contraindications to breast conserving therapy, some relative contraindications, and some factors that are not contraindications, but are wrongly thought to be. The American College of Surgeons, the American College of Radiology, the College of American Pathologists, the Society of Surgical Oncology and the Canadian Steering Committee on Clinical Practice Guidelines for the Care and Treatment of Breast Cancer have developed consensus standards of care for BCT. The evaluation of the breast cancer patient to determine whether she is a suitable candidate for BCT includes:

- A complete history and physical examination before treatment. This includes a complete past medical history, present medications, and family history of cancer.
- Bilateral mammographic evaluation, with appropriate magnification views, within 3 months of surgery. The tumor size, whether the mass is associated with microcalcifications, and the extent of the calcifications within and outside the mass should be included in the report.
- Accurate histologic assessment of the primary tumor, including histologic subtype and hormone receptor status. Thus a core-needle biopsy or excisional biopsy rather than fine-needle aspiration is the optimum choice for making a tissue diagnosis when BCT is considered.
- The most difficult part of the evaluation is the assessment of the patient's needs and expectations. This requires that the patient and her physician discuss the benefits and risks of mastectomy compared to BCT in regard to long-term survival, the possibility and consequence of local recurrence, and the impact on cosmetic outcome and psychosocial adjustment.

Recently, the use of magnetic resonance imaging (MRI) to determine eligibility for BCT has become more popular. Proponents state it can more accurately determine the extent of the tumor as well as identify multicentricity. However, the use of MRI is not without controversy. MRI of the breast is highly sensitive, but has limited specificity (see Chapter 2). As such, MRI will detect many benign lesions that would otherwise not preclude breast conservation. MRI is also limited in its ability to detect ductal carcinoma in situ (DCIS), which is often a reason why negative margins are not attainable. Most importantly, many institutions have the ability to perform MRI but not the technology to perform MRI-guided biopsy. If a woman undergoes a preoperative MRI and other lesions are detected, then she may undergo additional mammograms or ultrasound to try to identify, and biopsy, the MRI-detected lesion. However, if the mammogram and ultrasound are unable to identify the lesion and MRI-guided biopsy is not available, the woman is placed in a difficult position. She can ignore the findings of the MRI and proceed with BCT (risking increased recurrence) or proceed with mastectomy knowing she might have been a suitable candidate for breast preservation. Many women naturally choose the latter, and even when MRI-guided biopsy is available, some women choose mastectomy rather than go through additional biopsies. Thus the use of MRI may be leading to an unnecessary increase in mastectomy rates without having a significant effect on local recurrence rates. Further prospective studies are necessary before MRI can be considered a routine part of the preoperative staging process, and a full discussion of the risks, benefits, and possible outcomes of preoperative MRI should be discussed in detail with the patient. Preoperative MRI may be a reasonable option in patients who have dense breast tissue, limiting the ability of mammography to detect the true extent of the cancer or second cancers, or in women with a high risk of synchronous cancers (such as women with BRCA mutations) who desire breast conservation rather than bilateral mastectomies.

Absolute Contraindications

Multicentricity is an absolute contraindication to BCT (Box 12–3). This means two or more tumors are located in separate quadrants of the

BOX 12–3 ABSOLUTE CONTRAINDICATIONS TO BREAST CONSERVING THERAPY

- Patient does not desire breast conservation therapy
- Unable to receive radiation therapy
  - First or second trimester of pregnancy (see Chapter 22)
  - Collagen-vascular disease
  - Previous chest wall radiation
- Diffuse suspicious microcalcifications on mammography
- Multicentric disease
- Inability to achieve negative margins

breast. In patients with a known breast cancer and a suspicious lesion on either physical examination or breast imaging, a biopsy should be performed on the second lesion before proceeding with breast conservation, even if this means an additional procedure. Multicentricity is not the same as multifocality, which implies multiple foci of tumor when examined histologically. This has more to do with the pattern of tumor growth. The presence of multifocality is not a contraindication to BCT, as long as negative margins can be obtained. Likewise, the presence of two masses within the same quadrant may not require mastectomy. This may represent a dumbbell-shaped tumor. If both masses can be excised in one excision, this is acceptable if the cosmetic result is reasonable. On the other hand, performing more than one lumpectomy for multiple tumors is associated with high rates of local recurrence (>30%) and poor cosmetic outcomes.

The presence of diffuse microcalcifications on mammography, often described as extending beyond one quadrant, is another contraindication to breast conservation. These often, but not always, represent DCIS extending beyond the invasive cancer. Unfortunately, the pathology report of the mastectomy specimen often does not reveal extensive DCIS associated with these calcifications, which can make the surgeon and the patient question the need for the mastectomy. However, the presence of the calcifications not only may indicate more extensive disease, but also may make surveillance of the breast for local recurrence extremely difficult.

Another contraindication is a history of prior therapeutic irradiation to the breast region, which when combined with the proposed treatment would result in an excessively high total radiation dose to the chest wall. This includes women who have already been treated for breast cancer in that breast with radiation and women who have had radiation for other reasons such as for Hodgkin's lymphoma (Fig. 12–2). Prior radiation to other body sites is not a contraindication. Sometimes in evaluating a patient with a history of radiation, there is a question as to the dose and exact fields used. In these cases, it is best to obtain the previous treatment record and consult with a radiation oncologist before proceeding with breast conservation.

Pregnancy in the first or second trimester is an absolute contraindication to the use of breast irradiation. It may be possible to perform breast-conserving surgery in the third

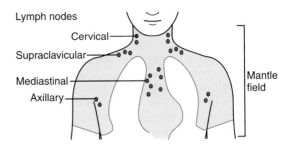

Figure 12–2. The field of radiation (including the mantle field) for Hodgkin's disease. (From Roses D. Breast Cancer. Philadelphia: Elsevier, 2005.)

trimester, deferring breast irradiation until after delivery. Breast cancer during pregnancy is discussed in more detail in Chapter 22.

Because lumpectomy and radiation go hand in hand, one must consider the morbidity of radiation therapy when one is discussing lumpectomy with the patient. Radiation often leads to fatigue, may lead to skin changes and inflammation of the breast, and can result in a temporary cough secondary to fibrosis of the lung. In the long term, radiation can lead to prolonged breast edema, shrinkage of the breast or induration of the cavity, fat necrosis, excessive fibrosis, irradiation pneumonitis, rib fractures, and pleural effusion. Cardiac effects and radiation-induced secondary neoplasms are also a concern. These are discussed in more detail in Chapter 15. However, it is important that the surgeon be able to discuss these with the patient when presenting the choice between BCT and mastectomy. On the other hand, the surgeon must be careful not to present mastectomy as "a way to avoid radiation"; depending on the pathology results, postmastectomy radiation may still be recommended.

Relative Contraindications

Some oncologists consider connective tissue disease to be an absolute contraindication to breast conservation because many of these patients tolerate irradiation very poorly. However, most consider it a relative contraindication, depending on the type of connective tissue disease and the relative risks and benefits of therapy. Scleroderma is an absolute contraindication. Systemic lupus erythematosus patients may also have a poor reaction to radiation therapy. For other types of collagen-vascular disease, such as Raynaud phenomenon, rheumatoid arthritis, Sjögren's syndrome, or polymyositis, the response to radiation has not been as severe, and these patients may still be considered for BCT.

The ideal candidate for breast conservation is the patient with T1 or T2 tumors and a breast large enough to encompass an adequate resection. However, this is subjective and size is not an absolute contraindication. Women with large breasts can undergo resection of a 4- or 5-cm tumor with a good cosmetic result and successfully undergo breast irradiation, although they may require radiation in the prone position to assure reproducibility of the patient set-up. Patients with large tumors who still want breast conservation may consider neoadjuvant chemotherapy to downstage the tumor (see Chapter 18).

Finally, there is the question of microscopic negative margins. Often described as a contraindication to BCT is the inability to obtain negative margins. If after a reasonable attempt at reexcision there are still diffusely positive margins, then a mastectomy is indicated. It is ideal that negative margins be obtained before proceeding to radiation, because the majority of studies have demonstrated a lower local recurrence rate with negative compared to positive margins. The impact of a close margin is less clear, and the decision whether to reexcise must be made on a case-by-case basis, taking into consideration the radiation planned and the use of systemic therapy. Close margins, which have been associated with an increased risk of recurrence in some series but not in others.

Not Contraindications

There are several features that may be associated with an increased risk of recurrence, but are not necessarily contraindications to breast conservation (Box 12–4). The most commonly misquoted contraindication is the presence of axillary nodal metastases, whether these are clinical or pathologic. Given the increased likelihood of systemic disease when the lymph nodes are positive, the impact of local control on overall survival diminishes. In addition, the risk of chest wall recurrence after mastectomy increases with the number of positive axillary lymph nodes. This is not true for breast conservation, possibly due to the use of radiation therapy. This is why chest wall radiation is considered after a mastectomy when the axillary nodes are positive (see Chapter 15).

Age is not a contraindication to BCT; physiologic age and the presence of comorbid conditions should be the primary determinants of local therapy in older women. It is also obviously wrong to assume that an older woman would be less concerned with her physical appearance or the effects of a

BOX 12–4 VARIABLES NOT CONSIDERED TO BE CONTRAINDICATIONS TO BCT

Variables Associated with an Increased Risk of Recurrence after Breast Conservation

- Tumor size
- Positive or close margins
- High grade
- Angiolymphatic invasion
- Excessive delay in radiation (>16 weeks)
- Young age (may be associated with higher grade or may be associated with surgeon willingness to compromise margins for cosmetic purposes)

Variables Associated with a Decreased Likelihood of Negative Margins but No Difference in Recurrence If Negative Margins Are Obtained

- Extensive intraductal component, defined as greater than 25% or more of the tumor composed of ductal carcinoma in situ both within and at the periphery of the margin
- Lobular carcinoma

mastectomy on her sexual image. Likewise, being young is not a contraindication. Even though some series have shown a higher risk of relapse in young women (defined as either younger than 35 or 40), some of these series have also shown that younger women have worse prognosis lesions (high grade, vascular invasion, ER-negative tumors) and a greater likelihood of distant disease.

Histologic subtypes other than invasive ductal carcinoma (e.g., invasive lobular cancer) are not associated with an increased risk of breast cancer recurrence, nor is the presence of an extensive intraductal component. This is defined as an invasive cancer associated with a large component of intraductal cancer (>25%) within the tumor and in the surrounding breast tissue. Both lobular carcinomas and noncalcified DCIS may extend beyond what is visualized on imaging studies, so it may take a wider lumpectomy or a reexcision to obtain negative margins. However, if negative margins can be obtained, then breast conservation is reasonable.

As with tumor size, tumor location must be considered on a case-by-case basis and is not in itself a contraindication to breast conservation. The surgeon should discuss with the patient the cosmetic implications of the position of the lumpectomy. Tumors in the 6-o'clock position of the breast will often cause downturning of the nipple after therapy. Tumors in the superficial subareolar location may require resection of the nipple-areolar complex to achieve negative margins. The patient and her physician need to assess whether each resection, and the effect on cosmesis, is preferable to mastectomy and reconstruction.

Breast implants previously placed for augmentation are not an absolute contraindication to lumpectomy. If a lumpectomy can be performed without violating the basic principles (complete tumor excision, accurate lymphatic mapping), then radiation can be delivered to the breast using standard techniques and doses. However, capsular contracture is a risk, causing the breast to become rounded, firm, and retracted upward. The suitability of BCT in women with breast implants in part depends on how the implant was placed. For example, if the implant was placed through an axillary incision, this may impact the accuracy of sentinel lymph node biopsy. Subcutaneous implants have a higher rate of capsular contraction with radiation than subpectoral. If negative margins cannot be obtained secondary to the tumor being in close proximity to the implant (cancers sometimes invade the fibrous capsule around the implant), the implant may need to be removed.

Finally, the patient's individual risk of developing a second cancer is not a contraindication to breast conservation, although a discussion should be held with these patients of their increased risk of a second breast cancer and the potential benefits of bilateral mastectomy. Thus breast cancer patients with a strong family history of breast cancer or with a known BRCA1 or BRCA2 mutation may opt for bilateral mastectomy; if they are not ready for that, then unilateral mastectomy as treatment of the known cancer is not warranted if they are candidates for, and desire, BCT.

Operative Management of Breast Cancer

Lumpectomy

Placement of the Incision

Lumpectomy may be performed either under general anesthesia or intravenous sedation with local anesthesia. The patient is placed supine on the operating room table and the entire breast and axilla is prepped and draped in an aseptic fashion. For a lumpectomy, the incision should ideally be placed directly over the mass. Excessive tunneling is not recommended because this may compromise margins and make a reexcision for positive margins unnecessarily difficult. Circumareolar incisions result in a superb cosmetic outcome and are appropriate for lesions located near the areola, but care should be taken in tunneling too far simply to use a circumareolar incision.

In the upper hemisphere of the breast, incisions should be curvilinear, following the normal lines of tension in the skin (Fig. 12–3). It is not necessary to routinely excise skin with the specimen; however, if the tumor is close to the skin, an ellipse over the tumor should be taken to ensure a negative anterior margin. In the lower hemisphere of the breast, either curvilinear incisions or radial incisions can be used. For small tumors in relatively larger breasts, where it will not be necessary to remove overlying skin and adequate breast parenchyma will remain around the cavity, curvilinear

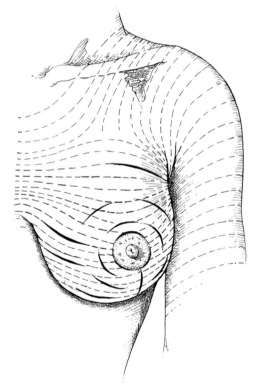

Figure 12–3. Planning the lumpectomy incision. Skin incisions should be placed within the Langer's lines when possible. Closer to the areola, circumareolar incisions are appropriate, but excessive tunneling should be avoided. In the lower hemisphere of the breast, radial incisions should be strongly considered, because these result in less distortion of the nipple-areolar complex. (From Roses D. Breast cancer. Philadelphia: Elsevier, 2005.)

incisions are acceptable. Otherwise, radial incisions should be used. Curvilinear incisions beneath the areola, where skin or a good amount of breast tissue is removed, will distort the breast in a way that the breast collapses inferiorly and the nipple points downward, resulting in an unacceptable cosmetic outcome. However, one must keep in mind how this would ultimately impact a mastectomy incision (particularly a skin-sparing mastectomy incision) in case the attempt at breast conservation fails (Fig. 12–4). The decision to use circumareolar or radial incisions in the lower hemisphere of the breast must be individualized to the patient, taking into account the size of the tumor, the size of the breast, and the pathology.

When the cancer is located in the upper outer quadrant of the breast, it may seem attractive to perform the sentinel lymph node biopsy or the axillary lymph node dissection through one longer incision. Even though this may be acceptable when the tumor lies high in the axillary tail of the breast, it should generally be avoided. It may result in a long suture line across normal skin creases, which leads to excess contraction and deformity. In addition, it complicates the planning and delivery of a boost to the tumor bed for the radiation oncologist. Thus two separate incisions for the lumpectomy and for the axilla are preferable, even if they are only 2 to 3 cm apart.

Lumpectomy

After creation of the skin incision, skin flaps are raised over the tumor. It is important that these skin flaps not be too thin. Thin flaps will result in excessive retraction of the cavity during radiation, resulting in a concavity at the site of the lumpectomy. On the other hand, thick flaps heal much better. The subcutaneous fat helps support the skin, and if left intact, helps preserve the natural contour of the breast (Fig. 12–5). For deep-seated tumors, after incising the skin, the breast tissue may be divided straight down to approximately 1 cm above the tumor mass before beginning the dissection around the tumor. For intermediate masses, the skin flaps should be created at a 45-degree angle. For more superficial lesions, an adequate amount of skin overlying the tumor should be taken so that thin skin flaps are not necessary for adequate margins.

Once appropriate flaps are raised peripherally around the tumor, the dissection should continue straight down toward the chest wall. The surgeon should keep one hand on the tumor at all times during the dissection to ensure adequate margins. A rim of normal breast tissue or fat of approximately 1 cm should be excised with the tumor centered in the specimen. The incision should be large enough to allow this. Removing a tumor

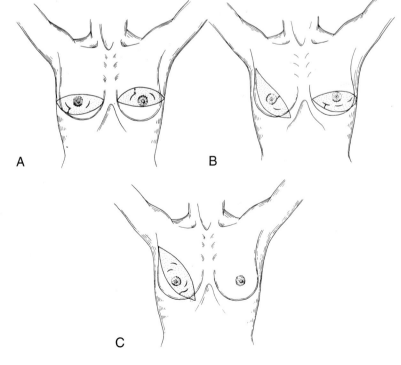

Figure 12–4. As with excisional biopsies, a subsequent mastectomy should be considered if the attempt at breast conservation fails. (From Bland KI, Copeland EM III. The breast, 3rd ed. Philadelphia: WB Saunders, 2004.)

A

B

C

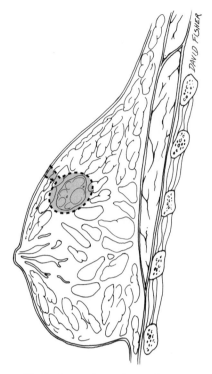

Figure 12–5. Preserving the subcutaneous fat between the skin and the tumor helps avoid excessive skin retraction and indentation. (From Bland KI, Copeland EM III. The breast, 3rd ed. Philadelphia: WB Saunders, 2004.)

through a small incision requires excessive manipulation of the tumor and an increased risk of positive margins on final pathology. Limiting yourself in an attempt to keep the incision small increases the need for a reexcision lumpectomy, which will have a worse cosmetic outcome than if the skin incision was simply lengthened. Excising even a small ellipse of skin with the tumor often allows for a wider operative field to work in. As the mass is freed peripherally, the tumor is grasped and retracted upward so that the posterior aspect may be completed. Exposure is aided by using small retractors. For deeper tumors, the pectoralis fascia should be included in the specimen. A portion of the pectoralis muscle should be included for very deeply situated tumors to ensure an adequate deep margin.

By working peripherally around the tumor and waiting until the tumor is circumferentially free to grasp the mass, the surgeon avoids excessive manipulation of the tumor. This is important because increased manipulation increases the likelihood of removing surrounding fat and tissue from the cancer. Exposing the tumor through excess manipulation results in ink approximating the cancer, and a pathologic finding of a positive margin, necessitating reexcision. When needed, a clamp can be used to grasp the normal tissue around the mass to assist in retraction, but care should be taken not to pull too aggressively. A clamp should never be placed directly on the tumor.

The lumpectomy may be performed with a scalpel, scissors, or cautery. Many surgeons prefer cautery to maintain hemostasis throughout the dissection, increasing visibility. However, the cautery effect on the specimen may obscure the ability of the pathologist to read the margins. Sharp dissection results in a clearer margin status and, with appropriate technique and retraction, bleeding can be kept to a minimum. Additional time can be taken once the specimen is out to ensure hemostasis.

As the tissue is removed from the lumpectomy cavity, it is important to note and maintain its orientation. Marking sutures are immediately placed on the specimen. A single stitch superiorly, a long stitch laterally, and a double stitch deep is an easily recalled method to orient the tissue the same way each time, and preprinted stickers can be created for the circulating nurse (Fig. 12–6).

If there is any concern clinically regarding the adequacy of any margin, an additional specimen can be taken from the wall of the lumpectomy cavity corresponding to the point opposite the area of concern. With the skin retracted anteriorly, the wall is grasped with a toothed pick-up or clamp and a new, adequate margin is obtained. This should be

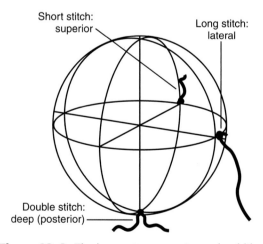

Short stitch: superior

Long stitch: lateral

Double stitch: deep (posterior)

Figure 12–6. The lumpectomy specimen should be oriented in three planes so that the pathologist can use a multicolor staining system to identify close or positive margins.

liberal, taking a generous portion of the wall of the cavity to ensure the margin of concern is truly excised. Otherwise, the pathologist may state that you obtained negative margins, but in reality left behind a close or positive margin. The new specimen should be marked appropriately with sutures so that the pathologist knows what the true margin is.

Wound Closure

After completion of the lumpectomy, hemostasis should be achieved to avoid a hematoma. Drains are never used after a lumpectomy. The surgeon should also never try to simply reapproximate the breast tissue. For large defects, there are methods to mobilize adjacent tissue (see later), but in general sutures should not be placed in the breast parenchyma to close the cavity. The lumpectomy cavity will fill with seroma and fibrin, and ultimately fibrous tissue, which maintains the normal, rounded contour of the breast.

Once hemostasis is achieved, surgical clips should be placed within the lumpectomy cavity in the six anatomic locations (anterior, posterior, medial, lateral, superior, inferior). This helps in the planning of the radiation therapy, specifically if a boost is planned or if partial breast irradiation is contemplated. The incision should then be reapproximated with absorbable deep dermal sutures followed by a subcuticular stitch or tissue adhesive. Interrupted nylon or silk sutures leave cross-hatching scars and are not necessary.

Wire-Localized Lumpectomy

With the increased use of screening mammography, many cancers are diagnosed by means of a stereotactic core biopsy of a mammographic abnormality. In these cases, a wire-localized lumpectomy will be necessary. Localization involves placing a rigid introducer needle with a flexible hooked wire inside of it at the site of the abnormality using either biplanar mammography or ultrasound (Fig. 12–7). Ultrasound is relatively simpler and more comfortable for the patient. In many cases, the original abnormality is gone, removed by the core-needle biopsy, and so a clip left by the radiologist is localized for excision.

Once the rigid needle is in place, it is withdrawn, leaving the hooked wire in place. The hook keeps the wire in place so it is not easily moved, although the external wire should still be secured to the skin so that it is not dislodged as the patient travels from radiology to the operating room. The craniocaudal and mediolateral views of the wire in place accompany the patient to the operating room.

The wire-localized lumpectomy is similar to the wire-localized biopsy except the surgeon is attempting to obtain negative margins. In some cases, more than one wire may be placed to bracket the mass or calcifications to give the surgeon a better idea of what needs to be excised to obtain negative margins. As with standard lumpectomy, an adequate skin incision should be used to allow adequate room to excise the entire region and not overly manipulate the tissue. The incision should be curvilinear in Langer's lines, and created with a subsequent lumpectomy or mastectomy in mind. The incision should be placed over the abnormality and not routinely made at the site of wire entry. The surgeon should use the wire and images to determine the site of the abnormality and place the incision directly over this.

The direction of the dissection is determined by the lesion size, direction of the wire, and the relative proximity of the wire to the lesion (Fig. 12–8). Wires placed just posterior to the lesion are helpful because the surgeon removes the lesion by staying deep to the localization needle. Once the incision is made, it is then necessary to identify the shaft of the lesion and retract it into the wound. Dissection in the plane facing the wire entry site allows for simple detection of the wire. Once identified, it is secured at the site of the parenchyma and the distal end of the wire is brought out into the wound. Failure to adequately secure the wire may result in accidental dislodgment. Once out, the tissue is grasped with an Allis clamp. It is preferable to grab the tissue near the wire but not the wire itself because pulling too hard on the clamp may pull the wire from the specimen. Resection of the tissue surrounding the wire proceeds. The relationship between the wire and the lesion, as demonstrated on mammography, helps guide how much tissue to take.

Immediately upon removal of the specimen, it is held in anatomic position and marked with orientation sutures. It is also helpful to place clips at the periphery of the specimen to allow for orientation of the specimen radiograph. These may help guide the excision of additional tissue of the lesion if there is any concern of a close radiographic margin. The specimen is sent to radiology for confirmation that the lesion in question was removed. If there is any

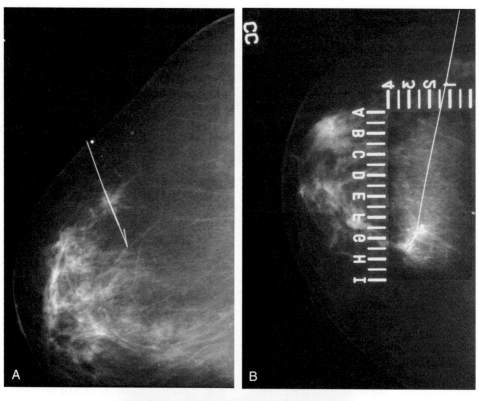

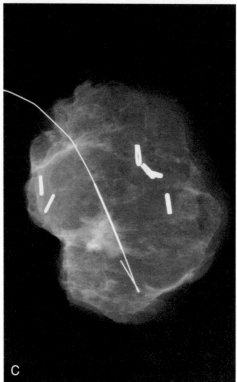

Figure 12–7. A and B, Mediolateral and craniocaudal views from wire localization using superior approach. **C,** Specimen radiograph demonstrates abnormality adjacent to the reinforced portion of the hookwire. Pathology demonstrated ductal carcinoma in situ. (Images courtesy of Dr. Alexis Nees, Department of Radiology, University of Michigan.)

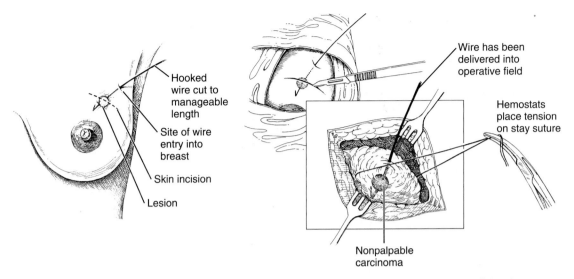

Hooked
wire cut to
manageable
length

Site of wire
entry into
breast

Skin incision

Lesion

Wire has been
delivered into
operative field

Hemostats
place tension
on stay suture

Nonpalpable
carcinoma

Figure 12–8. The wire-localized lumpectomy. The placement of the incision and direction of the dissection are determined by the lesion size, direction of the wire, and the relative proximity of the wire to the lesion. Once the incision is made, it is best to identify the shaft of the wire and retract it into the wound. Once out, the tissue is secured and resection of the tissue surrounding the wire proceeds. (From Roses D. Breast cancer. Philadelphia: Elsevier, 2005.)

clinical concern of a close or positive margin, that should be excised as a separate specimen. The specimen radiography may also suggest a margin that appears close and requires reexcision. Because wire-localized lumpectomies tend to have a higher rate of close or positive margins than lumpectomies for palpable masses, a more generous approach to reexcising margins at the first operation is warranted.

Reexcision Lumpectomy

Reexcision lumpectomy should be performed in any patient with unknown or positive margins. It is also strongly recommended in patients with close margins, approximately 2 to 3 mm. Reexcision is necessary in one fourth to one third of lumpectomies. Failure to reexcise close or positive margins stands a high chance of leaving residual disease and increases local recurrence rates.

The standard approach to a reexcision lumpectomy is to remove the entire cavity. An ellipse of skin is drawn around the previous skin incision so that the previous scar is removed with the specimen. Skin flaps are then raised. The previous cavity is usually readily palpable, and the approach to the reexcision is similar to that of a lumpectomy. As with a lumpectomy, the surgeon should keep one hand on the cavity at all times during the dissection to ensure adequate margins. It is important not to violate

the cavity because this complicates the inking and evaluation of the new margins.

This approach is necessary when the initial lumpectomy was not oriented and inked with the six-color system. In this setting, the surgeon does not know where the close or positive margins are, so the entire cavity needs to be excised. This approach, however, results in a large volume of resected breast tissue, often beyond what is necessary to achieve negative margins. If the original lumpectomy was oriented and the margin in question is known, an alternative approach might be to enter the previous biopsy cavity and excise only the involved margin. This minimizes the volume of tissue excised, and studies have shown that this approach is oncologically sound, with no increased risk of local recurrence. This stresses the importance of orienting and using the six-color inking system on all breast biopsies and lumpectomies.

To reexcise just the involved margin, the previous incision may be excised completely or reopened using a scalpel. The seroma fluid is suctioned out. If too much time elapses between the original lumpectomy or biopsy and the reexcision lumpectomy, the cavity may no longer be evident. In this case, it is preferable to excise the entire cavity as described earlier. However, if there is still a cavity, the margin in question can be grasped at the top with an Allis forceps and that margin reexcised to a depth of approximately 1 cm. The entire hemisphere in question should be reexcised because it is not possible to know precisely where the margin was involved. A positive lateral margin may have been at the anterior-lateral margin, posterior-lateral margin, superior-lateral margin, or inferior-lateral margin. Depending on the pathology report, more than one margin may need to be excised.

Lumpectomy in the Prosthetically Augmented Breast

With the increased popularity of breast augmentation, surgeons are increasingly facing the management of a breast cancer within an augmented breast. Many surgeons have routinely recommended mastectomy in this situation, with reconstruction to be performed immediately or at a later date. Arguments for this include fear of rupture of the implant, the need to radiate the implant, and the impact of the implant on mammographic surveillance. However, mastectomy is not absolutely indicated in this situation. Several series describe reasonable outcomes in patients who underwent BCT in the face of a previously placed implant. Several factors must be considered. It is true that capsular contraction will occur with radiation of the implant, no different than in women who undergo implant reconstruction followed by chest wall radiation. While rates of contracture are higher, this may still be an acceptable alternative to mastectomy. This is particularly true if the implant was placed submuscularly rather than subcutaneously. The size of the tumor and the ability of the surgeon to obtain negative margins without injuring the implant must also be considered. Careful attention should be paid to treatment technique, both surgical and radiation, and a balanced discussion must be held with the patient regarding the impact on cosmesis. However, in appropriately selected patients, BCT is a reasonable option in the face of prior augmentation.

Postoperative Care after Lumpectomy

The morbidity of a lumpectomy is relatively minimal. The most common complications are seroma, hematoma, and infection. Seromas are frequent but often cause no difficulty for the patient; if they are symptomatic, they are relatively easy to manage by needle aspiration. Hematomas and infection are relatively rare.

Both are typically managed conservatively, although incision and drainage is sometimes necessary. Altered sensation to the nipple can also occur depending upon the location of the incision.

The use of a support brassiere in the postoperative period bolsters efforts to sustain hemostasis and relieves tension on the skin closure imposed by the weight of the breast. This can be especially important with large, pendulous breasts, in which blood vessels running alongside the cavity can be avulsed mechanically if the heavy breast is allowed to suspend unsupported. The patient should be encouraged to wear the support brassiere day and night for several days.

Simple Mastectomy

After the induction of general anesthesia, the patient is positioned supine with the arm abducted to 90 degrees and secured to an armboard. To avoid a brachial plexopathy related to stretch injury of a malpositioned patient, the American Society of Anesthesiology recommends upper extremity positioning such that the arm is no greater than 90 degrees, with neutral forearm position, and use of padded armboards. The chest, axilla, and upper arm is prepped and draped in sterile fashion. The prep should extend sufficiently beyond the breast so that the landmarks can be easily identified; across the midline, to the costal margin, the base of the neck, and laterally to the operating room table.

The standard incision for a mastectomy is an elliptical skin incision including both the nipple-areolar complex and the previous biopsy incision. The ellipse may be oriented either transversely or obliquely. The choice of incision must be based on the size of the breast, body habitus of the patient, and size and location of the tumor (or biopsy cavity). Care should be taken to make the ellipse wide enough that redundant skin is avoided, including dog-ears, but not so wide that the closure is excessively tight. Undue tension may lead to vascular compromise of the flaps. Bear in mind that the patient's back is perfectly straight on the operating room table, something that is rarely maintained normally, so what seems tight will be less so once the patient is awake. The ideal ellipse has equal lengths of the superior and inferior lines. This may be facilitated by using a silk suture on a hemostat to measure both lines.

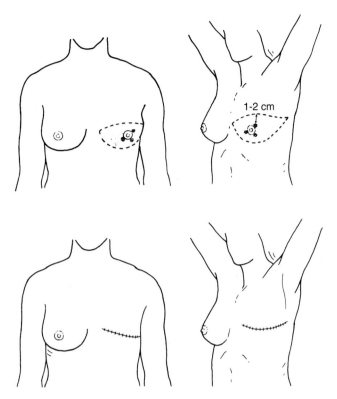

Figure 12–9. The classic Stewart elliptical mastectomy incision. The medial aspect is at the lateral edge of the sternum and the lateral aspect overlies the latissimus dorsi muscle. (From Bland KI, Copeland EM III. The breast, 3rd ed. Philadelphia: WB Saunders, 2004.)

There are several options for how this ellipse is oriented. The classic Stewart incision results in a transverse scar (Fig. 12–9). It should begin at the lateral margin of the sternum and end at the anterior margin of the latissimus dorsi. The Stewart incision may be modified to lie obliquely, so the final incision extends superiorly at the lateral margin. The Stewart incision is particularly good for central tumors, although it may be applicable for most tumors. It is often preferred by plastic surgeons when delayed reconstruction is planned, especially if postmastectomy radiation is to be employed.

The other popular incision is the Orr oblique incision. As opposed to the modified Stewart incision, which extends slightly superiorly in the lateral margin, the Orr incision is an oblique incision (Fig. 12–10). This approach is ideal for upper, outer quadrant incisions but, as with the Stewart incision, can be used for most tumors. Other less common variations may be appropriate for tumors in other quadrants. Alternatively, a skin-sparing incision should be used when immediate reconstruction is planned (Fig. 12–11). The skin-sparing mastectomy is described in more detail in Chapter 14.

In addition to marking the elliptical incision, the boundaries of the breast should be marked preoperatively. These include the lateral margin of the sternum medially, the

second rib superiorly, and the inframammary crease. This provides guidance as to how far to raise the flaps, which and can sometimes be lost during the operation.

The skin incision is then made with a scalpel, dividing the skin and superficial fascia just until the breast tissue is evident. Several superficial veins need to be cauterized. Once the skin incision is completed, the superior flap is raised.

The key to raising the skin flap is adequate retraction (Fig. 12–12). Although several instruments may be used to grasp the skin (Adair clamps, skin hooks, temporary silk sutures placed in the dermis), it is imperative that they be placed evenly along the flap and the retraction is directly anterior. It is not uncommon for the assistant to retract the flap anteriorly and superiorly. This allows the assistant a better view of the dissection but distorts the view of the surgeon and greatly increases the chance of being too close to dermis or even going through the skin. With the assistant retracting straight up, the surgeon pulls the breast tissue away from the flap with the opposite hand. A gauze pad should be kept on the breast tissue to not only prevent the hand from slipping but also maintain hemostasis if sharp dissection is used. This is the key maneuver during a mastectomy and the most common error by junior

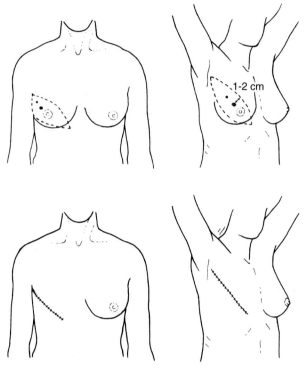

Figure 12–10. The classic Orr oblique elliptical mastectomy incision. (From Bland KI, Copeland EM III. The breast, 3rd ed. Philadelphia: WB Saunders, 2004.)

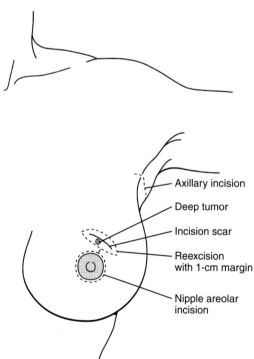

Figure 12–11. Skin-sparing mastectomy incisions incorporating the previous scar and nipple-areolar complex while preserving as much skin as possible. A separate incision is used for the lymph nodes. (From Bland KI, Copeland EM III. The breast, 3rd ed. Philadelphia: WB Saunders, 2004.)

residents when learning the procedure. The surgeon should be continuously repositioning the opposite hand closer to the plane between the breast and the flap, as well as assessing the thickness of the flap.

With the right retraction by both the surgeon and the assistant, the plane is readily apparent. Skin flaps should be elevated at the subcutaneous tissue level, not the subdermal level. This preserves the subcutaneous vascular plexus, which nourishes the overlying skin. Done properly, this can be relatively bloodless. The flap can be raised by the use of a scalpel, scissors, or cautery depending on the surgeon's preference. Several studies have compared scalpel to cautery, both retrospectively and prospectively, and found little difference with the exception of blood loss, which is lower with electrocautery. If cautery is used, it should not be maintained in one position for too long a period of time to avoid thermal injury to the flap. Once in the right plane, the superior flap can be developed quickly to the level of the subclavius muscle, from the lateral aspect of the sternum to the lateral edge of the pectoralis major and axillary fascia. The inferior flap is then raised in an identical manner to the inframammary crease. If the white undersurface of the dermis is seen, the subcutaneous plexus

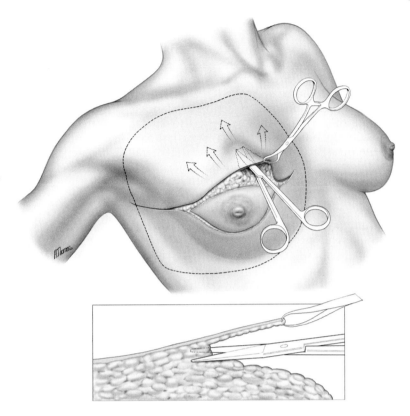

Figure 12–12. Elevation of skin flaps during a mastectomy using Metzenbaum scissors. (From Bloom N, Beattie E, Harvery J. Atlas of cancer surgery. Philadelphia: Elsevier, 2000.)

has been injured and there may be a question of flap viability. This is usually not a problem if immediate reconstruction is not planned, but may lead the plastic surgeon to delay reconstruction to a later date. As the inferior flap is raised, the inframammary crease is lost. This is why it is important for the surgeon to mark the crease preoperatively and to not go past this line while raising the inferior flap.

With the borders of the breast identified circumferentially, it is time to remove the breast. The breast and fascia is dissected off of the pectoralis major muscle. The plane is started at the cephalad portion of the breast. The breast is retracted inferiorly and the plane is developed. It may be helpful to grasp the superior-most aspect of the breast with clamps to assist with retraction when first developing the plane. The dissection proceeds inferiorly. The cautery should be moved parallel to the fibers of the pectoralis major muscle as the breast is removed. Small perforator vessels should be grasped with a pick-up and cauterized as they are identified. Medially, there are some larger perforating branches of the internal mammary vessels. If these are bleeding, it is important not to try to directly cauterize them, but rather to grasp them with a pick-up or hemostat first because they sometimes retract beneath the

muscle and can be difficult to control. If this is the case, they can easily be controlled with a figure-of-eight suture ligation. Excessive cautery or dissecting against the direction of the fibers (with lateral retraction of the breast) can cause separation of the pectoralis from the sternum, which can impact immediate reconstruction (see later). In addition, chasing these bleeding vessels deeper could lead to pneumothorax if the parietal pleura is violated.

While removing the breast, it is easy to slip from the plane between the muscle and the fascia, into the plane between the breast and the fascia, leaving the fascia behind. It is important to remove the fascia with the specimen to ensure an adequate resection. As the surgeon moves inferiorly, the breast is removed from the pectoralis, and the serratus anterior muscle is exposed. In contrast to the pectoralis, the fascia over the serratus anterior should be left intact, and care should be taken not to injure this muscle. If the patient is to undergo immediate reconstruction with an expander, these will be placed within a pocket beneath the pectoralis muscle, with closure to the serratus fascia to provide soft tissue coverage of the implant or expander. Injury to the pectoralis medially, or the serratus anterior inferiorly, compromises the ability to provide adequate coverage and may force the plastic surgeon to abandon plans for immediate reconstruction. Even if immediate reconstruction is not planned, these mistakes can still complicate delayed reconstruction, and proper technique should be employed in all cases.

Although no axillary dissection is planned as part of a simple mastectomy, the lateral aspect of the breast is traditionally the last part of the breast to be removed. Once the lateral border of the pectoralis major muscle is cleared, the axillary fascia is evident, marking the transition from the breast tissue to the axillary fat, and the mastectomy is completed. It is important to not terminate the mastectomy before encountering the axillary fascia, so that the axillary tail is not left behind. Sutures are placed to orient the breast before sending it off the operative field.

After the breast is removed, hemostasis is assured and the field is irrigated with copious amounts of warm saline. The skin margins are examined for any areas of devascularization. Any concerning areas should be debrided before closure. Through a separate stab incision in the inferior flap along the anterior axillary line, a single 10-French closed-suction Silastic catheter is placed along the inferomedial aspect of the wound bed to drain the space between the skin flaps and chest wall. This is secured in place with a 2-0 nonabsorbable suture. The wound is aligned and the deep dermal layer closed with interrupted 3-0 absorbable synthetic suture. A subcuticular 4-0 absorbable suture is then used to close skin, although tissue adhesives are gaining popularity. Suction catheters are connected to bulb suction.

One frustrating aspect of the mastectomy, particularly in heavyset patients with thick axillary fat pads, is "dog-ears," the triangular or cone-shaped flaps of redundant skin and fatty tissue at the ends of the incision. These are usually more prominent at the lateral aspect of the mastectomy incisions. Frequently the incisional dog-ear will not be readily apparent while the patient is lying supine on the operating room table, but when she sits or stands upright postoperatively, these unsightly protrusions become obvious. These can be quite uncomfortable for the patient because the upper arm rubs against them. If recognized intraoperatively, there are several surgical approaches to eliminate dog-ears. Sometimes the redundant axillary skin and fatty tissue can be resected by elongating the standard elliptical mastectomy wound. However, this often lengthens the scar while only moving the dog-ear more

laterally. It is better to excise the tissue using a broad "tear-drop" incision, with the point of the tear-drop oriented medially. Another option is to bring the redundant axillary tissue forward and create a "T" or "Y" configuration at the lateral aspect of the transverse mastectomy incision. When the dog-ear cannot be reasonably corrected at the time of surgery, or if it is not recognized in the supine position but becomes apparent in the postoperative setting, the best solution is to resect it at a later date in the outpatient setting.

Modified Radical Mastectomy

The MRM is becoming a less commonly used operation with the increased use of breast conservation and the decreased need for axillary dissection in the era of sentinel lymph node biopsy. Today, the MRM is used primarily for women who require or desire mastectomy and have documented nodal metastases.

After the induction of general anesthesia, the patient is positioned supine with the arm abducted to 90 degrees on an armboard (Fig. 12–13). Unlike the simple mastectomy, the arm is not secured to the armboard for the MRM so that it may be brought into the operative field during the case. The chest, axilla, and entire arm are prepped and draped in sterile fashion. The prep should extend sufficiently beyond the breast so that the landmarks can be easily identified: across the midline, to

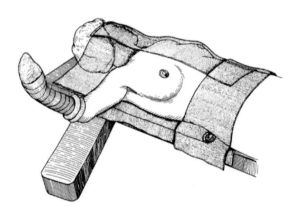

Figure 12–13. Patient position for a right modified radical mastectomy. The patient is positioned supine with the arm out at 90 degrees, never hyperextended. The entire arm is prepped to the wrist and the shoulder and lateral chest are prepped down to the table. The armboard is covered with a sterile drape and the arm sheathed to above the elbow with a sterile impervious stockinet, keeping it within the sterile field. (From Bland KI, Copeland EM III. The breast, 3rd ed. Philadelphia: WB Saunders, 2004.)

the costal margin, the base of the neck, and laterally to the operating room table, including around the shoulder. The forearm and hand are isolated in a stockinet dressing wrapped with a Kerlix roll.

The incision for the MRM is the same as for a simple mastectomy. It is not necessary to extend the incisions further into the axilla; a complete axillary dissection can be performed through the standard incisions. A skin-sparing mastectomy can still be performed when an MRM is necessary. In addition to the incision around the nipple-areolar complex, with a keyhole extension laterally, a second incision is made in the axilla to complete the axillary dissection.

After the patient has been marked, the superior and inferior skin flaps are raised as described for the simple mastectomy, and the procedure follows the same steps except for the lateral margin. As the lateral aspect of the inferior flap is completed, it is an ideal time to identify the latissimus dorsi muscle because this landmark is crucial to defining the borders of the axilla. Once identified, this can be cleared superiorly along the anterior border of the muscle. Dissecting medially along the muscle may result in injury to the thoracodorsal bundle.

The breast and fascia are removed from the pectoralis major muscle as described earlier (Fig. 12–14). As the breast is removed from the

lateral border of the pectoralis major muscle, the space between the pectoralis major and minor muscle can be developed so that palpation of the interpectoral (Rotter's) nodes can be undertaken (Fig. 12–15). Some surgeons only remove this tissue when palpable nodes are detected; other surgeons routinely include the fibroareolar tissue in the interpectoral space, which can be swept laterally and included with the specimen. However, excessive dissection in this area can lead to injury of the lateral pectoral nerve and is unlikely to be of added benefit if grossly involved nodes are not present. The axillary nodes are then removed en bloc with the breast. The steps of the axillary dissection are outlined in Chapter 13.

Once the breast and axillary contents are removed, the closure is the same as for a simple mastectomy, except two closed-suction drains are typically placed through two different stab incisions. In addition to one drain along the inferomedial aspect of the chest wall, a second drain is laced in the axillary space. The tip of the drain should be 2 cm below the axillary vein and should lie on the ventral surface of the latissimus dorsi.

Postoperative Care

The patient should be given a binder with adequate fluffs to provide adequate but not excessive compression. Tight pressure dressings are

Figure 12–14. Elevation of the breast and pectoralis major fascia off of the underlying muscle. Dissection should proceed superior to inferior and medial to lateral. (From Bloom N, Beattie E, Harvery J. Atlas of cancer surgery. Philadelphia: Elsevier, 2000.)

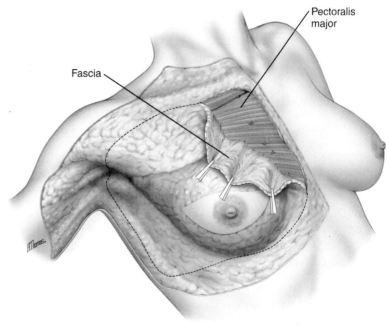

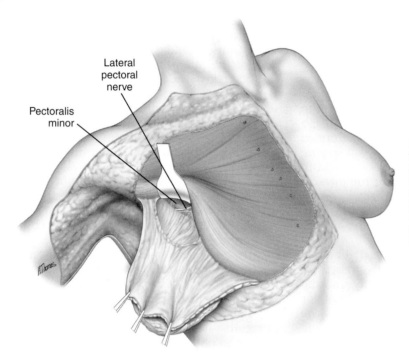

Figure 12–15. Retraction of the pectoralis major muscle, allowing the interpectoral (Rotter's) nodes to be removed en bloc with the specimen. (From Bloom N, Beattie E, Harvery J. Atlas of cancer surgery. Philadelphia: Elsevier, 2000.)

not necessary. The dressings should remain undisturbed for 48 to 72 hours after the surgery, unless concerns for flap viability warrant taking down the dressings to examine the flaps. Patients are encouraged to sit upright and avoid slouching so as to avoid excessive skin flaps. Range-of-motion exercises for the arm and shoulder are given to the patient preoperatively, with instructions to begin them on day 1. Particularly in the case of the MRM, it is important for the patient to use her arm rather than keep it at her side in a sling because this will lead to stiffening of the shoulder and limited range of motion. The drains remain in place until the output drops below 30 cc per 24-hour period for 2 consecutive days. Typically this takes 1 to 2 weeks, with the chest wall drain usually ready to remove before the axillary drain. Drains are removed at 4 weeks even if the output remains high secondary to infectious risks.

Complications of Breast Surgery

Breast surgery is relatively safe surgery, with low rates of major complications. Wound complications are typically minor and frequently managed on an outpatient basis, but can occur in up to 30% of cases. These include breast infections, seromas, and hematomas. Very rarely, more serious complications can occur. Deep venous thrombosis and pulmonary embolism (PE) are potential complications of any major surgery. Pneumothorax has been described as a result of wire localization or inadvertently deep dissection. Brachial plexopathy may occur related to a stretch injury of a malpositioned patient.

Wound Infections

Rates of postoperative infections in breast and axillary incisions have ranged from fewer than 1% of cases to nearly 20%. A metaanalysis on 2587 surgical breast procedures found an overall wound infection rate of 3.8% of cases. Wound infections of the breast are primarily related to skin flora, usually staphylococcal organisms. Increased risk factors for wound infection include obesity, tobacco use, older age, and diabetes mellitus. Second operations in the breast also appear to have a higher risk of wound infection.

Whether or not lumpectomies require preoperative antibiotic coverage is still controversial. Multiple retrospective and prospective studies have yielded disparate results. Although many retrospective series suggest a benefit of antibiotics, these results are slightly biased by the increased use of antibiotics among higher-risk cases. A reasonable approach, with a side benefit of reducing costs, is to limit antibiotic prophylaxis to high-risk patients and cases. It is also reasonable to use preoperative antibiotics in cases involving wire localization because this is a foreign body, although this has not been specifically identified as a wound infection risk factor. Antibiotics are also recommended in patients having a second breast operation (e.g., a mastectomy after an excisional biopsy or a reexcision lumpectomy).

If an infection does occur, it usually manifests as an incisional cellulitis. Mild incisional cellulitis can be treated with oral antibiotics. However, nonresponding or more extensive soft tissue infections require hospitalization and intravenous antibiotics. A minority of breast wound infections progress into a fully developed abscess. These most commonly appear 1 to 2 weeks postoperatively. Patients present with a fluctuant, erythematous, tender mass at the surgical site. If it is unclear whether this represents a cellulitis or abscess, ultrasound may be helpful, although it is often difficult to differentiate between a consolidating seroma or hematoma and an abscess. As with primary breast abscesses, aspiration and antibiotics may avoid the need for incision and drainage. However, postoperative abscesses are often complex and difficult to aspirate completely. Thus they usually reaccumulate. Definitive management therefore requires incision and drainage by reopening the original surgical wound and leaving the cavity open to heal by secondary intention.

Seroma

Seromas are extremely common after breast surgery secondary to the rich lymphatic drainage of the breast and possibly the low fibrinogen levels and net fibrinolytic activity within lymphatic fluid collections. In the case of a lumpectomy, the seroma may be desirable because it preserves the normal breast contour, even after a large-volume resection. This cavity is eventually replaced by scar formation as the cavity consolidates. In rare cases, the lumpectomy seroma is quite large, causing discomfort from a bulging fluid collection. In these cases, simple aspiration of the excess usually is adequate management.

Seroma formation under the skin flaps of mastectomy wounds impairs the healing process, which is why drains are usually left in place. After 1 to 3 weeks, the skin flaps heal and adhere to the chest wall, as evidenced by diminished drain output. Seroma collections that develop after drain removal can be managed by percutaneous aspiration. Aspiration is usually well tolerated because the mastectomy and axillary incisions tend to be insensate; these procedures can be repeated as frequently as needed to ensure that the skin flaps are densely adherent to the chest wall. In rare cases when the seroma continues to recur, a Seroma-Cath may be considered.

Hematoma/Bleeding

Bleeding complications can be diminished by meticulous hemostasis, but even in the best hands, they will occur. The risk is higher in patients using aspirin-containing products and nonsteroidal antiinflammatory drugs (NSAIDs) such as ibuprofen in the preoperative and postoperative period. These drugs have well-known antiplatelet activity, and these medications should be avoided for 1 to 2 weeks before surgery (the life span of the affected platelets). In addition, several over-the-counter medications and supplements that are widely used also have anticoagulant properties and are recognized for contributing to bleeding complications; these include vitamin E, ginseng, ginkgo biloba, and garlic.

A minority of patients may present with excessive bruising or a small hematoma at the site of the lumpectomy. These cases resolve spontaneously. However, an expanding hematoma, either at a lumpectomy site or underneath the skin flaps of a mastectomy, must be recognized as quickly as possible because significant blood loss can occur. Postoperative hemorrhage is often secondary to arterial perforators of the thoracoacromial vessels or internal mammary arteries. In some cases, these can be managed by reestablishing the patency of the suction catheters (which often clot when draining blood) and applying a compression dressing. However, in many cases the patient should be returned to the operating room for evacuation of the hematoma and hemostasis. Even if a large hematoma is controlled with pressure, it will take a long time to resolve and may be associated with significant discomfort. Thus in the long run, an early return to the operating room to evacuate the hematoma may simplify the recovery period.

Chronic Pain

Patients are often surprised that the immediate postoperative pain is less than they expected after both a lumpectomy and mastectomy, and that this pain usually resolves quickly. However, a small number of breast cancer patients experience chronic incisional pain. This can be quite debilitating, last for months to years, and not resolve with standard analgesics. The pain is often described as "burning" or "constricting," suggesting a neuropathic cause, although the exact etiology remains unknown. Surprisingly, it seems to occur more commonly after lumpectomy rather than mastectomy cases. Standard analgesics may not provide relief, recently successful management has been reported with use of serotonin uptake inhibitors, such as the antidepressants amitriptyline and venlafaxine.

Chronic Breast Lymphedema/ Cellulitis

It is well known that lymphedema of the upper extremity is a common complication of axillary surgery. Less known is that the breast can also experience chronic lymphedema as well as fibrosis and atrophy after breast cancer surgery. These are often due to a combination of surgery and radiation therapy. The European Organization for Research and Treatment and the Radiation Therapy Oncology Group have proposed a grading system for the late effects of BCT known as the Late Effects of Normal Tissue—Subjective, Objective, Management, and Analytic (LENT-SOMA) scales. The LENT-SOMA system stratifies breast symptoms on the basis of pain magnitude as reported by the patient, measurable differences in breast appearance, intervention requirements for control of pain and/or lymphedema, and presence of image-documented breast sequelae (e.g., photos, mammography, CT/MRI studies).

Chronic breast lymphedema can be frustrating for both the patient and the physician in that it is often difficult to differentiate between lymphedema and cellulitis. Recurrent episodes of breast cellulitis occurring several months to years after lumpectomy and/or breast radiation therapy have also been reported, although rarely. The patients usually return with a red, swollen, and tender breast. Although an infrequent cause, the first step is to rule out an inflammatory recurrence. At a minimum this requires breast imaging and possibly a skin punch biopsy. Any abnormalities on imaging should also be biopsied. If everything appears benign, a standard course of antibiotics should be initiated. Failure to respond should prompt a change in antibiotics (and a skin punch biopsy if not already done). Persistent edema and erythema may be lymphedema and not cellulitis, and physical therapy with a lymphedema specialist can often help dramatically. However, for fear of spreading infection, many physical therapists will not treat until cellulitis has been ruled out. Most cases eventually resolve, although occasionally patients have persistent pain and inflammation, prompting mastectomy.

Suggested Readings

1. Fisher B, Anderson S, Bryant J, et al. Twenty-year follow-up of a randomized trial comparing total mastectomy, lumpectomy, and lumpectomy plus irradiation for the treatment of invasive breast cancer. N Engl J Med 2002;347:1233–1241.
2. Haffty BG, Harrold E, Khan AJ, et al. Outcome of conservatively managed early-onset breast cancer by BRCA1/2 status. Lancet 2002;359:1471.
3. Janz NK, Wren PA, Copeland LA, et al. Patient-physician concordance: Preferences, perceptions, and factors influencing the breast cancer surgical decision. J Clin Oncol 2004;22(15):3091–3098.
4. Metcalfe K, Lynch HT, Ghadirian P, et al. Contralateral breast cancer in BRCA1 and BRCA2 mutation carriers. J Clin Oncol 2004;22:2328.
5. Newman LA, Kuerer HM. Advances in breast conservation therapy. J Clin Oncol 2005;23(8):1685–1697.
6. Punglia RS, Morrow M, Winer EP, et al. Local therapy and survival in breast cancer. N Engl J Med 2007; 256:2399–2405.
7. Sabel MS. Locoregional therapy of breast cancer: Maximizing control, minimizing morbidity. Exp Rev Anticancer Ther 2006;6(9):1281–1299.
8. Vitug AF, Newman LA. Complications in breast surgery. Surg Clin N Am 2007;87:431–451.
9. Warner M, Blitt C, Butterworth J, et al. Practice advisory for the prevention of perioperative peripheral neuropathies. A report by the American Society of Anesthesiologists' Task Force on the prevention of perioperative peripheral neuropathies. Anesthesiology 2000;92:1168–1182.

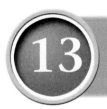
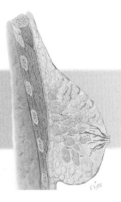

Regional Management of Breast Cancer

Key Points

- Understand the implications of regional metastases on surgical management, adjuvant systemic therapy, and radiation therapy.
- Develop an algorithm for evaluating the lymph nodes (N stage) in the patient who is clinically node negative and clinically node positive.
- Describe the technique for the performance of a sentinel lymph node biopsy, including the options for the type and site of injection of the tracers.
- Know the indications for an axillary lymph node dissection and describe the technique.

- Understand the pros and cons of internal mammary sentinel lymph node biopsy and describe the technique.
- Be familiar with the arguments for and against the performance of a completion node dissection when the sentinel lymph node is positive.
- Be familiar with the complications of sentinel lymph node biopsy and axillary lymph node dissection and their management.
- Describe the management of lymphedema after breast surgery.

Introduction

Ever since the lymphatic system was identified in the 17th century, scientists have surmised an important association between the regional lymph nodes and the development and progression of cancers of the breast. At that time, René Descartes proposed a lymph theory for the origin of breast cancer in direct contrast to the prevailing theory of the time: Galen's theory that cancer arose from an excess of black bile in the body. The lymph theory of cancer gained significant momentum in the 18th century when it was advocated by John Hunter, the "Father of Scientific Surgery," suggesting that a coagulative defect in the lymph ultimately led to the appearance of breast cancer. Hunter called for the removal of the cancer along with the potential areas of lymphatic spread nearly 100 years earlier than William Halsted.

The formal axillary lymph node dissection (ALND) was introduced by Lorenz Heister in the 19th century, although it was not quickly adopted. In 1867, Charles Hewitt Moore wrote a treatise titled, "On the Influence of Inadequate Operations on the Theory of Cancer," in which he described the importance of removing involved axillary lymph nodes en bloc with the cancer. He later went on to prescribe full axillary dissection for all patients with breast cancer, noting that involved nodes may not be detected clinically. The routine use of axillary dissection was adopted by notable surgeons such as Ernst G. F. Küster, Richard von Volkmann, Joseph Lister, and Samuel D. Gross, who reported a virtual elimination of axillary recurrences when axillary clearance was routinely performed.

Of course, it was Halsted who most radically changed the surgical management of breast cancer when he first described the radical mastectomy in 1882. This operation called not only for the removal of the breast and both pectoral muscles, but also, based on the reports of the aforementioned surgeons, an extensive axillary dissection incorporating levels I through III. Although the radical mastectomy was associated with significant postoperative deformity and diminished upper extremity function, and the operative procedure itself resulted in significant intraoperative blood loss, it had a dramatic impact on locoregional control and was quickly adopted. The modified radical mastectomy (MRM), popularized by D. H. Patey in the 1930s, spared the pectoral muscles while removing the breast and axillary contents (levels I and II). Much less morbid than the radical mastectomy, this operation eventually replaced the radical mastectomy when long-term followup failed to demonstrate any breast cancer recurrences in the preserved pectoral muscles, rarely in the level III or interpectoral nodes, and no difference in survival compared with radical mastectomy.

When it became apparent that the radical mastectomy dramatically lowered locoregional recurrence rates but had no significant impact on overall survival, the relative impact that local or regional control had on survival was called into question. To help address these questions, the National Surgical and Adjuvant Breast Project (NSABP) was established by Dr. Rudolph Noer under the supervision of the National Cancer Institute (NCI). One of the first trials that the NSABP conducted, NSABP B-04, sought to specifically address the controversy surrounding the ideal management of the axillary lymph nodes (NSABP B-06 would address the ideal local management of breast cancer, see Chapter 12). The NSABP B-04 trial, conducted between July 1971 and September 1974, took patients with operable invasive breast cancers and clinically negative nodes ($n = 1079$) and randomized them to one of three arms: (1) total mastectomy with ALND; (2) total mastectomy with postoperative radiation; and (3) total mastectomy with a delayed axillary dissection only if clinically positive axillary nodes developed. An additional 586 women with clinically positive nodes were randomized to either radical mastectomy or

TABLE 13–1 • Results of the NSABP B04 Trial

		Node negative		Node positive	
	RM	TM	RM + XRT	RM	TM + XRT
Number of patients	362	365	352	292	294
OS at 25 yrs	25%	26%	19%	14%	14%
OS at 10 years	58%	54%	59%	38%	39%
OS at 5 years	75%	74%	75%	62%	58%

Of patients who were clinically node negative 19% underwent delayed axillary lymph node dissection for axillary
relapse (median time to development of positive axillary nodes 14.8 months).
Of patients who were clinically node positive randomized to TM + XRT, 11.9% developed axillary relapse compared
to 1% in RM arm.
OS, overall survival; RM, radical mastectomy; TM, total mastectomy; TM + XRT, total mastectomy and external
beam radiation.)

total mastectomy without axillary surgery, but with postoperative radiation. Twenty-five-year followup of the B-04 trial has demonstrated no survival difference among either the node-negative treatment groups or the node-positive treatment groups (Table 13–1).

The NSABP B-04 trial did demonstrate the necessity of surgical lymph node dissection in identifying regional disease (clinical axillary staging was incorrect in 25% to 40% of cases) and also the superiority of surgical lymph node dissection compared with axillary radiation for local disease control among patients who were clinically node positive. However, the trial also revealed that the ALND as part of the surgical management of breast cancer was not associated with any survival benefit. Despite this finding, surgical management did not change and axillary dissection remained the standard of care. There were several reasons for this. Critics of the study point out that the study was not powered to detect a small survival benefit to ALND, and in the mastectomy alone, many of surgeons still included a large number of axillary nodes with the specimen. But the strongest reason that ALND remained standard despite no evidence of therapeutic benefit was that the prognostic information provided by ALND was still crucial for adjuvant therapy decisions. So while NSABP B-06 dramatically altered the local management of breast cancer NSABP-04 did not, as it was still necessary to perform routine ALND to identify patients who were node positive. However, this, too, would change dramatically when sentinel lymph node (SLN) biopsy for breast cancer emerged.

In the 80s and 90s, axillary sampling was being investigated as a means of staging the axilla without subjecting patients to the complications of axillary clearance. During this time, the use of intraoperative lymphatic mapping was being investigated for other cancers as a method of accurately identifying the first lymph node(s) that received drainage from the site of a tumor. This was not a new concept. In the mid-19th century, Virchow described the concept of lymphatic drainage from a given body site to a specific lymph node. Based on studies in cats and humans with vital dye, Braithwaite first described the "glands sentinel" as the lymph node that drains a particular area. In 1960, Gould described a "sentinel node" that directly drained the parotid gland and proposed that a radical neck dissection should be performed if this node contained micrometastatic disease. And in 1976, Cabanas suggested that the sentinel node of the penis could be used to determine the need for regional node dissection for penile cancer. However, the use of intraoperative lymphatic mapping to identify the sentinel node was truly brought forward by Donald Morton for the treatment of malignant melanoma, where it was demonstrated to be highly accurate in predicting the status of the regional basin. In 1994, Giuliano first described the use of SLN biopsy in breast cancer, prompting great interest in using this technique in breast cancer and numerous studies of SLN biopsy followed by completion axillary lymph node dissection.

Management of the Patient with Clinically Node-Negative Breast Cancer

Although there are still several controversies that exist regarding the ideal use of SLN biopsy, it has become the standard method of identifying regional metastases in patients with clinically node-negative breast cancer. The ALND should no longer be considered for this

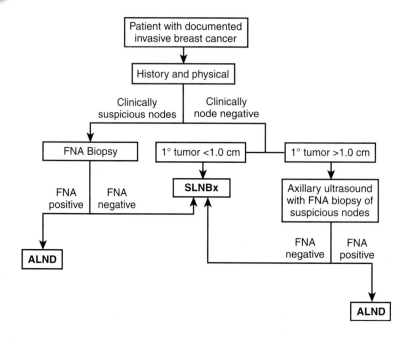

Figure 13–1. Clinical staging of the axilla. Patients with palpable axillary lymph nodes should undergo fine-needle aspiration (FNA) biopsy to confirm metastases. Because palpable nodes are not always involved by cancer, a negative FNA should prompt a sentinel lymph node (SLN) biopsy, taking care to excise any suspicious nodes regardless of whether they take up the tracer. For patients who are clinically node negative, axillary ultrasound and ultrasound-guided FNA biopsy will identify many patients who have regional metastases, allowing them to proceed to axillary lymph node dissection (ALND) or neoadjuvant chemotherapy. The size cutoff for the routine use of axillary ultrasound varies among institutions. At the University of Michigan, all patients with an invasive cancer greater than 1 cm undergo routine axillary ultrasound.

purpose, except in cases in which SLN biopsy is not possible. Outside of this scenario, the ALND should be thought of as a therapeutic procedure for patients with documented lymph node involvement. However, before proceeding with surgical management, a thorough evaluation should be completed to identify patients with regional involvement so that these patients may be spared SLN biopsy and proceed directly to axillary clearance (Fig. 13–1).

Noninvasive Axillary Assessment

If it has not already been done as part of the initial evaluation, any patient diagnosed with breast cancer requires a detailed examination of the regional lymph nodes, including the axilla, supraclavicular, and cervical basins. With the patient sitting up, the examination should begin with the cervical lymph nodes along the anterior border of the sternocleidomastoid muscle. As the examiner moves downward, adenopathy should be sought in the supraclavicular fossa and possibly some infraclavicular nodes within the deltopectoral groove. To examine the axillary nodes, the examiner should face the patient or stand slightly to his or her side. The examiner uses the nonpalpating hand to either steady the patient's shoulder or support his or her arm, asking him or her to let it go loose to relax the pectoralis major and axillary fascia (Fig. 13–2). Examining the axilla

without relaxation of the fascia will severely limit the ability to detect palpable adenopathy. Physical examination of the axilla involves palpation of the anterior, deep, and posterior axillary surfaces. Enlarged or firm nodes may sometimes be detected on firm compression of the axillary tissues against the smoother surface of the pectoral muscles, the lateral chest wall, or the subscapular musculature. The examination should start high in the axilla. In this way, the axillary nodes are trapped lower rather than initially pushed upward. Gently palpate back and forth to feel if any nodes are apparent. Several passes should be made from top to bottom, both anteriorly and posteriorly in the axilla. If any lymph nodes are detected, their size, consistency, and fixation should be noted.

It is important to acknowledge that physical examination alone is highly inaccurate for clinical staging, lacking in both sensitivity and specificity. Obviously micrometastatic disease will not be identified on physical examination. However, it is also possible to have a false-positive finding. Normal lymph nodes can sometimes be palpated depending on the body habitus of the patient, and sometimes enlarged lymph nodes are present in response to a previous breast biopsy. As many as 40% of clinically positive examinations may be inaccurate, even in experienced hands. Given that today women who are node negative can be spared the morbidity of ALND, the impact of a false-positive

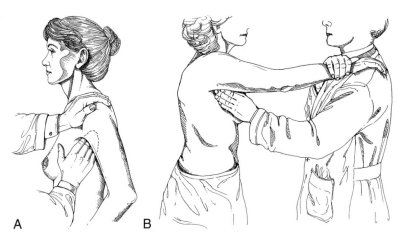

Figure 13–2. A, B: Axillary examination. The examiner should face the patient or stand slightly to his or her side. The examiner uses the nonpalpating hand to either steady the patient's shoulder or support his or her arm, asking him or her to let it go loose to relax the pectoralis major and axillary fascia. (From Roses D. Breast Cancer. Philadelphia: Elsevier, 2005.)

physical examination can be significant. Therefore, fine-needle aspiration (FNA) biopsy should be used to confirm the presence of metastatic disease in any patient with breast cancer with palpable axillary lymph nodes. This can be done freehand or with ultrasound guidance.

If FNA confirms the presence of metastatic disease, then when the patient proceeds to lumpectomy or mastectomy, a level I and II ALND should be performed. If the FNA is negative, however, ALND should not be the next step. If the examiner is highly suspicious of lymph node involvement and believes the negative FNA is secondary to sampling error, it may be worth performing an ultrasound-guided biopsy. In other cases, surgical lymph node excisional biopsy can be performed if the presence or absence of lymph node metastasis is a key component of the therapeutic algorithm.

If the examiner is confident that the node was sampled correctly, or the image-guided biopsy is also negative, the patient should undergo SLN biopsy at the time of their lumpectomy or mastectomy. It is crucial that the surgeon also remove the palpable node at the time of SLN biopsy, even if it does not demonstrate uptake of either the radioactive tracer or blue dye and consider frozen section analysis or imprint cytology to evaluate for metastases.

Axillary Ultrasound

In the patient with documented breast cancer and no palpable adenopathy, imaging of the axilla with ultrasound is rapidly becoming standard practice for preoperative axillary assessment. Sensitivity of axillary ultrasound in identifying abnormal nodes ranges from 50% to 70%; specificity is between 85% and 95%. When axillary FNA biopsy of abnormal lymph nodes is added to axillary ultrasound, the sensitivity increases to nearly 100% in some studies. The preoperative diagnosis of axillary metastasis is extremely helpful in the staging and operative planning of the patient with breast cancer. As SLN biopsy is not an inexpensive procedure, sparing patients with known lymph node metastases from the procedure not only simplifies their treatment but also saves health care dollars. It is also helpful in the preoperative staging and patient selection of patients considered for neoadjuvant chemotherapy. Several institutions consider it common practice to routinely obtain axillary ultrasounds on all patients with invasive cancers greater than 1.0 cm.

There are several criteria by which a lymph node is deemed suspicious on ultrasonography (Table 13–2). Abnormal lymph nodes are identified by either their size or a change in their general appearance on ultrasound (Figs. 13–3, 13–4, 13–5). Size is felt to be the weakest predictor of abnormality; normal nodes generally measure between 4 and 6 mm in length, and although nodes greater than 10 mm in length are generally considered abnormal, changes in morphology are significantly more useful in diagnosing metastasis. Rounding of the normal elliptical shape is considered an indication of neoplastic infiltration. Obliteration of the normally hypoechoic nodal cortex, irregularities of the cortical or medullary contours, and

TABLE 13-2 • *Features of a Suspicious Lymph Node on Ultrasound*

- Increased size
- Abnormal node adjacent to normal node (less likely to be inflammation)
- Rounded shape as opposed to normal ovoid shape
- Hypoechoic cortex
- Loss of echogenic outer capsule and angular margins
- Cortical thickening: uniform versus eccentric
- Hilar compression: uniform versus eccentric
- Hilar indentation ("rat bite")
- Hilar displacement or obliteration
- Hypervascular flow patterns

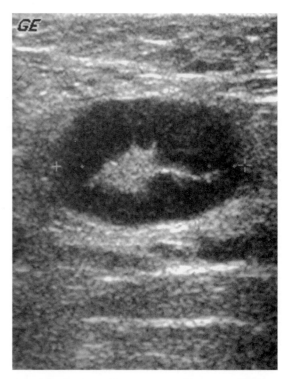

Figure 13-4. Axillary lymph node demonstrates asymmetric cortical thickening with flattening and compression of the hilum. (Image courtesy of Dr. Alexis Nees, Department of Radiology, University of Michigan.)

eccentric compression of the hyperechoic nodal medulla are also suggestive of metastatic disease. Loss of the nodal capsule is also an indicator of tumor invasion. The addition of color-flow Doppler may also enhance the diagnostic sensitivity of axillary ultrasound; hypervascularity and visualization of multiple feeding vessels for a single lymph node are strong indicators of neoplastic activity. Any abnormal lymph nodes identified on axillary ultrasound should undergo ultrasound-guided FNA to confirm the presence of metastases.

Patients with FNA-proven regional disease can be spared the time and expense of SLN biopsy and proceed directly to ALND at the time of their lumpectomy or mastectomy.

Contraindications to Sentinel Lymph Node Biopsy

Patients with invasive cancer and no clinical evidence of axillary disease are candidates for SLN biopsy. As stated, patients with palpable axillary nodes or suspicious lymph nodes on axillary ultrasound should be initially evaluated by FNA, with or without ultrasound guidance (Box 13–1 and Box 13–2).

Besides the patient who is clinically node positive, are there other indications when SLN biopsy is contraindicated? When SLN was first introduced clinically, its use was limited to small, unicentric invasive cancers. However, the success rates and accuracy of the procedure have subsequently been described in patient populations in which SLN biopsy was considered contraindicated. These include patients with multicentric cancers, patients with large

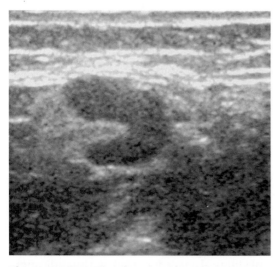

Figure 13-3. Axillary lymph node with symmetric cortical thickening. (Image courtesy of Dr. Alexis Nees, Department of Radiology, University of Michigan.)

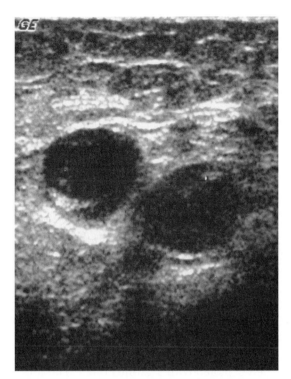

Figure 13–5. Lymph node on right demonstrates round shape with compression of the fatty hilum. Lymph node on left demonstrates loss of fatty hilum. Ultrasound-guided fine-needle aspiration (FNA) confirmed metastatic disease. (Image courtesy of Dr. Alexis Nees, Department of Radiology, University of Michigan.)

(>5 cm) primary tumors, and even patients with previous axillary surgery or breast irradiation. Many of these changes were prompted by alterations in the method of injection of the tracer. For example, tumor size had been considered a possible contraindication to SLN biopsy. Most surgeons recommend SLN biopsy for patients with clinically node-negative breast cancers with T1 and T2 tumors (less than 5 cm). However, SLN biopsy has been shown to be accurate for patients with larger tumors. On one hand, most of these patients (as high as 75%) will have regional metastases, so most will inevitably proceed to complete node dissection. On the other hand, even if it is a minority of patients, it is worth sparing these patients from the morbidity

BOX 13–1 ABSOLUTE CONTRAINDICATIONS TO SENTINEL LYMPH NODE BIOPSY

Clinically involved lymph nodes (confirm by fine-needle aspiration)
Inflammatory breast cancer

BOX 13–2 CONTROVERSIES IN THE USE OF SENTINEL LYMPH NODE BIOPSY

Prophylactic mastectomy	Pro: Staging of axilla if incidental cancer is detected. Con: Low likelihood of incidental cancer does not justify the cost of the procedure.
Ductal carcinoma in situ	Pro: Staging of axilla if incidental invasive cancer is detected after mastectomy. Con: If invasion is detected after lumpectomy, a sentinel lymph node (SLN) biopsy can still be performed.
Multicentric breast cancer	Con: Accuracy of SLN biopsy is not verified for multicentric cancer. Pro: Studies of periareolar injection suggest a common drainage pattern for all quadrants.
Pregnancy	Blue dye is contraindicated because of an allergic reaction. Methylene blue has not been studied. Tc99 appears safe, although some surgeons are hesitant to use it.
Previous axillary surgery	Con: Disruption to lymphatic pathways makes the accuracy of the procedure questionable. Pro: Several studies have demonstrated feasibility of the approach.

of an ALND. These patients are obviously ideal candidates for preoperative axillary ultrasound with ultrasound-guided FNA biopsy of any abnormal lymph nodes. If negative, a subset of these patients will still benefit from SLN biopsy. Many women with T3 tumors will be candidates for neoadjuvant chemotherapy. How the sentinel node procedure should be incorporated with neoadjuvant chemotherapy is discussed in detail in Chapter 18. In any such case, however, it falls on the judgment of the surgeon as to whether SLN biopsy will give an accurate representation of the nodal status. If there is reasonable concern, either before or during the procedure, then ALND should be performed.

Another area of controversy is the use of SLN with noninvasive breast cancer. Although SLN biopsy is primarily indicated in patients with invasive breast cancer, there are some situations in which it may be considered in patients with ductal carcinoma in situ (DCIS; see Chapter 11). Patients undergoing mastectomy for DCIS are candidates for SLN biopsy. This is primarily done as a method to stage the axilla should an unexpected invasive component be identified within the mastectomy specimen. If invasive cancer is incidentally identified in a patient with DCIS undergoing a simple mastectomy without SLN biopsy, the only option for staging the axilla is a complete ALND. Patients undergoing lumpectomy for DCIS do not require SLN biopsy; if an invasive component is discovered, they may return to the operating room. It is not unreasonable, however, to consider SLN biopsy in patients with DCIS undergoing breast conservation for whom there is a strong clinical suspicion for an invasive component, such as patients with DCIS presenting as a palpable mass or those with extensive high-grade DCIS with comedonecrosis.

Sentinel Lymph Node Biopsy

Surgical Technique

Injection of Tracers and Patient Preparation

Sentinel node biopsy is a multistep procedure, involving perioperative localization followed by intraoperative nodal excision. The method of nodal localization has been a subject of much investigation, using different timing sequences, agents, and injection techniques to determine the optimum procedure for identifying the sentinel node.

The initial description of the sentinel node procedure used blue dye only as a method of localizing the SLN. Today, the most common approach to SLN biopsy is the use of a combination of tracers, which had most commonly consisted of technetium 99-m (Tc99) and Lymphazurin (isosulfan blue dye). With recent difficulties in obtaining Lymphazurin, many surgeons have shifted to the use of Methylene blue dye. The application of both a nuclear tracer and blue dye does increase the sensitivity, specificity, and accuracy of sentinel node identification. However, use of blue dye alone has a sentinel node identification rate ranging from 77% to 92%, making sentinel node biopsy feasible in facilities that lack nuclear medicine capabilities.

The timing and technique of the injection of these tracers for sentinel node localization has been extensively researched. The procedure typically begins with the injection of the Tc99; a radiotracer bound to a colloid substance that travels through the lymphatic system. Sulfur colloid is the molecule commonly used in the United States; albumin is often the preferred compound overseas. In the United States, Tc-99m sulfur colloid is available as unfiltered or filtered, having been passed through a 22-μm filter. The uptake and travel time depend on the size of the labeled carrier and the amount of carrier fluid used. Larger particles may never make it to the nodes, whereas small particles may go too quickly, possibly resulting in multiple positive nodes. Filtration eliminates much of the heterogeneity found in the sulfur colloid molecules, theoretically producing a more concentrated and easily localized radioactive signal when explored with a gamma probe. Filtration through 100- or 220-nm filters has been studied, with goals of particle sizes ranging from 50 to 200 nm. A number of studies have been performed, examining the clinical benefit of using filtered versus unfiltered Tc-99m. The results have failed to demonstrate a clear advantage of one over the other. Selection may depend on the relative advantages and disadvantages, including when the injection is performed (day of versus night before).

Often the injections are performed the morning of the surgery, with lymphoscintigraphy performed 2 hours after injection. This can complicate surgical scheduling because cases involving SLN biopsies cannot begin until late morning. Several studies have demonstrated no difference in node identification rates using Tc-99m between 2 and 24 hours after injection, a fact that often simplifies the logistics of scheduling surgery by allowing the injection to take place the night before.

The technique of injection for sentinel node localization has also been examined by several institutions for both the radioactive colloid and the blue dye. Originally, injections were always performed peritumorally based on the concept that this would be the most accurate anatomically. The peritumoral injection involves injection of the tracer in the breast parenchyma surrounding the tumor or the cavity from the excisional biopsy. However, this requires that the person injecting the tracer (often a nuclear

TABLE 13–3 • *Relative Advantages of Different Injection Techniques*

	Pros	Cons
Intraparenchymal (peritumoral)	Conceptually the "purest" mapping route in replicating intramammary lymphatic path from breast tumor to sentinel node(s) More likely to map to internal mammary lymph nodes (IMNs)	Difficult for nonpalpable tumors Risk of injecting into breast cavity Where to inject for multiple tumors Shine-through effect for Tc99 for upper outer quadrant tumors
Dermal	Rapid lymphatic uptake Easier with nonpalpable tumors, but requires marking of skin overlying lesion less shine through	Where to inject for multiple tumors May require image-guided marking of skin site overlying nonpalpable tumor Blue tattooing of skin Risk of necrosis with methylene blue dye Less identification of internal mammary nodes
Subareolar or periareolar	Rapid lymphatic uptake Less shine through Can be used for cases of multiple breast tumors Does not require knowledge of tumor location Possibly more physiologic, based on embryologic lymphatic system development	"Blue breast" syndrome Risk of necrosis with methylene blue dye Less identification of IMNs

medicine technician) knows where the tumor is, which for nonpalpable lesions can be an issue. In addition, accidental injection into the cavity results in a failure of localization. Subsequent studies have shown that other methods of injection are equally accurate, if not more so. Periareolar, subareolar, and intradermal injections have all been used in various studies with both blue dye and radioactive colloid (Table 13–3). Intradermal injections still require knowledge of the tumor location, and unless the skin overlying the tumor is resected, will leave residual radiation and blue dye. For tumors in the upper outer quadrant, false gamma countersignals, colloquially referred to as "shine through" from a peritumoral or intradermal Tc99 injection can make identification of the SLN difficult. Many

surgeons advocate periareolar or subareolar injections for the radioactive colloid. This simplifies the procedure because the person injecting the tracer does not need to know where in the breast the tumor is. This also avoids the shine through phenomenon for upper outer quadrant tumors.

Lymphoscintigraphy

The use of routine lymphoscintigraphy is controversial in breast cancer lymphatic mapping (Fig. 13–6). If the surgeon is prepared to go after internal mammary lymph nodes should they take up the tracer, then lymphoscintigraphy is essential. The tracer should also be injected peritumorally because intradermal and periareolar injections rarely demonstrate

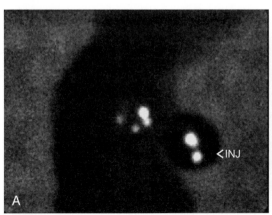
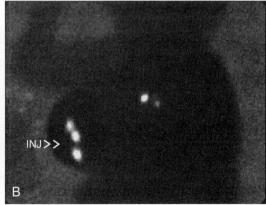

Figure 13–6. A, B: Lymphoscintigrams showing uptake in ipsilateral axillary lymph nodes after periareolar injection of Tc99.

internal mammary lymph nodes. Otherwise, the lymphoscintigraphy does not appear to be necessary or helpful in identifying the sentinel node. Cost and reimbursement issues, however, dictate that if nuclear medicine is going to be doing the injection of the radioactive colloid, then they must also perform lymphoscintigraphy. If lymphoscintigraphy is to be eliminated, then in most cases the surgeon will have to assume the responsibility for the storage and disposal of the radioactive substances and waste.

Sentinel Lymphadenectomy

Once the patient is in the operating room, injection of the blue dye takes place. Although many surgeons use isosulfan blue dye for this, the recent difficulties in obtaining Lymphazurin have led to many surgeons to use methylene blue instead, and in many cases liking it better than Lymphazurin, citing lower cost, fewer allergic reactions, and similar efficacy. If isosulfan blue dye is used, allergic reaction is an important complication of the procedure for the surgeon to keep in mind during this portion of the procedure and to discuss preoperatively with the patient. Allergic reactions can occur in 1% to 2% of patients. Most of these involve urticaria, blue hives, or pruritus, however about 0.5% may have bronchospasm and hypotension. If the patient is undergoing general anesthesia, it is reasonable to delay the injection of the blue dye until the airway is secured. Allergic reaction should be considered in any patient experiencing hypotension in which blue dye was used and is readily managed with fluid resuscitation and short-term pressor support.

Methylene blue does not carry the same risk of allergic reaction, however, it does carry the risk

of skin necrosis. For this reason, it should be diluted with normal saline. The recommended dilution is 2 ml of methylene blue dye and 3 ml of normal saline. It is also advisable to not perform an intradermal injection of the methylene blue dye, using peritumoral injections only.

The method of injection for the blue dye can be peritumoral, intradermal, or subareolar. Multiple studies suggest the superiority of intradermal injection compared to subdermal or deeper peritumoral breast injections. Injection of the dermal lymphatics is felt to drain the marker faster to the axilla than injection into the breast parenchyma. However, intradermal or subareolar injections of blue dye may cause tattooing of the nipple or skin, which may persist for months in patients undergoing breast conservation. In the case of methylene blue dye, skin necrosis is a significant complication as well. In a patient undergoing a mastectomy, either an intradermal or subareolar injection of the blue dye seems ideal. For the patient undergoing lumpectomy, intradermal injection can be used if the overlying skin will be resected with the tumor. Otherwise a peritumoral injection of the blue dye will provide adequate localization without leaving the breast tattooed for an extended period of time. Care must be taken to avoid injecting the blue dye into a cavity after an excisional biopsy. After injection, the breast is gently massaged for approximately 5 minutes.

Nodal excision is typically performed via a small axillary incision, posterior to the lateral border of the pectoral muscle. Preoperative scanning with the gamma probe is often helpful in planning the incision. The incision should be easily incorporated into an incision for a subsequent ALND (Fig. 13–7). Nodes that stained blue or with attached blue lymphatic

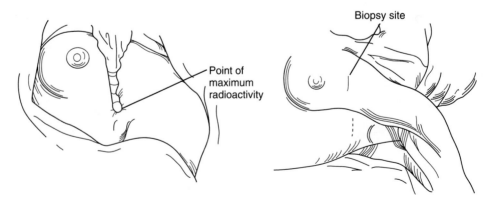

Figure 13–7. The gamma probe is used to identify the point of maximum counts. A small incision should be made here, being sure it can be easily incorporated into an incision for a subsequent axillary lymph node dissection.

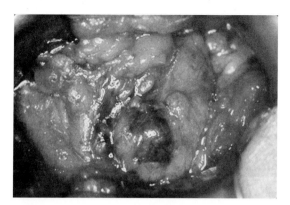

Figure 13-8. In vivo image of a sentinel lymph node taking up blue dye. A node is considered a sentinel lymph node if it is blue, partially blue, or has a blue stained lymphatic leading to it. (Image courtesy of Dr. Tara Breslin, Department of Surgery, University of Michigan.)

channels, or with evidence of radioactivity on the gamma probe, are excised intact and sent in formalin for pathologic review (Fig. 13–8). In addition, nodes that are palpably firm or enlarged should also be excised. The procedure is considered complete after scanning with the gamma probe fails to reveal further radioactive counts greater than 10% of the highest count detected.

In some cases the lymphoscintigraphy will demonstrate uptake in the internal mammary lymph nodes (IMNs; Fig. 13–9). The routine

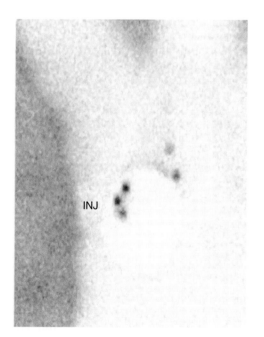

Figure 13-9. Lymphoscintigraphy showing uptake in the internal mammary nodes.

BOX 13-3 ARGUMENTS FOR AND AGAINST ROUTINE EXPLORATION AND BIOPSY OF INTERNAL MAMMARY LYMPH NODE UPTAKE ON LYMPHOSCINTIGRAPHY

For:

- The presence of metastases in the internal mammary lymph node (IMN) provides critical staging information and may impact adjuvant therapy.
- Possibly more prognostic than axillary nodes.
- Preventing IMN recurrence is crucial as this can be difficult to manage clinically.

Against:

- Technically challenging, risk of pneumothorax.
- Many patients with IMN uptake on lymphoscintigram will not have identifiable sentinel lymph node (SLN) at surgery.
- Few patients with IMN uptake have tumor involvement (0% to 6%) and many also have axillary involvement, hence impact on adjuvant therapy decisions is negligible.

biopsy of these nodes has become a point of much contention. Between 5% and 10% of patients undergoing lymphoscintigraphy will have evidence of radioactivity at the ipsilateral IMN chain. This is partly dependent on the method of injection. Internal mammary drainage is more commonly seen after peritumoral injection and much less so after subareolar or intradermal injection. In patients who drain only to the IMN, or to both the IMN and axillary nodes, the surgeon should consider each patient individually, considering the possible impact on subsequent therapy decisions should IMN metastases be identified (Box 13–3). A further discussion of the IMNs is presented later in this chapter.

Intraoperative Evaluation of the Sentinel Lymph Node Biopsy

Intraoperative evaluation of sentinel nodes has been investigated in a number of studies, in hopes of sparing patients from multiple operations for axillary staging and clearance. Frozen section analysis of SLNs has proved to be accurate for identifying macrometastatic lesions, however, this adds considerable time

BOX 13–4 RELATIVE ADVANTAGES AND DISADVANTAGES OF INTRAOPERATIVE SENTINEL LYMPH NODE ANALYSIS IN BREAST CANCER

	Advantages	Disadvantages
No routine intraoperative analysis	Less operating time Improved scheduling	All patients who are sentinel lymph node (SLN) positive require a second operation
Touch-prep cytology	Quick, minimal impact on operating time. Allows for simultaneous axillary lymph node dissection (ALND).	Adds some time to each case. More difficult to schedule cases if each case has possible ALND. Requires an experienced cytopathologist to read. Possibility of false-positives.
Frozen section	Highly accurate. Allows for simultaneous ALND. Read by pathologist.	Adds some time to each case. More difficult to schedule cases if each case has possible ALND.

to the procedure, and there is some concern that frozen section significantly decreases the subsequent detection of micrometastases. Touch-prep protocols provide a rapid approach to sentinel node diagnosis, with sensitivity ranging from 40% to 95.7%. Combining immunohistochemistry (IHC) with intraoperative touch-prep plus IHC increases the sensitivity to around 80%. Although a negative SLN intraoperatively does not completely preclude a return to the operating room for subsequently discovered metastases, it will spare many women the need for a second operation (Box 13–4).

Postoperative Care of the Sentinel Lymph Node Biopsy

The morbidity of SLN biopsy is dramatically less than with ALND, but this is not to say the procedure is without complication. Many surgeons are under the impression that SLN biopsy eliminates the risk of lymphedema, but this is not the case, with lymphedema rates reported between 1% and 7%. This partly depends on how one defines lymphedema. Lymphedema is more common for upper outer quadrant tumors and may be exacerbated by removing the sentinel node through the same incision used for the wide excision of an upper outer quadrant tumor (this also may complicate the radiation planning). Obesity is also a risk factor for lymphedema after SLN biopsy. Trauma or infection in the extremity in the postoperative period will increase the risk of lymphedema, and so patients should be cautioned to take care.

Seroma and infection are also possible complications of SLN biopsy. With the use of prophylactic antibiotics, wound infections are rare. Patients with a symptomatic seroma after biopsy can be easily managed by needle aspiration. Patients with asymptomatic seromas will typically resolve on their own, although this may take a few weeks. Hematoma formation is also a possible, albeit rare, complication of SLN biopsy. Any expanding hematoma should return to the operating room for evacuation and identification of any bleeding points. Delayed hematomas will resolve with time. Any attempt to aspirate a hematoma should be avoided because it is unlikely to work and may introduce infection. A large or symptomatic hematoma should be removed in the operating room.

A temporary sensory neuropraxia can occur after SLN biopsy from irritation of the intercostobrachial nerve. This can vary in intensity, from numbness of the region under the arm and along the inner aspect of the arm, to dysesthesias. Patients often describe a sunburnlike sensation or an itching that is not relieved by scratching. Patients should be reassured that these symptoms will resolve with time, although it may take several weeks. For the most severe cases, Neurontin may be of benefit. Injury to the motor nerves or to the brachial plexus is extremely uncommon after SLN biopsy.

Histopathologic Examination of the Sentinel Lymph Node

When an ALND is performed, the pathologist typically takes each node and bisects it, staining each half with hematoxylin and eosin (H&E) to identify tumor cells. Only a small area of each lymph node is examined because subjecting each lymph node to a more meticulous search, considering there may be from 10 to 30 lymph nodes in the specimen, is time and cost prohibitive. However, with SLN biopsy, the pathologist typically has only 1 to 4 lymph nodes to examine. This allows for serial sectioning for a more thorough examination of the nodes and the identification of metastases that would have otherwise been missed (Fig. 13–10). The nodes should be examined by H&E at a minimum of 2-mm intervals. With this technique, SLN biopsy is more sensitive at finding lymph node metastases than ALND.

A key feature of SLN biopsy is the detailed pathologic review. By focusing on a few nodes, rather than the entire axilla, a more thorough examination of each node in the sentinel node specimen is feasible (Fig. 13–11). As compared with bivalving the SLN, several studies have demonstrated the importance of obtaining multiple sections in detecting axillary metastases. Many centers also examine nodal sections with IHC, a more sensitive method of detecting metastatic cells. The use of IHC staining will be discussed in further detail later in the text.

With increased scrutiny of the SLN, smaller and smaller metastases can be identified. Although it would seem quite reasonable to presume that the discovery of any disease in the lymph node would portend a worse prognosis, this is not necessarily the case. Several retrospective studies of patients with negative ALND have involved reexamining the lymph

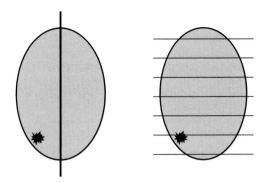

Figure 13–11. Step-sectioning the sentinel lymph node as opposed to bisecting it, allows for evaluation of a greater cross-sectional area of the lymph node and improves the accuracy of axillary staging. In this example, a micrometastasis would have been missed by bisection (false-negative) but is detected by step-sectioning.

nodes by serial sectioning and IHC, and the outcomes of patients with occult metastases compared to those without. Although some studies found a worse outcome associated with micrometastases, most found no negative impact on prognosis.

The significance of micrometastases detected by IHC is further called into question by the DCIS literature. Micrometastatic disease can be detected in as many as 10% of patients undergoing SLN biopsy for DCIS, which has a nearly 99% survival and for which axillary recurrences are extremely rare. In addition, three studies have demonstrated that micrometastases detected by IHC correlate more with the method of biopsy than with the biology of the cancer, suggesting they may be an artifact rather than a biologic phenomenon. Thus, the available evidence does not support the routine use of IHC in the evaluation of the SLN. IHC may be used selectively, such as in the case of lobular carcinoma, which may be difficult to identify in the lymph node. If metastases are detected by IHC, their presence should be confirmed on H&E.

Patients with micrometastases less than 0.2 mm are considered node negative (current American Joint Committee on Cancer [AJCC] staging stages these patients as N0mic) and should not be considered for completion dissection or adjuvant chemotherapy based solely on their nodal status. Patients with metastases greater than 0.2 mm should continue to be treated as node positive. Pending data from recent prospective trials will hopefully help clarify these issues.

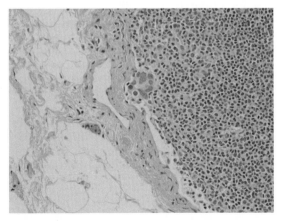

Figure 13–10. Micrometastases identified on sentinel lymph node biopsy. (Image courtesy of Dr. Maria Braman, Department of Pathology, University of Michigan.)

Management of the Clinically Positive Axilla

Axillary Lymph Node Dissection

Whether the disease was identified by physical examination, axillary ultrasound, or SLN biopsy, ALND remains the standard of care for patients with known involvement of the axillary lymph nodes. The few patients in whom a sentinel node cannot be identified, even intraoperatively, are also candidates for primary complete axillary lymphadenectomy for staging purposes. The axillary dissection for breast cancer involves en bloc resection of the level I and level II lymph nodes. The axilla is anatomically defined posteriorly by the subscapularis and latissimus dorsi muscles, medially by the chest wall and the overlying serratus anterior muscle, laterally by the skin and subcutaneous tissue of the underarm area, and superiorly by the axillary vein. These anatomic boundaries do not imply that lymph nodes do not reside above the axillary vein, and these nodes can be included in the specimen by pulling the fatty tissue above the vein inferiorly with the specimen, taking care not to injure the brachial plexus. However, aggressive dissection above the vein exposes the brachial plexus to injury. This area encompasses the intercostobrachial nerve(s), thoracodorsal bundle, and the long thoracic nerve, which are often intimately involved with the soft tissue and lymphatics of the surgical specimen.

The thoracodorsal bundle, consisting of a nerve, artery, and vein, contains the major blood supply and innervation to the latissimus dorsi. Disruption of the thoracodorsal nerve results in weakness during abduction and medial rotation of the shoulder. The long thoracic nerve is the sole motor nerve to the serratus anterior, a thin, flat muscle primarily responsible for anchoring the scapula to the posterior chest wall. Injury to the long thoracic nerve results in "winging" of the scapula, in which the medial edge of scapula protrudes involuntarily and uncomfortably from the posterior thorax.

Axillary dissection is accomplished in concert with mastectomy (a MRM) via an oblique elliptical mastectomy incision or in concert with a lumpectomy using a separate curvilinear incision connecting the anterior and posterior axillary lines, just inferior to the axillary hairline.

Technique

Patient Position

Before being brought back to the operating room, the correct arm for dissection should

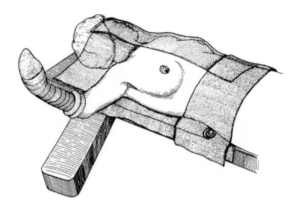

Figure 13–12. The patient is positioned supine with the arm out at 90 degrees, never hyperextended. The entire arm prepped to the wrist and the shoulder and lateral chest are prepped down to the table. The armboard is covered with a sterile drape and the arm sheathed to above the elbow with a sterile impervious Stockinette, keeping it within the sterile field. Bland KI, Copeland EM 111. The Breast, 3rd ed. Philadelphia: WB Saunders, 2004.

be marked in the preoperative area. This is not only to avoid performing a lymph node dissection on the wrong side, but also so that the nurses and anesthesia team place all intravenous lines, blood pressure cuffs, and monitors on the contralateral arm. Long-acting muscle relaxants should be avoided so that motor nerves can be identified during the procedure. Short-acting muscle relaxants during intubation are okay because these typically wear off before nerve identification.

The patient is positioned supine with the arm out at 90 degrees (Fig. 13–12). The arm should not be hyperextended at any point in the operation. The armboard should be padded appropriately to avoid subluxation of the shoulder because this can stretch the brachial plexus. Standard skin prep is used, with the entire arm prepped to the wrist. The shoulder and lateral chest are prepped down to the table because these will be exposed when the arm is brought across the chest. The armboard is covered with a sterile drape and the arm sheathed to above the elbow with a sterile impervious Stockinette. The arm is brought through a lap sheet, with the drapes underneath the shoulder so that the arm is within the operative field.

Procedure

The surgeon stands below the arm with a first assistant above the arm. If available, a second assistant can be positioned on the contralateral side. A curvilinear incision is made just inferior to the hair-bearing area, extending from just posterior to the pectoralis major muscle and just anterior to the latissimus dorsi muscle. The first step is to raise superior and inferior skin flaps. A common error is to make these flaps too thin. This does not increase the number of lymph nodes removed and can lead to a more pronounced cosmetic defect in the axilla. The incision should be carried straight down to just above the axillary fascia and then flaps created. Once the flaps are raised, the next step is to identify three landmarks; the pectoralis major and minor muscles, the axillary vein, and the latissimus dorsi muscle (Fig. 13–13). Although these can be identified in any order, the pectoralis muscle is usually the easiest to expose. Once identified, the lateral aspect of the pectoralis major muscle is exposed with electrocautery along its length. With the pectoralis major muscle retracted medially, the pectoralis minor muscle is exposed, and the investing fascia can be opened in a similar manner. During the exposure of the muscles, it is important to identify and preserve the medial pectoral neurovascular bundle. There is typically a small vascular branch coursing toward the axillary contents

that will need to be divided. However, cutting the nerve will cause atrophy of a portion of the pectoralis muscle and can be easily avoided with careful surgical technique.

The latissimus dorsi muscle can then be identified at the inferior aspect of the axilla and then exposed superiorly, staying on the anterior edge of the muscle to avoid injury to the thoracodorsal bundle. The latissimus dorsi muscle should be exposed to the point where the axillary vein crosses it. During this dissection, the lateral aspect of the intercostobrachial nerves will be encountered. Preserving these nerves, although adding time to the procedure, will avoid numbness of the upper inner arm.

Finally, the axillary vein needs to be exposed. The vein is often encountered during the exposure of the muscles. If it was not seen, careful exploration and dissection should be used to identify it. It is important not to dissect superior to the level of the axillary vein because an injury to the brachia plexus can be one of the most debilitating complications

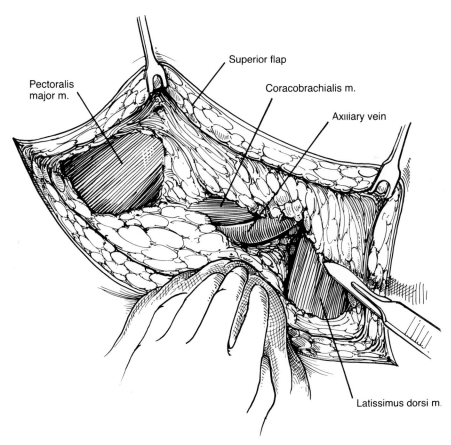

Figure 13–13. Superior and inferior flaps are raised, and the pectoralis major, latissimus dorsi, and axillary vein are identified.

of an ALND. Once the vein is identified, dissection should be on its inferior aspect. Skeletonizing the entire anterior surface of the vein may increase the potential for lymphedema. This dissection is greatly facilitated by retracting the axillary contents caudally. As the fat is dissected from the vein, small superficial branches of the axillary vein are divided and ligated with 3-0 silk sutures. As the vein is cleared laterally to medially, the next step is to identify the thoracodorsal bundle. The thoracodorsal vein is usually the first *deep* branch off of the axillary vein as one moves medially. The artery is often seen in close proximity. At this point, the nerve is not typically running with the vein, but rather located more medially (Fig. 13–14). It will eventually join the vein and artery as they course toward the latissimus dorsi muscle. Once the entire bundle is identified, the fibrofatty tissue can be cleared from the neurovascular structures so that they may be seen entering the latissimus dorsi muscle. Although this portion of the dissection may be deferred until the end of the case, with the optimal exposure it is worth

completing. During this dissection, it is important not to divide this tissue to reveal the bundle, but rather retract the tissue medially and dissect it off of the underlying subscapularis, sparing the thoracodorsal bundle. Otherwise the node-bearing tissue between the latissimus dorsi muscle and the thoracodorsal bundle is left behind.

As the thoracodorsal vein is cleared, a branch is noted heading toward the chest wall. This "crossing branch" can often provide a clue to the location of the long thoracic nerve. Some surgeons will routinely follow this branch to the serratus anterior at this point in the dissection to identify the long thoracic. Others identify the long thoracic after the dissection of the level II nodes. Either way is acceptable, but regardless of when the long thoracic is identified, this crossing branch should be preserved.

For a level I and II dissection, the pectoralis minor muscle must be raised to allow access to the level II nodes. Division of the fascia and ligation of the external mammary vessels found near the lateral border of the pectoralis

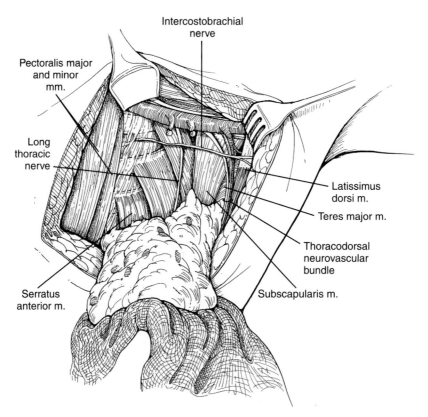

Figure 13–14. The thoracodorsal neurovascular bundle is seen laterally. Near the axillary vein, the thoracodorsal nerve is more medial than the artery and vein. As they course toward the latissimus dorsi, they are in closer proximity. (From Roses D. Breast cancer. Philadelphia: Elsevier, 2005.)

minor muscle allows for mobilization. Again, care is taken not to injure the medial pectoral nerve. The pectoralis minor is then retracted upward and medially to allow removal of the nodes beneath it. This is greatly facilitated by rotation of the arm medially. The exposure of the axillary vein can then be continued under the pectoralis minor muscle with inclusion of this fibrofatty tissue with the specimen. During this portion of the dissection, an aggressive use of suture ligation should be employed to avoid bleeding in a difficult to visualize area. In the patient with grossly involved lymph nodes, especially when level II involvement is suspected, a level III dissection should be included. This can be accomplished by dividing the pectoralis minor muscle near its origin. This should be done distal to the pectoral nerve so that innervation to the pectoralis major is preserved. With this added exposure, the node-bearing tissue medial to the pectoralis minor (the level III nodes) are easily included in the specimen.

The axillary contents are now dissected from medial to lateral off of the serratus anterior muscle. During this portion of the dissection, the medial aspect of the intercostobrachial nerve is identified, and the entire nerve can be freed from the specimen if the decision was made to preserve it. The long thoracic nerve is also identified. Unless disturbed by previous axillary surgery or tumor, the long thoracic nerve is in the same anteroposterior plane as the thoracodorsal nerve (Fig. 13–15). Knowing where the thoracodorsal nerve is will help the surgeon identify the long thoracic. The crossing branch of the thoracodorsal vein will serve the same purpose. The most common mistake is to look for the nerve directly on the serratus anterior, thus actually retracting the nerve into the specimen. The nerve is actually a few millimeters off of the muscle in the encapsulating fascia. Once identified, it is cleaned off along its length. With the intercostobrachial, thoracodorsal, and long thoracic nerves identified and cleared, all that remains is to free the axillary contents from the underlying subscapularis muscle between the nerves. With both nerves visualized, the tissue between the nerves may be clamped at the inferior margin of the vein and suture ligated. The tissue may now be dissected free from the muscle. It is important not to rush through this portion because excessive retraction of the

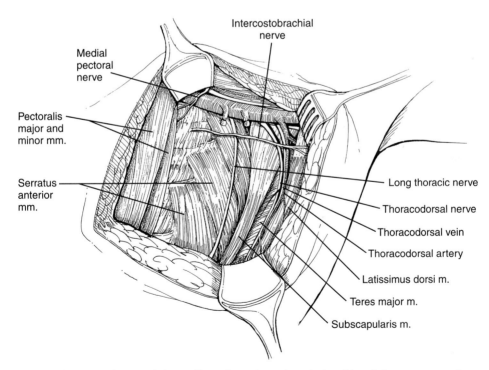

Figure 13–15. After completion of the axillary dissection, the relationship of the nerves can be seen. The intercostobrachial nerve can be identified and preserved. The long thoracic nerve is identified slightly lateral to the serratus anterior, in the encapsulating fascia. The long thoracic nerve is in the same anteroposterior plane as the thoracodorsal nerve, so knowing where the thoracodorsal nerve is will help the surgeon identify the long thoracic. (From Roses D. Breast cancer. Philadelphia: Elsevier, 2005.)

specimen inferiorly can pull either the thoracodorsal or long thoracic nerve into the specimen and lead to an inadvertent injury. The nerves should be visualized throughout this portion of the dissection.

Once the specimen is removed, hemostasis is assured and a closed suction catheter is placed through a separate incision lower on the chest wall. Do not place this stab incision too far posterior because this will inconvenience the patient. The drain is secured with a Nylon suture and attached to a suction reservoir. The wound is closed with absorbable subcutaneous sutures and the skin may be reapproximated with a subcuticular stitch or tissue adhesive.

Postoperative Care

The patient is discharged after being instructed on drain management (Box 13-5). The patient should be taught to care for the drain and to record the amount of drainage. When the volume in the reservoir is less than 30 ml/24 hours, the drain can be removed. All patients will have some limited abduction of the shoulder after ALND, but this will return to normal with routine exercises or physical therapy once the wound is completely healed. Some patients will completely avoid use of the arm or keep the arm in a sling after the operation. This should be strongly discouraged because this can result in capsular contracture and a frozen shoulder. Exercises are given to the patient to encourage mobility; some are to be performed immediately, and others to be included after the drain is removed. Physical therapy may be necessary to return to a full range of motion. An orthopaedic consult may be needed in those rare cases in which full range of motion does not return with physical therapy.

Management of the Internal Mammary Lymph Nodes

The breast drains predominantly to the axillary lymph nodes, but also drains to the supraclavicular, infraclavicular, cervical, and IMNs. Anatomically, 75% of the breast lymphatics drain toward the axilla, and 25% drain into the IMNs. Going back to the early part of the last century, attempts to improve on the Halsted radical mastectomy included attempts to include the IMN with the resection (known as the extended radical mastectomy [ERM]). This failed to improve survival, and momentum shifted toward less radical surgery, the MRM. The ERM did, however, give us information on the incidence of IMN metastases in breast cancer. Contrary to what many surgeons believe, metastases to the IMN do not come only from the inner quadrants of the breast, but rather from all quadrants. The likelihood of IMN drainage does decrease as one moves from medial to lateral. Overall, there appears to be a low risk of metastases to the IMN in the absence of metastases in the axillary lymph nodes. In a study of over 7000 patients who had ERM, the overall incidence of IMN metastases was 22%, but only 10% when the axillary lymph nodes were negative. Of those patients with negative axillary nodes, the risk of IMN metastases for medial lesions was 14%, but only 6.5% for lateral lesions.

Given the morbidity of IMN dissection and the low likelihood of finding disease in the IMNs that would change adjuvant chemotherapy decisions, few surgeons advocated routine IMN biopsy for breast cancer. However, with the advent of SLN biopsy, the question of how to best handle the IMN has returned.

Lymphatic mapping with lymphoscintigraphy may identify IMN in as high as 25% of cases, depending on the method of injection of the Tc99. When Tc99 is injected peritumorally, there will be drainage to the axilla in 99% of cases. In 76%, this is the only drainage. In 10%, there is primary drainage to the axilla with secondary drainage to the IMNs. In 5% there was drainage to the IMNs primarily, with secondary drainage to the axilla. The remaining cases include combinations of drainage to the axillary, IMNs, and clavicular lymph nodes. Other studies have shown slightly higher rates of IMN-only drainage, as high as 4%. However, if the Tc99 is injected in a subareolar or intradermal manner, drainage to the IMNs is a relatively rare occurrence.

Studies of IMN metastases in the age of SLN biopsy show patterns similar to that in the age of the ERM, with metastases in the IMNs in 27% of patients who have axillary node metastases but only in 7% of patients who are negative in the axilla. As one would expect, the presence of disease in the IMNs is independently prognostic. Patients tumor-free in both basins have a higher survival than that of patients with disease in either the axillary or IMNs. The survival is the lowest for patients with disease in both basins.

Whether or not to biopsy these nodes if they light up on lymphoscintigraphy remains controversial. Unidentified disease in the IMNs

BOX 13–5 PATIENT INSTRUCTIONS ON DRAIN MANAGEMENT

Care of Your Drain

After your surgery you will go home with a bulb drain in place. The drain will remove fluid that builds up under your wound to promote healing. The drain generally does not cause pain.

1. For the first 3 days, it is recommended that you clean the area where the drain tubing enters your body and change the gauze. Clean the insertion site using cotton-tipped swabs and a solution of one-half water and one-half peroxide.
2. Apply a clean drain sponge around the insertion site daily. You may it more often if it becomes heavily soiled.
3. After 2 days you may shower or gently wash the area where the drain tubing enters your body.
4. You may use nonperfumed soaps (Ivory or Neutrogena).
5. Always pat dry, never rub.
6. Reapply gauze after cleansing.
7. Women should continue to wear their bra.

Notify your doctor or the breast care center if:

- The reservoir cannot be reactivated (it quickly reexpands).
- The drain falls out or the stitch holding the drain tube comes out.
- The drainage fluid in the reservoir becomes foul smelling.
- You have a fever or there is any increased redness, swelling, or drainage from the site.
- There is an air leak, fluid leak, or malfunction of the drain bulb.
- Clots form in the tubing and block drainage and cannot be cleared by "milking" the drain tubing.

Emptying the Drain (Reservoir)

You will need to empty and reactivate the drain bulb (reservoir). You will also need to record the amount of fluid collected in the reservoir. Empty the reservoir as many times a day as directed by your doctor or nurse or if full. Wash your hands before and after handling the reservoir. Empty the reservoir into the measuring container when the fluid collected reaches the 100 ml mark or before. Do *not* let the reservoir completely fill because the drainage will stop.

Keep a record of the amount of fluid collected in the reservoir. Record the date, time, and amount of fluid that has accumulated from *each* reservoir. If the drainage stops within the first few days after your surgery there may be a clot in the drain tubing. Try milking or "stripping" the drain if this is the case.

Attach the reservoir (using the plastic strap) to your bra or shirt, usually with a safety pin. Do not disconnect, kink, or puncture the tubing that is connected to the reservoir. You will notice the amount of drainage decreasing over time. The color of the drainage will also lighten over time.

Milking or Stripping the Drain Tubing

To keep the drain working well you will be shown how to milk the drain tubing three times per day. You should always wash your hands before handling the drain.

- Grasp the tubing close to your body with one hand and pull toward your body.
- With your other hand, grasp the tubing below the first hand.
- Using an alcohol swab, pinch tubing tightly, sliding your fingers down the tubing and away from your body, repeat this two or three times.
- Be sure that the drainage is flowing into the bulb. It is okay if the tube becomes flat from the suction. *Never* disconnect the tubing from the bulb at any time.

could potentially account for the poor prognosis of patients falsely labeled as node negative based on the axillary sentinel node. Identifying disease in the IMNs could potentially upstage patients and change adjuvant therapy decisions, especially for patients with smaller tumors who, based on T stage alone, would not receive chemotherapy if their axillary nodes were negative. In addition, the presence of microscopic disease in the IMNs might change the radiation fields to include the internal mammary chain, although this is associated with increased morbidity. Excising sentinel nodes from the IMN that harbor microscopic disease might also decrease the risk of parasternal recurrences. For these reasons, some surgeons advocate the routine biopsy of these nodes when performing SLN biopsy. If this is to be done, peritumoral injections of Tc99 are mandatory.

On the other hand, the increasing use of chemotherapy for patients who are node negative and the availability of Oncotype DX to make adjuvant therapy decisions (see Chapter 16) lessens the impact of a positive IMN on decision making. The decision to radiate the IMN is often made on the tumor size, location, and presence of disease in the axillary nodes. Recurrent disease in the IMN is not a common occurrence. Given the additional morbidity of excising an internal mammary SLN, including the risk of pneumothorax, many surgeons opt not to go after SLN in the IMN, and inject the Tc99 in a manner that is unlikely to demonstrate IMN drainage on lymphoscintigraphy.

Internal Mammary Sentinel Lymph Node Biopsy

The internal mammary lymph node biopsy often takes breast and general surgeons outside their area of comfort. For surgeons who feel that biopsy of the IMN should be performed when the lymphoscintigraphy shows uptake, but do not feel comfortable performing the procedure themselves, it is not unreasonable to do so in conjunction with a thoracic surgeon. The drawback to this approach is obviously that of scheduling because it is usually not known whether the thoracic surgeon is needed until the day of (or night before) the surgery.

The internal mammary sentinel node can be excised through the same incision as the mastectomy, and in many cases, (because most tumors that drain to the IMNs are medial) the lumpectomy incision. In the rare case in which a more lateral tumor drains to the IMNs, a separate incision can be made parallel to the sternum, approximately 3 cm from the lateral sternal margin. The pectoralis muscle needs to be exposed for approximately 2 to 3 cm over the interspace identified by the gamma probe. When performing the biopsy through a lumpectomy incision, this may require raising the breast parenchyma off of the underlying muscle.

The pectoralis major muscle fibers are split to expose the superior intercostal space, exposing the external and internal intercostals muscles. These need to be divided transversely from the sternal border for approximately 3 to 4 cm. The two potential injuries during this part of the procedure are to the anterior intercostal vessels and to the inferior parietal pleura, leading to pneumothorax. The vessels course along the inferior aspect of each rib and are avoided by dividing the muscles in the middle. Care must be taken not to injure the parietal pleura when dividing the internal intercostals muscle. If it does occur, it can be closed with a fine absorbable suture, and postoperative chest tubes are rarely necessary.

After dividing the intercostals, the internal mammary vessels should be identifiable. The artery is approximately 1 to 1.5 cm from the lateral sternal border. They are located in an extrapleural space, surrounded by fibrofatty tissue and lymphatics. This tissue is divided and small vessels coagulated. A vessel loop should be placed around the artery and vein (either together or separately). This not only helps keep the vessels in view, but it helps prevent major bleeding in the case of accidental transection. While encircling the vein, coagulation or clipping of some small venous branches might be needed.

If excessive bleeding from the vein occurs, it can be ligated. The artery should be preserved in case it is needed in the future for pedicled transverse rectus abdominis myocutaneous (TRAM) flap reconstruction or coronary artery bypass graft (CABG). However, if transection does occur, the rib may need to be either disarticulated or transected to obtain control.

Once the vessels are controlled, the probe is used to identify the node within the surrounding adipose tissue. The SLN may be either medial or lateral to the vessels. The node is excised, taking care to clip or coagulate the small surrounding vessels.

The wound is irrigated and on the final irrigation, the water left within the wound and observed for small air bubbles that would be indicative of an injury to the pleura. The fibers of the pectoralis muscle are reapproximated using 2-0 Vicryl sutures, although pulling these too tightly will transect the muscle fibers. If the procedure was performed through a lumpectomy incision, the breast parenchyma can be reapproximated to restore the shape of the breast.

In the recovery room, a chest x-ray should be obtained to rule out a pneumothorax, if there is any question regarding the pleura.

Internal Mammary Node Dissection

An internal mammary node dissection is an extremely rare operation, typically done in conjunction with a mastectomy when there are grossly involved internal mammary lymph nodes. The surgeon identifies the attachment of the pectoralis major muscle to the sternum

and the first rib. In the first intercostals space, the medial fibers of the pectoralis major are split, and the intercostal muscles are identified (Fig. 13–16). The intercostal muscles are divided from the sternal border to about 3 cm laterally. Underneath this, the internal mammary vessels can be identified. These are ligated. The fifth rib is then identified, and the intercostal space between the fifth and sixth rib is entered in a similar manner, identifying the internal mammary vessels and ligating them. A tunnel can be established underneath the pectoralis major muscle. A sternal knife is placed into the first interspace, directed medially to the mid sternum, and directed down through the mid sternum to the level of the fifth intercostal space, and then directed laterally to come out in the fifth intercostal space. The chondral portion of the second, third, fourth, and fifth ribs are transected lateral to

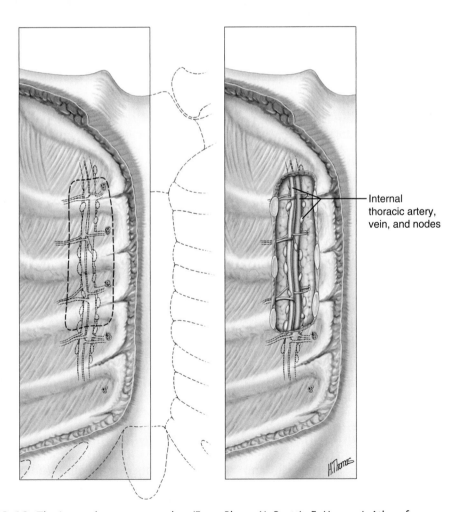

Internal thoracic artery, vein, and nodes

Figure 13–16. The internal mammary nodes. (From Bloom N, Beattie E, Harvey J. Atlas of cancer surgery. Philadelphia: Elsevier, 2000.)

the origin of the pectoralis muscle. When transecting the ribs, care is taken to secure the intercostal vessels at the lower margin of each rib. The entire internal mammary lymph node chain can be removed in this manner, along with the pleura underneath. Chest tubes are placed through the skin distal to the lower skin flap and within the chest wall defect to manage the pneumothorax.

Is Axillary Lymph Node Dissection Necessary for a Positive Sentinel Lymph Node Biopsy?

Just as lumpectomy greatly minimized the morbidity of breast surgery compared to mastectomy, SLN biopsy has done the same for axillary surgery compared to ALND. As described previously, ALND may be safely avoided in the 80% of women with negative sentinel node biopsies. What about the 20% of patients with a positive sentinel node biopsy? As many as one half of patients with a positive SLN will have additional disease detected in the nonsentinel lymph nodes (NSLNs). Documenting the number of involved nodes provides further staging information that may impact adjuvant chemotherapy and radiation decisions because multiple involved lymph nodes are associated with increased recurrence rates and decreased survival. In many patients, however, simply knowing the patient is node positive or node negative may be enough information to determine the remainder of their therapy. In these patients, is there a therapeutic benefit to gaining regional control, or can these patients be observed, with ALND performed, only if they recur?

As almost all patients with node-positive SLN will receive adjuvant systemic therapy, regional recurrence in this situation may be extremely low. But even if recurrence did occur, and the patient undergoes a delayed ALND, would this impact their survival? As mentioned, the NSABP B-04 trial specifically addressed this issue, and after a 25-year follow-up, did not demonstrate any difference in overall survival among patients undergoing axillary dissection, axillary radiation, or delayed axillary clearance for recurrence. This is the strongest evidence against the need for ALND. However, the study was not large enough to detect a small but meaningful difference in survival, and many surgeons, in the habit of routinely performing MRMs, still removed a substantial number of axillary lymph nodes when performing a simple mastectomy, clouding the

results. There are also other studies suggesting there is a survival benefit to the early removal of micrometastatic disease in the lymph nodes.

One of the largest of these studies was conducted at the Institut Curie from 1982 to 1987. The Curie study randomized 658 patients to either lumpectomy and axillary dissection or lumpectomy with postoperative radiation. Enrollment was limited to patients who were clinically node negative with tumors less than 3 cm in size. Five-year follow-up demonstrated a 4% survival benefit ($p = 0.014$) for patients undergoing axillary dissection compared with those with axillary radiation only. A meta-analysis of six randomized controlled trials examining axillary node dissection in early breast cancer demonstrated a 5.4% overall survival benefit for patients who were clinically node negative undergoing axillary dissection.

However, these studies have limitations. The meta-analysis included several sizable European studies (including the Institut Curie study) conducted from the 1950s to the 1980s. Since that time, there have been significant advances in screening, surgical management, and adjuvant therapy. It is unclear whether these results translate to today. More importantly, in some of these studies, patients who were found to be node positive were treated with adjuvant chemotherapy, an option not available to women who did not undergo ALND. Thus, there is a significant treatment bias between the two groups.

Although these data suggest a possible benefit to controlling regional disease, one cannot assume that the results obtained with the omission of ALND among patients who were clinically node negative from years ago would be the same as among patients who are SLN positive today. Neither the risk of distant disease, nor the amount of residual disease in the axillary nodes, is directly comparable. The only way to determine whether ALND may be safely omitted for patients with a positive SLN would be a randomized trial, which was initiated by the American College of Surgeons Oncology Group (ACoSOG), but unfortunately closed prematurely as a result of poor accrual. Therefore, the therapeutic benefit of completion ALND remains unknown.

Rather than declaring whether ALND is or is not necessary, if one could accurately predict which patients are so unlikely to harbor additional disease in the remaining nodes, a selective approach to complete ALND could be applied. Although some clinicopathologic features such as the size and grade of the primary tumor, the size of the lymph node metastases, or the ratio of positive SLN to the number of SLN removed may help stratify risk, no factor appears sufficient to select patients who may avoid dissection. Even the lowest risk groups have a 10% to 20% chance of harboring additional disease. Although the use of statistical models or nomograms may better select patients with a low likelihood of harboring disease in the NSLN, it must be cautioned that these studies underestimate the risk of additional disease, as the NSLN are not subjected to the histologic scrutiny to which the sentinel node is subjected.

Complete ALND is not the only option available to patients with a positive SLN. Axillary radiation may be a reasonable alternative, as evidenced by data from before the emergence of SLN biopsy. In a series of 418 women treated with axillary radiation therapy after either no or limited ALND, only 1.4% developed a regional failure after 8 years of follow-up. Of the subset of patients who had a limited ALND with positive nodes, the regional failure rate was 7% (3 of 42 cases). A randomized trial in Italy of ALND versus axillary radiation therapy accrued 435 patients, and after a mean follow-up of 66 months, recorded only one axillary recurrence in the radiation arm and two axillary recurrences in the surgery arm. Although these data suggest that axillary radiation may be effective in obtaining regional control, it is again difficult to transpose these numbers to the population who is SLN positive. A randomized trial of axillary radiation versus ALND for patients who are SLN positive is presently accruing patients and will not only answer these questions, but also help determine whether axillary radiation truly decreases the morbidity of treatment compared with surgery.

Complications Associated with Sentinel Lymph Node Biopsy

Sentinel node biopsy has greatly reduced the morbidity of breast cancer surgery, sparing 80% of women from the morbidity of an axillary node dissection. However, sentinel node biopsy is not without morbidity. While the complications of sentinel node biopsy are relatively minor compared with a full node dissection, there can be serious complications that must be discussed with the patient. In addition to the surgical complications of the procedure, there are also technical complications, specifically a failure to find the sentinel lymph node at all or a false negative finding.

Inability to Find the Sentinel Node

Being unable to find the sentinel node is a relatively rare occurrence. A meta-analysis of SLN biopsy, reveals overall identification rate of 96% and overall false negative rate of 8.4%; this analysis included data from 69 studies involving 10,454 patients. Many of these occurred when surgeons had just started using sentinel node biopsy (early on the learning curve) and when surgeons were using a single mapping agent in comparison to using both blue dye and isotope. With more experience and more surgeons using the dual-tracer technique, the identification rate is likely higher and the false-negative rate lower. Older age, obesity, previous excisional biopsy, tumor location, and tumor size have been implicated as other factors leading to either a failure to find the SLN or a false-negative finding, although these have been variable across studies, and many decrease as significant factors with increased experience. For example, if the mapping procedure is being performed after a prior excisional biopsy, there is a risk of inadvertent injection into the biopsy cavity and the mapping agent will not reach the nodal basin. As experience with lymphatic mapping grew, these technical failures declined and investigators have specifically documented the ability to reliably identify the SLN in the setting of prior excisional biopsy. The method of injection of the tracers may also impact the ability to find the SLN biopsy, as previously discussed.

Given the importance of the axillary nodal status on guiding adjuvant therapy decisions and the potential benefit of removing nodal disease early, if a SLN is not identified, a level I and II axillary lymph node dissection should be performed. Patients should be warned and consented for this possibility.

Allergic Reaction to Blue Dye

A rare, but serious, risk of sentinel node biopsy is the potential allergic reaction to isosulfan blue or patent blue dye. Allergic reactions to methylene blue have not been described. This complication requires rapid recognition and intervention. Within a few minutes to an hour following blue dye injection, 1% to 2% of patients may experience sudden hemodynamic instability and other sequelae of intraoperative anaphylaxis. It is therefore prudent to alert the anesthesiologist when beginning the injection of the blue dye. Although it can be a shocking moment to have a young healthy woman suddenly drop her heart rate and blood pressure, these episodes are usually readily responsive to supportive care, which includes discontinuation of the gaseous anesthetics, 100% oxygen, aggressive fluid resuscitation, and pressor support. In most cases the anesthesia and surgical procedure can be resumed and completed uneventfully after the patient has been stabilized. If there is any question, it is not unreasonable to abandon the procedure, let the patient recover, and schedule it at a later date using radiocolloid only. Either way, patients should be monitored closely for 24 hours because continued uptake of the blue dye from skin and soft tissue can result in protracted or delayed secondary (biphasic) reactions.

Surgeons and anesthesiologists should also be aware that blue dyes can also cause a spurious decline in pulse oximetry measurements, related to intravascular uptake and interference with spectroscopy; arterial blood gases in these circumstances will reveal normal oxygenation. Although the impact of the blue dye should be recognized as the most likely cause, a sudden drop in pulse oximetry measurements should still prompt verification that the pulse oximetry is working, the endotracheal tube is in place, and the patient is ventilating well. A less severe form of allergic reaction to the blue dye that can occur is "blue urticaria" or "blue hives."

Allergic reactions to isosulfan blue dye or patent blue dye do not seem to correlate with past allergy history. A history of sulfa allergy does not preclude the use of isosulfan blue dye, but a known allergy to triphenylmethane is a contraindication to blue dye use. It is believed that prior sensitization from exposure to industrial dyes in cosmetics, textiles, detergents, and such may be the cause, but preoperative skin testing is unreliable in identifying high-risk patients. Some anesthesiologists prefer to premedicate patients before the injection of blue dye with steroids, antihistamines, or histamine receptor blockade, although the true benefit of this approach is unknown.

Methylene blue dye does not appear to carry the same risk of allergic reaction, and there are several reports that methylene blue dye is just as reliable as isosulfan or patent blue dye. However, methylene blue dye does carry a risk of skin necrosis after dermal injection. If methylene blue dye is to be used, it should not be injected intradermally or subareolarly unless that area will be widely resected (as with a mastectomy), and it should be diluted with normal saline before injection (2 ml of methylene blue with 3 ml of saline).

Surgical Complications of Sentinel Lymph Node Biopsy

As with any incision, the SLN biopsy can be associated with bleeding (hematoma) and wound infection, although both of these are rare complications. Seroma formation after SLN biopsy can occur and is readily treatable by needle aspiration. Other complications of SLN biopsy are similar to those seen in ALND, including axillary web formation, neurosensory disturbances, and lymphedema. Although it is rare, and certainly less common than with ALND, it is a mistake to believe that SLN biopsy completely avoids the risk of lymphedema. Lymphedema rates have been described in as many of 5% to 7% of SLN biopsy procedures.

Complications of Axillary Lymph Node Dissection

Nerve Injuries

Nerve injuries can occur during ALND that can result in a variety of neuropathies (Box 13–6). The most severe is a brachial plexopathy, which can occur from direct injury to the brachial plexus during dissection, or from extreme manipulations of the arm during positioning or during the procedure. This can result in both numbness and tingling of the fingers and dysesthesias of the arm. It can also

BOX 13–6 MAJOR COMPLICATIONS OF AXILLARY LYMPH NODE DISSECTION

Seroma
Infection
Paresthesia
Chronic pain
Shoulder immobility
Axillary vein thrombosis
Thoracodorsal nerve injury
Long thoracic nerve injury (winged scapula)
Brachial plexopathy
Arm lymphedema
Breast lymphedema

cause weakness of the upper extremity, and in the most severe of cases, paralysis. All of these are temporary. Physical therapy is helpful in this situation.

The most common neuropathy comes from ligation of the intercostobrachial nerve, which is often done routinely during an ALND (although it can be preserved). This causes numbness in the inner side of the upper arm. Sometimes this is simply an absence of sensation. Other patients may describe pain similar to that of a sunburn or a dull ache. The painful sensations will resolve, although it does take some time. In severe cases, Neurontin may be of benefit. When the intercostobrachial nerve is cut, the size of the anesthetic area may get smaller with time, although there may always be some areas without sensation.

Motor nerve injuries are less common with ALND. Injury to the long thoracic nerve results in paralysis of the serratus anterior and the "winged scapula." This presents as a posterior shoulder bony protrusion. Patients will often complain of discomfort sitting up against a hard surface. Asking the patient to extend her arms in front of her will exaggerate the deformity. Often, the nerve is intact but overstimulation or stretching causes a temporary paralysis. In this case, return of normal muscle function (and alleviation of the winged scapula) will occur in a few weeks. If the nerve was transected, this will be a permanent deformity.

The thoracodorsal nerve innervates the latissimus dorsi muscle. Atrophy of this muscle after injury to the nerve will make the tip of the scapula more prominent. It will also limit the patients from abducting and internally rotating the humerus. Patients may notice an inability to reach posteriorly as high on the back as before. Injury to the medial pectoral nerve will deprive the lateral half of the pectoralis major muscle of innervation. This may not be noticed by a patient who had breast conservation or reconstruction, but it may detract from the cosmetic results of a mastectomy.

Cording or Limited Range of Motion

Cording (axillary web syndrome) can occur after ALND and is defined as visible cordlike bands in the chest wall and axilla that may run down the upper arm. They can sometimes reach as far as the thumb. These restrict the motion of the upper arm and can occasionally be tender. The reported occurrence of cording is between 5%

and 10% after ALND, although neither the true incidence nor the pathophysiology is well understood. Cording will eventually resolve in about 2 months, particularly with physical therapy, which includes passive stretch and soft tissue mobilization. Other patients may have stiffness and limited range of motion of the shoulder, without cording or axillary webs. These patients also often respond rapidly to a program of exercises and physical therapy.

Lymphedema

The most significant complication of an ALND is lymphedema of the upper extremity. Approximately 10% to 30% of patients who have an ALND will experience lymphedema. This increases dramatically if the axilla is irradiated after an ALND. The risk of lymphedema also increases with obesity and the extent of the dissection (Box 13–7). The standard ALND is limited to levels I and II. A level III dissection is generally considered unnecessary (unless there is grossly apparent disease present in the axillary apex) because skip metastases to level III only occur in 2% to 3% of cases.

The greatest risk of lymphedema occurs within the first 3 years after surgery; however, there is a lifelong risk and even a minor trauma can trigger lymphedema many years after ALND. Often a precipitating event cannot be identified. Axillary irradiation alone can cause lymphedema, as can the regional recurrence of disease. Any patient who develops lymphedema years after ALND should be evaluated for signs of recurrent disease.

Lymphedema occurs when increased protein leakage into the interstitial fluid increases the osmotic pressure and draws more water into the tissue spaces. Normally, there is a balance between the hydrostatic pressure and colloid osmotic pressure as one goes from the

BOX 13–7 RISK FACTORS FOR LYMPHEDEMA AMONG PATIENTS UNDERGOING AXILLARY SURGERY

Extent of surgery
Radiation
Regional recurrence
Infection
Inflammatory diseases (rheumatoid arthritis, chronic dermatitis)
Venous obstruction
Obesity
Air travel

arteriole to the capillary and then to the venule. However, obstruction to the outflow of lymph (as occurs with ALND) will increase the leakage of plasma protein into the tissue. Other factors that accelerate protein leakage include venous obstruction, injury, infection, or arteriolar dilation (as with heat or exercise).

Early in its development, lymphedema is reversible (see Box 13–7). However, untreated it can progress to fibrosis and nonpitting edema. Fibroblasts organize the excess proteins within the tissues, and this process cannot be reversed. Long-standing lymphedema can result in limited mobility of the arm, brachial plexus stretch injury from the increased weight, and Stewart-Treves syndrome. This is one of the most serious long-term sequelae of chronic lymphedema and describes the development of angiosarcoma in the affected arm. Although frequently referred to as "lymphangiosarcoma," the cancer arises in the endothelial cells of blood vessels, so this term is technically incorrect. Angiosarcoma of the involved extremity often presents as bluish-reddish macular lesions nodules on the skin of the arm and can be difficult to treat, sometimes requiring amputation of the extremity. Unfortunately, most patients who develop angiosarcoma will die of distant disease, with a median survival of only 2 years.

Given the difficult in treating lymphedema and the long-term risks, great emphasis is placed on prevention and early intervention if lymphedema occurs. Prevention of lymphedema begins with educating the patient on what to avoid (Box 13–8). Any patient who has had an ALND will need to minimize the chance of injury to that extremity for life. The patient needs to inform all doctors and nurses that they have had an ALND so that blood pressures, intravenous lines, or blood draws can be done on the opposite arm. The patient should wear protective clothing (long sleeves or gloves) to avoid cuts or scratches when gardening or doing household projects. If a minor injury does occur, it should be treated promptly with antiseptics. A compression garment should be worn prophylactically when on an airplane. Extremes in temperature should also be avoided, as with sunburns, hot tubs or saunas, or reaching into hot water or ovens and dryers.

Management of Lymphedema

The onset and presentation of lymphedema may be quite variable. Some patients may have a transient lymphedema within the first

BOX 13–8 RECOMMENDATIONS AFTER AXILLARY LYMPH NODE DISSECTION TO MINIMIZE LYMPHEDEMA

- Use the opposite arm for intravenous catheters, blood draws, injections, or blood pressure measurements. Always inform all doctors and nurses that you have had a lymph node dissection on that side.
- Avoid cuts, scratches, or burns to your hand and arm by wearing long sleeves and/or gloves when doing cooking, gardening, household projects, etc. If you do cut yourself, wash immediately with soap and water and apply an antiseptic. Notify your physician of any redness or swelling.
- Do not wear tight or constricting jewelry or clothing. Bra straps should be wide, padded, and not cut into the skin.
- Avoid heavy lifting with that arm. Try not to carry a purse or suitcase on that side when possible. Avoid repetitive heavy lifting in particular, and wear a compression sleeve if lifting is necessary.
- Avoid sunburn of the arm by wearing long sleeves and sunscreen.
- Do not pick at cuticles or hangnails.
- Use insect repellents.
- Avoid high temperatures (saunas or hot tubs, reaching into hot ovens or clothes driers).
- Shave under the arm with an electric razor rather than a blade.
- Wear a compression sleeve on the arm when traveling on an airplane.
- Maintain an ideal body weight.

2 months of treatment (surgery or radiation) that resolves on its own. Other patients may go months to years without any signs or symptoms of lymphedema, and then notice its onset after air travel, excessive use of the arm, minor trauma, or sitting in a hot tub. Other triggers include venipuncture or cellulitis. In some cases this may be reversible, or at least manageable, whereas in others, the disease will progress to a morbid and irreversible situation (Box 13–9).

Patients with lymphedema may have symptoms of lymphedema before the onset of a notable swelling. These may include a sensation of fullness or heaviness of the arm. When swelling does occur, it may occur anywhere in the upper extremity. It may start in the hand

BOX 13–9 SYMPTOMS ASSOCIATED WITH EARLY LYMPHEDEMA

- Pain, dull aching
- Tightness
- Stiffness or limited range of motion
- Heavy feeling
- Decreased strength

TABLE 13–4 • *International Society of Lymphology Staging of Lymphedema*

Stage	Description	Severity based on limb volume
0	Lymphostasis: A subclinical condition in which swelling is not evident despite impaired lymph transport.	None
I	An early accumulation of fluid relatively high in protein content. Edema decreases with elevation. Pitting may occur.	Minimal (<20% increase)
II	Edema that does not significantly reduce with elevation. In late stage II the tissues are increasingly fibrotic.	Moderate (20% to 40% increase)
III	Lymphostatic elephantiasis: Pitting is absent, and there are trophic changes (acanthosis, fat deposits, verrucous hyperplasia).	Severe (>40% increase)

or forearm and then progress up the arm, or it may begin in the upper arm or trunk. Left untreated, lymphedema can cause multiple adverse effects.

Lymphedema is typically not painful, but it is associated with uncomfortable feelings such as the arm being "achy," "heavy," or "tight." The most common consequence of lymphedema is limited range of motion of the upper extremity. Depending on the location and severity of the swelling, this can involve any of the joints of the arm. Lymphedema can be particularly hard on the shoulder joint as a result of the increased weight of the arm and the traction it places on the joint. This can lead to tendonitis or bursitis.

Patients with lymphedema have an increased risk of developing cellulitis or erysipelas (a superficial cellulitis with lymphatic vessel involvement). This can begin as a few red blotchy areas that spread and coalesce and trigger fever, chills, and myalgias. Management of cellulitis requires rest, elevation, and antibiotics. The most common organism associated with cellulitis in patients with lymphedema is *Streptococcus pyogenes* (Group A β-hemolytic strep). Less common are *Staphylococcus aureus*, *Escherichia coli*, and *Pseudomonas*. If the case is mild, oral antibiotics are appropriate; however, a severe infection or signs of systemic disease should prompt admission and intravenous antibiotics. Patients who are prone to recurrent episodes of cellulitis may require prophylactic antibacterial therapy. The most worrisome consequence of chronic lymphedema is the development of an angiosarcoma of the involved extremity (Stewart-Treves syndrome). Any new blue or reddish blue nodules on the arm that grow rapidly and bleed easily should be biopsied.

Risk Reduction

Because lymphedema is difficult to manage and the consequences can be dramatic, significant energy is placed on risk reduction. Several precautions should be explained to patients who have undergone ALND to reduce the risk of both infection and any increased lymphatic load in the extremity (Table 13–4). These are lifelong recommendations because lymphedema can occur decades after the surgery. It is also important that these precautions be described to the patient before undergoing an ALND so that patients may make truly informed decisions regarding the risks and benefits of ALND. It is not adequate to simply explain that lymphedema may occur as a risk of the procedure because all patients undergoing the surgery will need to make these lifestyle changes to reduce their risk.

Because even transient infections or mild cellulitis can incite lymphedema, patients are cautioned against behaviors that may result in nicks or cuts. These include cutting cuticles, or gardening or other hobbies without gloves or long sleeves. Mild burns can occur with cooking or ironing, so care should be taken. Sunscreen should be used to avoid sunburns and insect repellent used to avoid bug bites. Increased temperatures for extended periods of time, such as occurs with hot tubs or saunas, can lead to an increased lymphatic load and should also be avoided. Air travel has been associated with the onset of lymphedema, presumably from the lower cabin pressure, dehydration, and stasis. Most reported cases have been on longer trips, and the swelling occurs while they are on the plane. It is therefore recommended that any patient who has had an ALND should wear a 20 to 30 mm Hg upper extremity support garment from departure to destination when flying. In addition, patients should remain adequately hydrated and move around during the flight.

Several studies have shown that an increased body mass index (BMI) among patients undergoing ALND is associated with an increased risk of lymphedema. Clearly, patients should be counseled on the importance of maintaining a healthy weight after surgery. Patients who are already overweight should be encouraged to lose weight, although this is a challenge in the patient with breast cancer. Many women actually gain weight during their adjuvant chemotherapy for breast cancer. However, increased exercise, weight loss, and decreased fat intake have been associated with a decrease in breast cancer recurrence and improved survival, so this should be strongly encouraged. In women who are overweight and who do develop lymphedema, weight loss should be a critical part of their treatment. Essential to weight loss is exercise, however, there is some concern that vigorous, repetitive exercises of the at-risk extremity may cause lymph overload and result in lymphedema. The literature is mixed on this subject.

Treatment

Women who develop upper extremity swelling should be thoroughly evaluated for both regional recurrence and deep vein thrombosis because this may be the cause of a sudden onset of lymphedema. Diagnostic studies such as venous Doppler ultrasonography, computed tomography (CT) scan, or magnetic resonance imaging (MRI) may be helpful. Lymphoscintigrams are rarely necessary.

The degree of lymphedema should be measured and documented, although there are multiple methods for doing so. Subjective reports by the patient or semiobjective reports by the physician are unreliable. The simplest method is to perform circumferential measurements. There is some normal variation between the two arms, and the degree of lymphedema may be underestimated in a woman who is obese or overestimated in a woman who is thin. However, this is inexpensive and easily performed on each physical examination. The upper and lower arms should be measured, and the measurement should be performed 10 cm above and below the crease of the elbow to assure the same area is measured each time.

Arm volume can also be measured by the water displacement method. Although this is more accurate than circumferential measurements (with a volume difference of 200 ml or more between the two arms considered lymphedema), it is not easily performed in an office setting, especially on every visit.

Once lymphedema has been identified, early treatment is recommended. This should be done by physicians with expertise in the area. As lymphedema can not typically be reversed, and the anatomic changes can not be corrected, the goal of treatment is to control swelling of the arm. The most common approach uses a combination of massage, exercise, external pressure, and physical therapy. The physical therapy departments associated with most major cancer centers typically have a dedicated lymphedema program, and prompt referral is recommended.

The mainstay of treatment is the graded compression garment. These elastic lymphedema sleeves can deliver pressures of 20 to 60 mm Hg, and the pressure decreases as one moves proximally, encouraging edema mobilization. Depending on the symptoms and degree of lymphedema, these can be worn 24 hours a day or only when awake or when the arm is in use. The garments do lose their elasticity over time and will need to be replaced every 4 to 6 months.

A specific form of upper extremity massage, known as manual lymphedema drainage (MLD), may be of benefit, although the results of randomized controlled trials are mixed. The technique uses light pressure to move fluid from distal to proximal. It should be performed by a trained practitioner. Massage should be avoided if there is concern of active infection or active neoplasm. These should be ruled out first, along with the possibility of an acute deep venous thrombosis.

More severe cases of lymphedema may require external pneumatic compression or complex physical therapy. Intermittent or sequential pneumatic compression can be achieved through the use of a plastic sleeve that is inflated sequentially by pumps in a distal to proximal direction. These must be used in combination with the other techniques if they are to be effective. As with massage, they should be avoided in the face of active injection, cancer, or thrombosis.

Complex physical therapy is a complicated combination of preventative care, compression wrapping, and manual lymphedema treatment. It should be initiated in any woman not responding to standard elastic compression therapy and needs to be coordinated by a dedicated multimodality lymphedema program.

Other therapies, such as diuretics, antibiotics, anticoagulants, laser therapy, and surgery have not been proven to be effective and are not recommended unless being used to treat a specific cause or complication of lymphedema.

Suggested Readings

1. Cabanes PA, Salmon RJ, Vilcoq JR, et al. Value of axillary dissection in addition to lumpectomy and radiotherapy in early breast cancer. The Breast Carcinoma Collaborative Group of the Institut Curie. Lancet 1992;339:1245.
2. Chagpar AB, McMasters KM. Treatment of sentinel node positive breast cancer. Expert Rev Anticancer Ther 2006;6(8):1233–1239.
3. Cox C, White L, Allred N, et al. Survival outcomes in node-negative breast cancer patients evaluated with complete axillary node dissection versus sentinel lymph node biopsy. Ann Surg Oncol 2006; 13(5):708–711.
4. de Kanter AY, van Eijck CH, van Geel AN, et al. Multicentre study of ultrasonographically guided axillary node biopsy in patients with breast cancer. Br J Surg 1999;86(11):1459–1462.
5. Degnim AC, Griffith KA, Sabel MS, et al. Clinicopathologic features of metastasis in nonsentinel lymph nodes of breast carcinoma patients. Cancer 2003;98(11):2307–2315.
6. Edge SB, Niland JC, Bookman MA, et al. Emergence of sentinel node biopsy in breast cancer as standard-of-care in academic comprehensive cancer centers. J Natl Cancer Inst 2003;95:1514.
7. Engel J, Kerr J, Schlessinger-Raab A, et al. Axilla surgery severely affects quality of life: Results of a 5 year prospective study in breast cancer patients. Breast Cancer Res Treat 2003;79:47–57.
8. Fisher B, Jeong JH, Anderson S, et al. Twenty-five year follow-up of a randomized trial comparing radical mastectomy, total mastectomy, and total mastectomy followed by irradiation. N Engl J Med 2002;347:567–575.
9. Giuliano AE, Kirgan DM, Guenther JM, et al. Lymphatic mapping and sentinel lymphadenectomy for breast cancer. Ann Surg 1994;220:391–398.
10. Goldhirsch A, Wood WC, Gelber RD, et al. Meeting highlights: Updated International Expert Consensus on the Primary Therapy of Early Breast Cancer. J Clin Oncol 2003;21:3357.
11. Guiliano AE, Dale PS, Turner RR, et al. Improved axillary staging of breast cancer with sentinel lymphadenectomy. Ann Surg 1995;222:394–401.
12. Katz A, Niemierko A, Gage I, et al. Can axillary dissection be avoided in patients with sentinel lymph node metastases? J Surg Oncol 2006;93:550–558.
13. Kim T GA, Lyman GH. Lymphatic mapping and sentinel lymph node biopsy in early stage breast carcinoma: A metaanalysis. Cancer 2006;106(1):4–16.
14. Krag DN, Weaver D, Ashikaga T, et al. The sentinel node in breast cancer: A Multicenter Validation Study. N Engl J Med 1998;339(14):941–946.
15. Kuerer HM, Newman LA: Lymphatic mapping and sentinel lymph node biopsy for breast cancer: Developments and resolving controversies. J Clin Oncol 2005;23(8):1698–1705.
16. Mamounas EP, Brown A, Smith R, et al. Accuracy of sentinel node biopsy after neoadjuvant chemotherapy in breast cancer: Updated results from NSABP B-27. Proceedings of the American Society of Clinical Oncology 2002;21:140.
17. Mansel RE, Fallowfeld L, Kissin M, et al. Randomized multicenter trial of sentinel node biopsy versus standard axillary treatment in operable breast cancer: The ALMANAC trial. J Natl Cancer Inst 2006;98(9):599–609.
18. Miltenberg DM, Miller C, Karamlou TB, et al. Meta-analysis of sentinel lymph node biopsy in breast cancer. J Surg Res 1999;84(2):138–142.
19. Naik AM, Fey J, Gemignani M, et al. The risk of axillary relapse after sentinel lymph node biopsy for breast cancer is comparable with that of axillary lymph node dissection: A follow-up study of 4008 procedures. Ann Surg 2004;240:462.
20. Newman L. Lymphatic mapping and sentinel lymph node biopsy in breast cancer patients: A comprehensive review of variations in performance and technique. J Am Coll Surg 2004;199(5):804–816.
21. Orr RK. The impact of prophylactic axillary node dissection on breast cancer survival—a Bayesian meta-analysis. Ann Surg Oncol 1999;6:109.
22. Sakorafas GH, Peros G, Cataliotte L. Sequelae following axillary lymph node dissection for breast cancer. Expert Rev Anticancer Ther 2006;6(11): 1629–1638.
23. Sapino A, Cassoni P, Zanon E, et al. Ultrasonographically-guided fine-needle aspiration of axillary lymph nodes: Role in breast cancer management. Br J Cancer 2003;88:702.
24. Sato K, Tamaki K, Tsuda H, et al. Utility of axillary ultrasound examination to select breast cancer patients suited for optimal sentinel node biopsy. Am J Surg 2004;187:679.
25. The American Society of Breast Surgeons. Consensus statement on guidelines for performing sentinel lymph node dissection in breast cancer. 2005. Available at www.Breastsurgeons.org
26. Van Zee KJ, Manasseh DM, Bevilacqua JL, et al. A nomogram for predicting the likelihood of additional nodal metastases in breast cancer patients with a positive sentinel lymph node biopsy. Ann Surg Oncol 2003;10:1140–1151.
27. Veronesi U, Paganelli G, Viale G, et al. A randomized comparison of sentinel-node biopsy with routine axillary dissection in breast cancer. N Engl J Med 2003;349(6):546–563.
28. Vitug AF, Newman LA. Complications in breast surgery. Surg Clin North Am 2007;87(2):431–451.
29. Wilke LG, McCall LM, Posther KE, et al. Surgical complications associated with sentinel lymph node biopsy: Results from a prospective international cooperative group trial. Ann Surg Oncol 2006; 13(4):491–500.

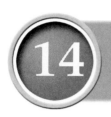

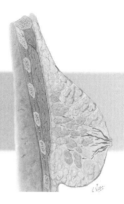

Principles of Breast Reconstruction

Principles of Breast Reconstruction: Key Points

- Describe the reconstruction options patients have after mastectomy.
- Know the implications of postmastectomy radiation therapy on breast reconstruction and the pros and cons of delayed versus immediate breast reconstruction.
- Be familiar with the techniques used for free and pedicled transverse rectus abdominis myocutaneous flaps and the deep inferior epigastric perforator flap.
- Understand other forms of free flaps for breast reconstruction.
- Describe the technique used for a skin-sparing mastectomy.
- Understand oncoplastic approaches to performing a lumpectomy.

The goals of the surgical therapy of breast cancer include not only local control of the tumor and accurate surgical staging of disease, but also the restoration of an acceptable cosmetic outcome. Although breast-conserving surgery has significantly improved the aesthetic result after breast cancer therapy, numerous women still undergo mastectomy. Many of these women will opt for breast reconstruction. It is becoming increasingly apparent that breast reconstruction can improve the psychosocial well-being and quality of life of the patient. Despite early concerns, breast reconstruction does not delay adjuvant therapy, increase the risk of local recurrence, or impact the ability to detect recurrence. Breast reconstruction has also been aided by advances on the health policy front. In 1998, Congress passed the Women's Health and Cancer Rights Act (WHCRA), guaranteeing insurance reimbursement for breast reconstruction or external prostheses, contralateral procedures for symmetry, and treatment for any sequelae of mastectomy.

There are several options for reconstruction, and the most appropriate choice and timing of reconstruction must be balanced with the need for adjuvant systemic therapy and postmastectomy radiation. It is imperative that the desire for the best possible cosmetic outcome not supersede the patient's oncologic treatment or carry unnecessary risk. The optimal management in this situation requires a collaborative effort between breast and reconstructive surgeons, radiologists, pathologists, and radiation and medical oncologists.

Types of Breast Reconstruction

Breast reconstruction can be divided into two categories according to the material used to recreate the breast: autologous tissue or prosthetics (Table 14–1). Autologous methods use tissue flaps. There are many types of flaps available (Box 14–1). These can be *pedicled* flaps, in which the tissue is rotated on the vascular supply, or *free* flaps, which involve a microsurgical vascular anastomosis. The most commonly used is the transverse rectus abdominal myocutaneous (TRAM) flap. This tends to give the

BOX 14–1 AUTOLOGOUS TISSUE FLAPS USED FOR BREAST RECONSTRUCTION
• Transverse rectus abdominis myocutaneous (TRAM) flap
• Latissimus dorsi myocutaneous flap
• Inferior and superior gluteal flaps
• Lateral transverse thigh flap
• Taylor-Rubens periiliac flap

best cosmetic result with the fewest complications. Prosthetic methods of reconstruction involve the use of implants—either saline or silicone. Often the patient has the implantation of a temporary tissue expander, followed by placement of a permanent implant.

Expander/Implants

Breast reconstruction can be obtained with either a silicone gel or saline-filled implant. Using implants for reconstruction is technically easier, requiring less experience on the part of the plastic surgeon. The initial recovery is also easier for the patient, making implant-based reconstruction an excellent choice for older patients and those with comorbidities, who may not be able to tolerate the longer time under general anesthesia.

Implants can be placed immediately after a mastectomy, without the use of expanders, although this is not common. This simple technique requires skin flaps that can sufficiently cover the implant, and this is not typical. There is also an increased risk of skin necrosis secondary to the tension. It is preferable to place implants beneath the pectoralis major muscle, in the submusculofascial space, rather than directly underneath the skin because there is increased soft tissue coverage over the foreign material. However, it is the rare woman who after a mastectomy has enough laxity to the pectoralis muscle to allow for an implant large enough to equal the size of their breast. It is typically not possible to insert an implant greater than 300 ml and provide adequate coverage. So unless the woman is an A or B cup or wants to undergo a reduction mammoplasty at the time of her reconstruction, the use of a tissue expander is necessary. In general, implant placement without tissue expansion is discouraged.

Instead, most patients will undergo tissue expansion followed by permanent implant

TABLE 14–1 • *Relative Advantages of Autologous versus Prosthetic Reconstruction*	
Autologous Reconstruction	**Prosthetic Reconstruction**
No foreign material	Less complex surgery
Improved cosmesis	Less expensive
Natural aging of breast	Quicker postoperative recovery
Less subsequent revisions necessary	Color match
	Intact sensation
	Less scarring and no donor site defect

placement. For the tissue expander, a balloon-like expander is placed beneath the pectoralis major muscle following the mastectomy. Intraoperatively, the goal is to provide complete coverage of the expander so that the implant is protected should the skin break down. If there is any question that the skin is at an increased risk of necrosis secondary to a compromised vascular supply, expander placement should be delayed. This underscores the importance of the surgeon in not devascularizing the skin while creating the skin flaps. In addition, it may be necessary for the plastic surgeon to raise the lateral portion of the serratus anterior and possibly the superior aspect of the rectus abdominis muscle to provide complete soft tissue coverage, and injury to these structures during removal of the breast may also compromise the ability of the plastic surgeon to perform an immediate expander placement (Fig 14–1).

Over the next 2 months, saline is intermittently injected into the expander to enlarge it and stretch the overlying skin and muscle (Fig 14–2) This is typically done once a week. The volume injected depends on patient comfort and the tightness of the skin. Once this has been accomplished (usually the expander is overexpanded by about 25% to improve the skin drape over the implant) and maintained long enough to become permanent (4 to 6 months), the patient returns to the operating room for removal of the expander

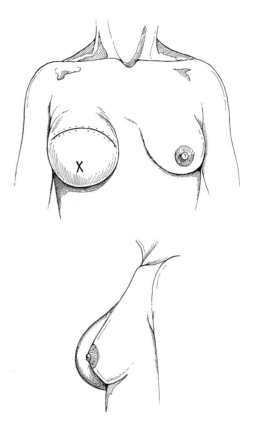

Figure 14–2. The expander is overexpanded by about 25% to improve the skin drape over the implant and maintained long enough to become permanent before the patient returns to the operating room for removal of the expander and placement of a permanent implant. (From Roses D. Breast cancer. Philadelphia: Elsevier, 2005).

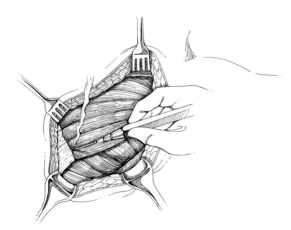

Figure 14–1. Transection of the pectoralis major for placement of the tissue expander. The plastic surgeon will create a pocket for the tissue expander under the pectoralis major muscle and may need to use the serratus anterior or rectus abdominis to provide complete soft tissue coverage. Injury to these structures during mastectomy may compromise that, precluding expander placement. (From Roses D. Breast cancer. Philadelphia: Elsevier, 2005).

and placement of a permanent implant, either silicone gel or saline (Fig 14–3). Although silicone-gel implants have a more natural feel to them, there is a higher risk of capsular contracture. There is always some degree of contracture around the implant; however, when this is severe, the breast can become hard and painful. There are also heightened concerns among patients regarding silicone leaks. For these reasons, many surgeons and patients prefer saline implants.

Complications include hematoma, seroma, or the need to remove the expander or implant for exposure, infection, malposition, or leak. Long-term complications can include capsular contracture, implant deflation, and visible wrinkling of the implant (especially in thin women).

There are several disadvantages to the expander/implant. Although it requires the least amount of initial surgery and less overall operative time, it does require weekly visits and a second surgery several months down the

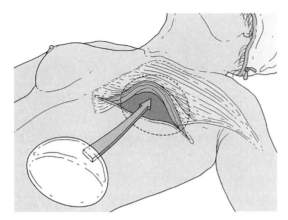

Figure 14–3. The expander is removed, and a permanent implant is placed beneath the pectoralis major muscle. (From Bland K, Copeland E. The breast, 3e. Philadelphia: Elsevier, 2004.)

road. Even the best contoured breast implants are rarely able to completely match the curves of the natural breast, and while the other breast changes over time, the implant side will remain unchanged, leading to an increasingly noticeable difference. The implant also will not move like the opposite breast, remaining upright when the woman lies down. Although the symmetry is often corrected by wearing a bra, many times surgery on the opposite breast will be necessary. This may involve a lift to decrease the ptosis or improve fullness in the upper aspect of the breast or a reduction so that a smaller implant can be used.

Reconstruction with Autologous Tissues

Although implant breast reconstruction remains the most common method for reconstructing the breast, there are problems previously described (capsular contracture, migration of the implant) and the difficulty in achieving a ptotic breast mound that matches the opposite breast. Reconstruction with autologous tissue solves some of these problems by reconstructing the breast with the patient's own tissues. The breast is softer and more natural than a breast reconstructed with an implant, and rather than deteriorating with time (as implant-based reconstructions usually do), they tend to improve. A successful breast reconstruction with autologous tissue often looks, moves, and feels much like a real breast.

Although the initial surgical procedure required to reconstruct a breast with autologous tissue is much longer and more complicated than that required for implant-based

reconstruction, subsequent surgical procedures are simpler, shorter, and less frequent. Thus, there are several advantages to autologous tissue breast reconstruction when that option is available. Several methods for reconstructing the breast using autologous tissue are available.

Transverse Rectus Abdominis Myocutaneous Flaps

The first successful method of breast reconstruction was the pedicled TRAM flap. The TRAM flap is based on the dual blood supply to the rectus abdominis muscle, allowing for either a pedicled TRAM based on the superior epigastric system or a free flap based on the inferior epigastric (Fig 14–4). The pedicled TRAM involves removing a wide ellipse of skin and fat from the lower abdomen left attached to one of the two rectus abdominis muscles. The flap is then tunneled between the abdominal dissection and the mastectomy defect, maintaining its blood supply from the superior epigastric artery and vein. The abdominal defect is closed primarily, and the flap is shaped to form the breast mound.

Patient selection is extremely important when determining whether a TRAM flap is appropriate. The ideal candidate is a generally healthy patient without significant medical comorbidities. Patients with medical problems that increase the risk of the additional operative time required for autogenous reconstruction

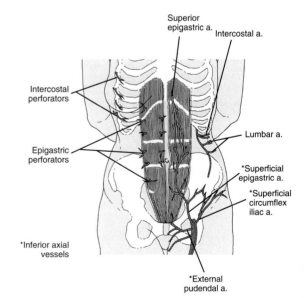

Figure 14–4. Blood supply to the rectus abdominis muscle and overlying skin. (From Bland K, Copeland E. The breast, 3e. Philadelphia: Elsevier, 2004.)

are a relative contraindication to a TRAM flap. The patient's body habitus and expectations regarding the size of the reconstructed breast are important considerations. They should neither be too thin or more than moderately obese. Patients without an adequate amount of lower abdominal soft tissue to reconstruct one or both breasts would be poor candidates. The biggest risk of the pedicled TRAM flap is loss of the flap secondary to an insufficient blood supply. Patients with comorbidities that compromise the blood supply (diabetes, heart disease, significant obesity, and smoking) are poor candidates for a pedicled TRAM. In these patients, either an implant reconstruction should be considered or the patients should undergo a free-flap TRAM because this technique provides for better skin island perfusion.

The donor site can be a source of problems for patients. Patients can have postoperative abdominal weakness, bulging, or hernia, although these risks are low. Patients who are active physically may be better served by a free-flap muscle-sparing technique so as to limit the donor site impact.

Pedicled Transverse Rectus Abdominis Myocutaneous Flap Procedure

In the preoperative area, the patient should be marked while in the upright position. Particularly important is the inframammary line. For the breast surgeon, this defines the lower limit of the dissection, however sometimes during a mastectomy, this may become detached. If this occurs, the plastic surgeon must reestablish this important aesthetic landmark or risk asymmetry of the breasts. The incision on the breast is marked out as either a standard mastectomy incision, or better yet, a skin-sparing incision. The general boundaries of the breast are also generally marked. The transverse skin island of the TRAM flap is marked out over the lower abdomen, encompassing as much redundant tissue as is available. A midline mark is made from above the umbilicus, through the TRAM skin island, and onto the pubis. This helps to close the defect symmetrically.

After the patient is placed under general anesthesia, he or she is positioned with each arm extended and secured. The patient should be positioned and secured on the table so he or she may be sat straight up. A lower extremity warming blanket is placed after insertion of a Foley catheter. The entire chest and abdomen is prepped and draped into a single operative field. It is possible, and desirable, that a two-team approach is used, so that the breast surgeon performs the mastectomy at the same time that the plastic surgeon is working on the TRAM flap.

The skin island is dissected to the first row of both medial and lateral perforators, preserving a lateral and medial band of muscle and fascia. The anterior rectus fascia is divided up to and over the costal margin, and then dissected off of the rectus abdominis muscle medially and laterally. This preserves the entire rectus fascia from the costal margin to the superior edge of the fascial defect for the skin island. Although the pedicled TRAM flap will be based on the superior epigastrics, it is a wise idea to dissect out the inferior epigastrics with the flap and ligate them distally. Preserving them allows for providing additional blood flow (supercharging) should the skin island appear compromised at the completion of the case. Once this is done, the inferior portion of the rectus abdominis muscle is divided with electrocautery, and the muscle is dissected off of the peritoneum and posterior rectus sheath. The muscle is freed to the costal margin and then transpositioned into the mastectomy defect (Fig 14–5). At this point, the skin island should be observed for a few minutes to look for evidence of venous congestion or poor arterial perfusion. If present, it is possible to anastomose the inferior epigastrics to the thoracodorsal system to provide additional blood flow.

The fascial incision in the upper anterior rectus fascia can be primarily repaired and an inlay mesh used to repair the defect from the flap harvest. The abdominal skin is reapproximated with replacement of the umbilicus. The patient is then repositioned upright, and the TRAM flap modeled so that it matches the contralateral breast. The final step is to deepithelialize the buried portion of the TRAM skin island and approximate the skin incisions.

If there is concern preoperatively about the blood supply to the pedicled TRAM flap, it is reasonable to take the patient to the operating room 1 to 2 weeks before the TRAM reconstruction to divide the blood vessels that enter the flap from below. Dividing the inferior epigastric vessels will encourage the superior epigastrics to be come larger. This is effective in reducing the risk of vascular insufficiency to the flap. Although it requires an additional minor procedure, it may be combined with a sentinel lymph node (SLN) biopsy in patients with clinically node-negative cancer. In this manner, it is known at the time of the

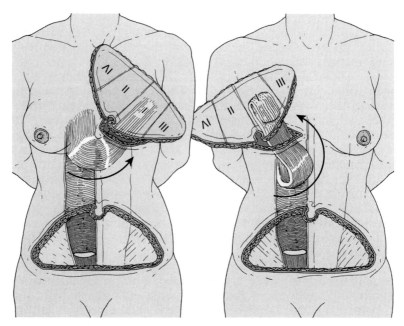

Figure 14-5. The transverse rectus abdominis myocutaneous flap rotation. **A,** Contralateral technique. **B,** Ipsilateral technique. (From Bland K, Copeland E. The breast, 3e. Philadelphia: Elsevier, 2004.)

definitive operation whether an axillary lymph node dissection (ALND) is necessary, which helps avoid a return to the operating room for a lymph node dissection in a patient who has already undergone reconstruction.

Free Transverse Rectus Abdominis Myocutaneous Flaps

The free TRAM flap gets its blood supply from below, from the deep inferior epigastric vessels (Fig 14-6). This requires the division and

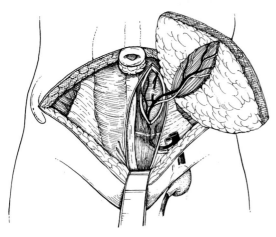

Figure 14-6. The blood supply to the free transverse rectus abdominis myocutaneous flap is based on the deep inferior epigastric vessels. (From Roses D. Breast cancer. Philadelphia: Elsevier, 2005).

microsurgical reanastomosis of these vessels. The main disadvantage of this approach is the total dependence of the flap on the anastomosed blood vessels. Should they become obstructed, the entire flap will die. In experienced hands, however, this occurs less than 2% of the time. If done correctly, however, there are several advantages to the free TRAM flap. The blood supply is stronger and less likely to cause partial flap loss or fat necrosis. Less of the rectus abdominis muscle needs to be sacrificed so that there is less postoperative pain and abdominal wall weakness. The aesthetic results tend to be better because the strong blood supply allows for more aggressive shaping of the flap.

The patient is marked, positioned, and prepped as previously described. The plastic surgeon must decide where the inferior epigastrics will be anastomosed to. For patients undergoing a simple mastectomy (with or without SLN biopsy), or when this is done as a delayed flap in a patient who already had an ALND, the internal mammary vessels are usually selected. If the patient is having an immediate reconstruction and an ALND is to be performed, the thoracodorsal vessels are often chosen.

In the case of a free TRAM flap, the inferior epigastrics are divided near their attachment to the external iliacs. Both the superior and inferior muscle is then divided and the entire flap is moved to the chest site, where the vascular anastomosis is performed. This can be done with either surgical loupes or the operating microscope. Once complete, the vessel clamps are removed and the flap assessed for anastomotic patency. The flap tissue is temporarily attached to the chest wall so that it does not move and disrupt the anastomosis while the abdominal defect is closed. Once that is completed, the patient is placed in the upright position and the flap modified appropriately. After removing the skin that would be buried under the natural skin and reapproximating the skin, it is wise to identify and mark a site on the exposed portion of the flap where a surface arterial Doppler signal is present. This is then used for postoperative monitoring.

After a TRAM flap, patients are transferred directly to their hospital bed and kept in a semi-Fowler position to limit the tension on the abdominal donor site. Close observation is used in patients who had a free TRAM flap, with frequent checking of the arterial Doppler signal (every 30 minutes for the first 24 hours, every hour on day 2, every two hours on day 3 and then every 4 hours until discharge). The Foley catheter remains in place for 24 to 48 hours. Patients typically are discharged on postoperative day 3 to 5. Drains can be removed before discharge depending on their output. At home, patients should avoid lifting anything greater than 10 lbs or do anything more athletic than walking. These restrictions are maintained for 6 weeks.

Deep Inferior Epigastric Perforator and Superficial Inferior Epigastric Artery (Perforator) Flaps

A new method of autologous breast reconstruction is the deep inferior epigastric perforator (DIEP) flap. The skin and fat island are the same as the TRAM flap, but the perforating blood vessels are dissected through the rectus abdominis muscle so that the muscle can be left behind (Fig 14–7). By not sacrificing the muscle, the patient has less postoperative pain and a stronger abdominal wall. The main disadvantages of this flap are the technical complexity and an increased risk of partial flap loss and fat necrosis as a result of a somewhat reduced blood supply. It is prudent to reserve the DIEP flap for patients who will not require the entire flap to reconstruct the breast. Contraindications to the DIEP flap are a history of abdominoplasty or abdominal liposuction, active smoking, or previous large transverse or oblique abdominal incisions.

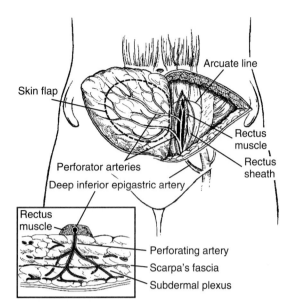

Figure 14–7. Mobilization of the deep inferior epigastric perforator flap. (From Roses D. Breast cancer. Philadelphia: Elsevier, 2005).

It is often preferable to use the contralateral abdomen because it is easier to inset the flap. The setup is similar as with a standard TRAM flap, but in addition to the standard preoperative markings, a Doppler probe is used to identify the main perforators of the medial and lateral branches of the deep inferior epigastric artery and the superficial inferior epigastric artery (SIEA). The internal mammary artery (IMA) and internal mammary vein (IMV) are the preferred recipient vessels, although the thoracodorsal vessels may be used as well.

The superior and inferior skin incisions are made and the superficial inferior epigastric vessels are identified. If the vessels are large enough, then an SIEA flap can be performed. The SIEA flap is preferable because there is less donor-site morbidity because no incision must be made in the abdominal fascia and no dissection performed through the rectus abdominis muscle. Unfortunately the SIEA is not always present, and often when it is present, it is not large enough. However, if it does have sufficient caliber, it is followed down to its origin from the common femoral artery and saphenous vein. The flap can be raised without opening the rectus abdominis fascia and transferred to the mastectomy defect.

More commonly, the SIEA is not adequate, and a DIEP flap will be necessary, but the vessels should still be dissected free for several centimeters to be used as a backup. The skin island is carefully elevated from lateral to medial until the lateral row of perforators is encountered. These are dissected and included with the flap. The medial row is approached in a similar fashion. As many perforators in the same row that can be preserved should be, as often more than one perforator may be necessary to perfuse the flap if there is not one dominant perforator. Once the perforators are chosen, the anterior rectus sheath is opened around these vessels and they are dissected down through the muscle to the deep inferior epigastric artery and vein. The muscle is spread apart in the direction of the fibers to expose the vessels. This dissection requires high-power loupe magnification and careful microsurgical technique and continues until the pedicle is of sufficient length (typically 8 to 10 cm). The artery and veins are ligated, and then the flap is transferred to the anterior chest wall. With great care not to twist or kink the vessels (this is aided by marking the anterior surface of the vessels), temporary stay sutures are placed in the flap and the operating microscope is used to anastomose the vessels. An anastomotic coupling device may be used to connect the veins. If an SIEA flap is being performed, it may be preferable to anastomose the vessels to smaller perforating branches of the internal mammary vessels to better match the size between the flap and recipient vessels.

Once the surgeon is sure that the flap is well perfused and not congested, the abdomen is flexed so that the wound can be closed. Mesh is not used, the abdominal fascia is closed primarily and then the skin. The flap is inset and sutured in place similar to the standard TRAM flap.

Extended Latissimus Dorsi Flaps

Another alternative for patients who are not good candidates for a TRAM flap is the extended latissimus dorsi flap (Figs. 14–8, 14–9). In this flap, the standard latissimus dorsi flap is modified so that additional skin and fat are removed from the back and transferred to the chest. The donor site on the back is more scarred than after a standard latissimus dorsi flap, but in many cases, the breast can be reconstructed without an implant. The breasts are therefore softer than after a standard latissimus dorsi reconstruction, and the risk of capsular contracture is avoided.

The main advantage of this flap over a TRAM flap is that it is a simpler technique and can be used in less healthy patients who might not be

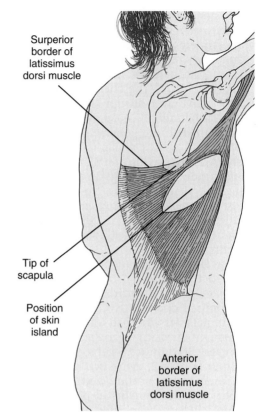

Figure 14–8. Skin and fat are removed from the back along with the latissimus dorsi muscle. (From Bland K, Copeland E. The breast, 3e. Philadelphia: Elsevier, 2004.)

good enough surgical candidates to have a TRAM flap. It is therefore particularly indicated in obese patients and in older patients. Although poor surgical candidates should not have any reconstruction, some patients who are not healthy enough to undergo a TRAM flap are acceptable candidates for an extended latissimus dorsi flap. This flap is also a reasonable choice for healthy patients who cannot have a TRAM flap because they have had a previous TRAM flap or abdominoplasty. Patients in this category may also be good candidates for a gluteal free flap. The choice between these donor sites is usually made after considering the relative laxity of tissues in the back versus the buttock in each individual and patient preference.

Gluteal Artery Perforator Flaps

The gluteal artery perforator (GAP) flaps are good choices for autologous reconstruction in women who have more skin and fat available

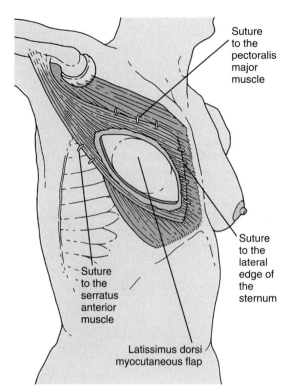

Figure 14–9. The extended latissimus dorsi flap is passed anteriorly through the axilla. (From Bland K, Copeland E. The breast, 3e. Philadelphia: Elsevier, 2004.)

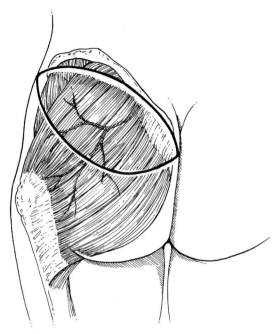

Figure 14–10. The superior gluteal artery perforator flap is based on the superior gluteal artery. (From Roses D. Breast cancer. Philadelphia: Elsevier, 2005).

in the buttock area than in the abdomen. Donor site morbidity is minimal and no muscle must be sacrificed. The GAP flaps may be based on either the superior gluteal artery perforator (S-GAP) or inferior gluteal artery perforator (I-GAP).

Superior Gluteal Artery Perforator Flap

The S-GAP flap is taken from the buttock and is based on the superior gluteal artery, which arises from the internal iliac artery and exits the pelvis superior to the piriformis muscle (Figs. 14–10, 14–11). It enters the gluteus maximus muscle approximately one third of the distance along the line between the posterior superior iliac spine and the greater trochanter. The S-GAP flap requires no muscle to be sacrificed because the flap is only skin, fat, and blood vessels. It is more difficult than a TRAM flap because the gluteal tissue is harder to shape into a breast, but is an excellent choice for patients who cannot undergo a TRAM but are otherwise good surgical candidates.

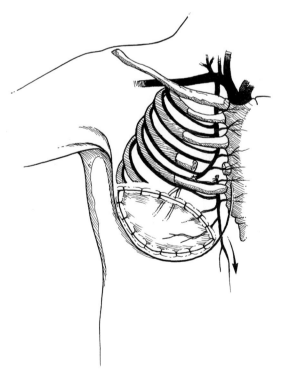

Figure 14–11. In the superior gluteal artery perforate flap, the superior gluteal artery is anastomosed to the internal thoracic artery. (From Roses D. Breast cancer. Philadelphia: Elsevier, 2005).

Preoperatively the patient is marked first in the lateral position, using the Doppler probe to identify the perforating vessels from the superior gluteal artery. The skin paddle is then marked in an oblique pattern from inferomedial to superolateral so that these perforators are included. The S-GAP flap has a short pedicle, and so anastomosis to the internal mammary vessels is preferred.

The patient is placed in the lateral decubitus position. The internal mammary vessels are prepared as previously described. The flap is divided down to the gluteus maximus, with significant beveling to ensure adequate tissue for reconstruction. The flap is elevated from the muscle in the subfascial plane and the perforators approached from lateral to medial. If present, a single large perforator is preferable, but sometimes multiple perforators in the same plan can be taken together. The muscle is spread in the direction of the fibers to allow dissection of the perforating vessels until the artery and vein are of sufficient length and diameter to be anastomosed. The patient is repositioned supine and the microvascular anastomosis is performed.

Inferior Gluteal Artery Perforator Flap

The I-GAP flap is taken from the lower buttock and is based on the inferior gluteal vessels (Fig 14–12). It requires sacrifice of a small amount of the gluteus maximus vessels. Like the S-GAP flap, it is more difficult than a TRAM but indicated in patients who cannot have a TRAM flap yet are otherwise good surgical candidates. The inferior gluteal artery is a branch of the internal iliac artery and leaves the pelvis through the greater sciatic foramen. The artery is accompanied by the greater sciatic nerve, internal pudendal vessels, and posterior femoral cutaneous nerve. Because the inferior gluteal vessel is more oblique through the gluteus maximus muscle than the superior gluteal artery, the length of the I-GAP pedicle is typically longer than the S-GAP and can be anastomosed to the thoracodorsals if the internal mammary vessels are not an ideal choice.

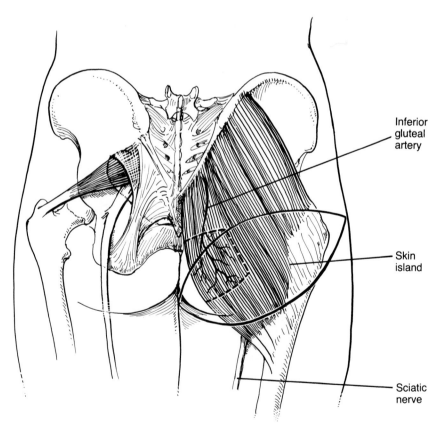

Inferior gluteal artery

Skin island

Sciatic nerve

Figure 14–12. The inferior gluteal free flap uses tissue from the lower buttock and is based on the inferior gluteal artery.

When marking the patient, the patient stands so that the gluteal fold may be marked. The inferior limit for this flap is marked 1 cm inferior and parallel to the gluteal fold. The patient is then placed in the lateral position and the Doppler probe is used to find the perforating vessels from the inferior gluteal artery. An ellipse is drawn for the skin paddle to include these perforators.

The Skin-Sparing Mastectomy

One of the cosmetic drawbacks to autologous flaps has been the difference in color between the skin of the flap and the skin of the chest wall. This has been greatly improved with the introduction of the skin-sparing mastectomy. Although there was initial concern regarding the oncologic appropriateness of this operation with early reports of increased local recurrence, subsequent studies have shown no increased local recurrence rates when proper technique is used. This technique allows for the preservation of as much uninvolved breast skin as possible, which provides improved symmetry (skin color and shape), form (cleavage), contour, and minimal scar. Any patient who does not require a significant amount of skin to be resected with the tumor is a candidate for a skin-sparing mastectomy. Skin-sparing technique can be used for both simple mastectomy and modified radical mastectomy (MRM).

There are several principles of the skin-sparing mastectomy that must be adhered to (Box 14–2). The breast and arm are prepped and draped as with a total or MRM. The key to the skin-sparing mastectomy is the choice of incision. If the cancer was diagnosed by needle biopsy, then only an incision is needed around the nipple and areola (another advantage to using needle biopsies for diagnosis). Depending on the size of the areola and the size of the breast, the entire mastectomy may be feasible through this incision. Otherwise, a keyhole approach can be used (Fig 14–13).

If a previous biopsy or lumpectomy has been performed, the skin surrounding the incision can be excised with approximately a 1-cm margin surrounding it. If the incision is near the nipple areolar complex, these can be incorporated into one incision (Fig 14–14). This may or may not require a keyhole for added exposure. If the previous incision is further away from the areola, any number of incisions can be used to incorporate both while preserving as much skin as possible (Figs. 14–15, 14–16, 14–17). These incisions should be designed by both the breast surgeon and the plastic surgeon in the preoperative area, to be sure that an appropriate oncologic operation can be performed with optimal reconstruction.

BOX 14–2 SURGICAL PRINCIPLES OF THE SKIN-SPARING MASTECTOMY

- Excision of the nipple-areolar complex
- Excision of the biopsy/lumpectomy incision
- Total glandular mastectomy, adhering to the same surgical principles of a total mastectomy
- Sentinel node biopsy or axillary node dissection through breast incision (with possible lengthening) or separate incision in the axilla

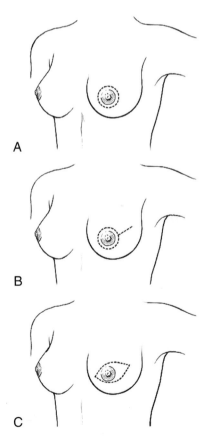

Figure 14–13. Skin-sparing mastectomy incisions can be periareolar **(A)**, periareolar with a keyhole extension **(B)** or elliptic **(C)**. (From Roses D. Breast cancer. Philadelphia: Elsevier, 2005).

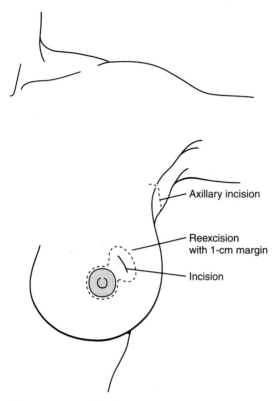

Axillary incision

Reexcision
with 1-cm margin

Incision

Figure 14–14. If the biopsy scar is close to the areola, they can be incorporated into one incision. (From Bland K, Copeland E. The breast, 3e. Philadelphia: Elsevier, 2004.)

A sentinel node biopsy can often be performed through a skin-sparing incision, but if there is any concern, a separate incision in the axilla can be performed. In patients who require a lymph node dissection, a separate, standard axillary dissection incision should be used.

After making the skin incision(s), flap elevation proceeds (Fig 14–18). The skin flaps are elevated widely to reach the same boundaries as with a standard mastectomy, and with the same technique to assure all breast tissue is removed. Compromising this for the sake of a skin-sparing mastectomy is oncologically inappropriate and likely the reason for increased local recurrence rates in some series. Care is taken not to compromise the vascular supply to the flaps. The main difference in technique with a skin-sparing mastectomy is that the surgeon needs to work circumferentially rather than raising the superior flap and then the inferior flap. Otherwise, the surgeon risks working deep in a hole, with limited visibility. It becomes more difficult to see the appropriate planes and if bleeding is encountered, it may

be difficult to control. Therefore, a part of the superior flap is raised, and once visibility diminishes, the retraction is relocated and the surgeon works on another part. This may require returning to the same location several times before the anatomic landmarks are reached.

The breast is then taken off of the pectoralis major muscle using the same technique as with a simple mastectomy, removing the pectoralis major fascia with the specimen. This may be slightly more challenging at first, given the limited space, but gets easier as the operation proceeds, particularly if the partially raised breast can be brought out the incision.

In patients who require an SLN biopsy, this can usually be done through the same incision with adequate retraction of the pectoralis major, allowing access to the axillary contents. If not, the keyhole incision can be extended or a separate incision can be made in the axilla. For patients who require an MRM, it is possible to remove the breast and axillary contents en bloc using two incisions. If, however, this proves technically challenging, it is not unreasonable to remove the entire breast and then perform the level I and II dissection through the axillary incision.

Nipple and Areolar Reconstruction

Nipple and areolar reconstruction is usually performed only after the breast shaping has been completed and the reconstructed breast form has stabilized (at least 6 to 8 weeks after reconstruction). The most important part of nipple reconstruction is its location. Even the best nipple will not look right if it is in the wrong place. It is also important to have comparable appearance and color to the contralateral nipple-areolar complex because even small discrepancies are obvious.

Although there are many techniques for nipple reconstruction, most modern techniques use local flaps of skin and fat to create a projecting nub (Fig 14–19). Full-thickness skin grafts can be performed to reconstruct the areola (with donor skin coming from the opposite areola, abdominal wall after a TRAM or medial thigh), although medical tattooing alone will usually result in an excellent cosmetic outcome. Nipple reconstruction can be performed in the office or clinic under local anesthesia. In this way it can be kept simple, inexpensive, convenient, and relatively painless. Although the results of nipple

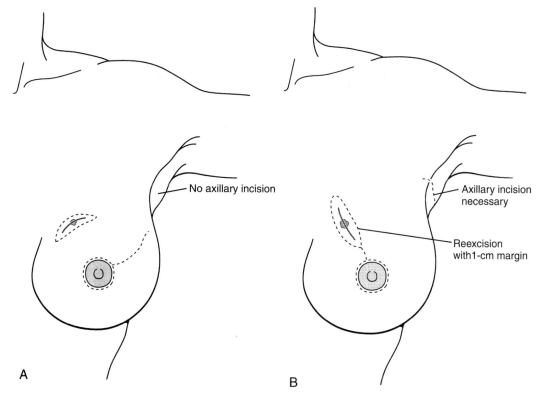

A

B

Figure 14–15. A, B, When the biopsy scar is further away from the areola, alternate incisions can be used to excise them together while still preserving a maximum amount of natural skin. (From Bland K, Copeland E. The breast, 3e. Philadelphia: Elsevier, 2004.)

reconstruction are not perfect, the presence of a reconstructed nipple does contribute significantly to the illusion of having recreated a normal breast. Patients are therefore encouraged to undergo nipple reconstruction and complete the process of breast reconstruction whenever possible.

Treatment of the Contralateral Breast

An important aspect of reconstruction is symmetry. Given the limitations of expander/implants and autogenous flaps, it may not be feasible to reconstruct the absent breast to the same size as the remaining breast. Or in a small-breasted woman, the reconstructed breast may be larger than the contralateral size. Therefore, women may require breast reduction, breast augmentation, or a breast lift (mastopexy) to create symmetry. This can be done at the same time as the reconstruction or at a later date. However, it is important to point out that breast reconstruction does not always produce a breast that is symmetrical to the contralateral side.

Timing of Breast Reconstruction

Historically, all reconstruction was delayed so that the reconstructed breast would not interfere with the detection of recurrent disease. Reconstruction was only performed in patients with early-stage disease and often delayed for 2 years because most recurrences occur within 2 years of mastectomy. These practices have been abandoned, and today patients may choose to have their reconstruction performed simultaneously with mastectomy ("immediate"), or they may wish to undergo mastectomy and then return for reconstruction after completion of their adjuvant therapies ("delayed"). Even in the more recent past, delayed reconstruction was preferred secondary to concerns that complications of reconstruction could delay adjuvant therapy, putting patients at increased risk of recurrence. Subsequent studies have failed to demonstrate any increased risk with immediate reconstruction, so this method is an appropriate choice. However, there are several relative advantages and disadvantages to immediate versus delayed reconstruction (Table 14–2).

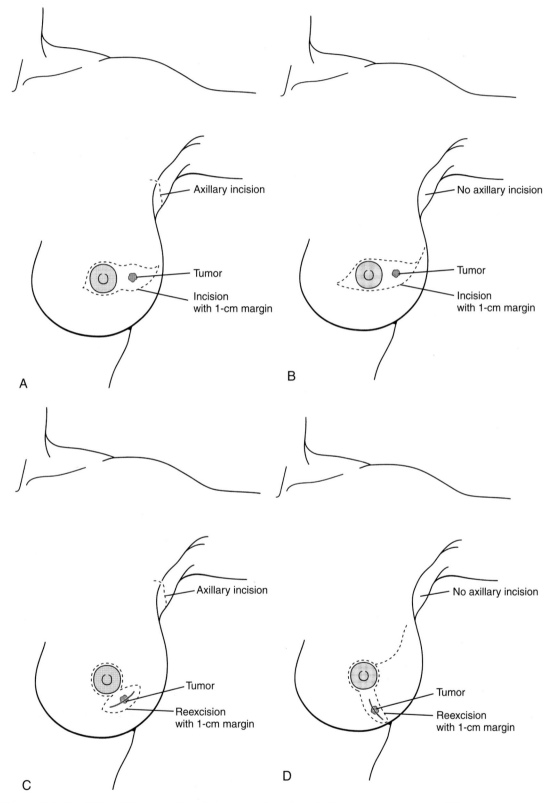

Figure 14–16. A-D, Additional options for excising both the nipple-areolar complex and biopsy scar for skin-sparing mastectomy. (From Bland K, Copeland E. The breast, 3e. Philadelphia: Elsevier, 2004.)

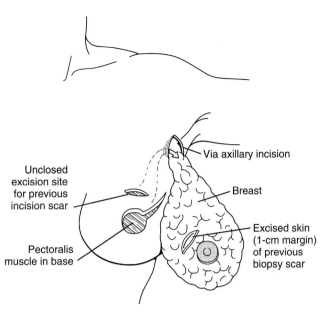

Figure 14–17. The biopsy scar may also be excised separately from the nipple-areolar complex. It is important that the island of skin between the two incisions be well perfused. (From Bland K, Copeland E. The breast, 3e. Philadelphia: Elsevier, 2004.)

Immediate reconstruction has the obvious benefit of avoiding the psychological impact of waking from surgery without a breast. It also reduces the number of times the patient needs to undergo general anesthesia. By using as much of the native skin of the breast as possible, this improves the cosmetic outcome. Immediate reconstruction can be an excellent option for patients with ductal carcinoma in situ (DCIS) or with early-stage disease. Autogenous tissue reconstructions performed at the time of the mastectomy tend to have better aesthetic results than delayed procedures because this allows for a skin-sparing mastectomy to be performed. Recovery is faster and overall cost is reduced.

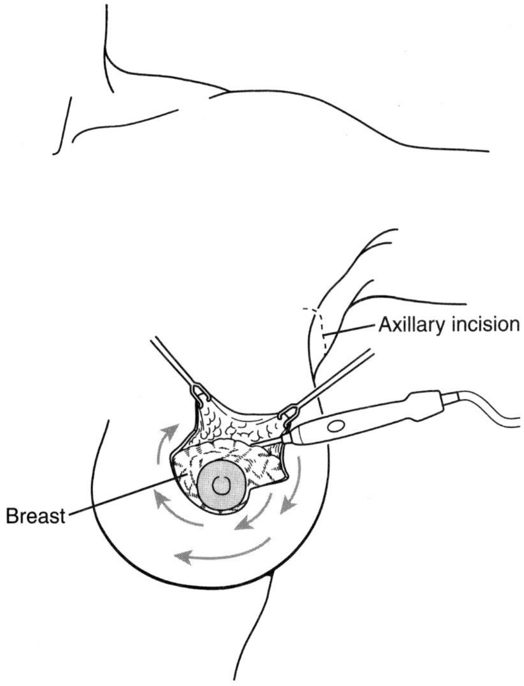

Delayed reconstruction has its advantages as well. For the patient who is unsure about reconstruction, it allows time to make the decision. Many patients are not as disappointed with the absent breast as they thought they might be and ultimately decide to forego reconstruction. The recovery period from the simple mastectomy is quicker. Patients do not typically have much choice about when they need cancer surgery, but they can delay the reconstruction until they have more time for recovery. In addition, it is usually easier and faster to schedule a simple mastectomy than for the breast surgeon and the plastic surgeon to find time for a combined procedure. Patients can also proceed quicker to adjuvant therapy, if necessary, after a simple mastectomy. It is important to point out, however, that most studies have shown no significant delay in adjuvant therapy with immediate reconstruction. With delayed reconstruction, the nodal status is known, so there is no chance of having to return to the operating room for an ALND after reconstruction or the need to irradiate the reconstructed breast.

Figure 14–18. Skin flap elevation during the skin-sparing mastectomy moves in a centripetal fashion to provide optimum exposure. (From Bland K, Copeland E. The breast, 3e. Philadelphia: Elsevier, 2004.)

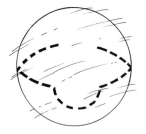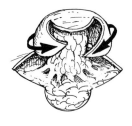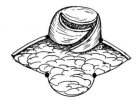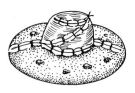

Figure 14–19. Local flap nipple reconstruction. **A,** Markings. **B,** Flap elevation, **C,** Flap rotation, **D,** Final appearance. (From Roses D. Breast cancer. Philadelphia: Elsevier, 2005).

TABLE 14–2 • Relative Advantages of Immediate versus Delayed Reconstruction	
Immediate Reconstruction	**Delayed Reconstruction**
Avoidance of second operation	Less complexity, shorter operations
Lower cost	No delay to adjuvant therapies
Possible better cosmetic outcome	Less need for integration of radiation and reconstruction
Better scarring, increased skin availability (skin sparing)	Allows additional time to consider reconstruction and what time
No period of time without breast	Increased satisfaction of reconstruction compared with absent breast, as compared to previous breast (some women expect an exact duplicate)

The avoidance of postmastectomy radiation to the reconstructed breast is one of the strongest arguments for delayed reconstruction.

Breast Irradiation and Reconstruction

The most challenging aspect of incorporating reconstruction in with breast cancer therapy is the interaction of radiation therapy and reconstruction. Over the past several years, the indications and use of postmastectomy radiation have risen (see Chapter 15). Indications for postmastectomy radiation include the size of the primary tumor (>5 cm), close margins after mastectomy, or four or more positive lymph nodes. The benefit of postmastectomy radiation for patients with one to three positive lymph nodes is still debated, but its use is increasing. It becomes obvious,

therefore, that a percentage of patients who are scheduled to undergo mastectomy may fall into one of these categories once the final pathology is known. If a patient opts to have immediate reconstruction, the situation may arise that radiation needs to be delivered to the reconstructed breast.

Delivery of radiation to the reconstructed breast may present some challenges to the radiation oncologist. Some reconstruction techniques distort the chest wall anatomy, so radiotherapy portals may need to be modified. A steeply sloping contour of the new breast may make it difficult to match fields. The foreign material may affect the radiation dose distribution within the breast. All of these factors must be taken into account during the radiation planning. With the use of computed tomography (CT) based planning and immobilizing devices, radiation can still be safely and effectively delivered to the reconstructed breast and chest wall, with no compromise of local recurrence rates or increased damage to the lung or heart. So in the hands of an experienced radiation oncologist, the reconstruction should not markedly affect the radiation dose distribution. However, the radiation may affect the reconstruction.

Effects of Irradiating a Tissue Expander/Implants

Postoperative radiation when an implant has been placed is generally contraindicated. However, there are situations where only after an expander has been placed does the possibility of postmastectomy radiation arise (such as a positive margin or positive lymph nodes). If it is known that radiation will be used, reconstruction can be delayed, although this is not without increased complications. If, however, the expander has already been placed (or the patient is strongly against delayed reconstruction but not a candidate for a flap), the options include performing the radiation before expansion, after tissue expansion but before placement of the permanent implant, or after placement of the implant. Radiation before expansion means expansion of the recently irradiated field. Radiating after the expansion process is complete means having to replace the expander with the implant in the face of acute radiation changes. The radiation should be delayed until the acute changes have settled but ideally before chronic radiation changes set in, or the radiation can be delayed until after the placement of the final implant. However, this means a delay in radiation, which may decrease its effectiveness. This will in part depend on whether the patient will be receiving systemic therapy. If chemotherapy is to be used, a good option is to expand during the chemotherapy and then do the exchange 3 to 4 weeks after chemotherapy finishes. The radiation is initiated, 3 to 4 weeks later.

Radiating an expander or permanent implant will increase the rate of capsular contracture. However, despite the fact that the radiation of an expander or an implant is often described as contraindicated, that is not the case. Despite an increased rate of contracture, successful reconstruction is still accomplished in most patients. Although aesthetic outcomes as graded by the surgeon or independent observers are less than when radiation is employed, these rates can still be acceptable. More importantly, the difference in patient opinions between implants after mastectomy alone and implants followed by radiation does not appear to be as significant as physician or third-party opinions, at least in the short term. Satisfaction rates do tend to separate more by 5 years, thought to be the result of progressive asymmetry between the natural and reconstructed breast, which tends to be more pronounced if the implant has been irradiated. It is also important to keep in mind that delayed expansion and implants after radiation also have a higher rate of complication rates.

Effects of Irradiating the Autologous Flap

If postmastectomy radiation is indicated, and the patient does not want a delayed reconstruction, the ideal reconstruction is an autologous flap. However, postoperative radiation after a flap reconstruction may be associated with increased wound complications and an altered cosmetic outcome. A well-vascularized TRAM flap should tolerate the 5000 to 6000 Gy typically delivered to the chest wall after a mastectomy. However, an individual patient's response to radiation may be quite variable, and the resulting edema and fibrosis can significantly alter the shape and softness of the reconstructed breast. The resultant volume, contour, and symmetry loss is unpredictable and may require additional surgeries to correct the radiation-induced changes, which may not always be as successful as hoped.

For this reason, many plastic surgeons would recommend that if it is known that the patient will need postmastectomy radiation, or it is suspected that this might be the case, consideration should be made to delaying the reconstruction until 3 to 6 months after the completion of radiation therapy. It is still debated by plastic surgeons whether delayed autologous reconstruction after radiation is truly superior to immediate autologous radiation followed by radiation. Many plastic surgeons report excellent outcomes with autologous flaps after post-mastectomy radiation.

Effects of Placing a Prosthesis after Irradiation

It is generally accepted that if postmastectomy radiation is necessary and expander/implant is the reconstruction of choice, then it is best to do the radiation first, followed by delayed placement of the expander. However, reconstruction of the irradiated chest wall after mastectomy still has complications. The effects of radiation limit the success of tissue expansion. The expansion process is associated with increased pain, less leeway in overexpansion, rib cage contour deformities, a greater infection rate, and expander extrusion. Compared to expander/implants in the nonirradiated breast, the resultant breast may be harder, asymmetric and lack projection. Some series have reported complication rates (including unfavorable aesthetic results) as high as 60% and an increased use of capsular contracture releases, additional tissue coverage and other additional procedures.

If, after the patient has recovered from radiation, the flaps show little evidence of radiation damage, or the amount of skin expansion needed is not excessive, expansion after radiation can be done safely with an increased but not unreasonable complication rate. If, however, the skin shows clear evidence of radiation induced changes, or a significant volume is needed for symmetry, it may be preferable to combine a latissimus dorsi flap with the tissue expander or breast implant. This allows the use of nonirradiated, well-vascularized tissue for reconstruction. The latissimus dorsi readily covers the device and expands nicely. In addition, the skin island that comes with the flap can replace heavily irradiated skin.

Effects of Performing an Autologous Flap after Irradiation

The ideal choice for reconstruction when post-mastectomy radiation is needed is a delayed autologous reconstruction using any of the aforementioned methods. It is worth noting that pedicled TRAM flaps have a higher rate of fat and skin necrosis when their pedicle has been exposed to radiation preoperatively. Free TRAM flaps have a lower complication rate than pedicled TRAM flaps in irradiated beds. There is a slightly higher rate of healing complications secondary to the irradiated tissue's ability to heal. To overcome this, it is prudent to use a larger amount of skin from the flap and excise a correspondingly wider area of the irradiated, fibrotic chest wall skin.

Sentinel Node Biopsy and Reconstruction

Two recent changes in the management of breast cancer have altered the clinical scenario; the introduction of SLN biopsy (see Chapter 13) and the suggestion that post-mastectomy radiation may be beneficial in patients who are node positive, including patients with one to three positive nodes (see Chapter 15). This has introduced the not uncommon scenario of a patient who is clinically node negative, requires (or desires) a mastectomy and is interested in immediate reconstruction. Those patients who turn out to be node positive, will not only need to return to the operating room for an ALND (which can be performed after immediate reconstruction) but will be candidates for postmastectomy radiation. This might mean radiating an expander or implant or radiating an autologous flap, both of which appear to have higher complication rates than performing the reconstruction after the radiation is complete.

The optimal management will depend on the stage of the primary cancer (and thus the likelihood of finding regional metastases), the chosen method of reconstruction,

the need for systemic therapy (thus delaying the radiation), the opinion of the plastic surgeon on radiating the reconstructed breast, and the opinion of the radiation oncologist on the relative benefits of chest wall radiation depending on the number of involved nodes. In some cases it may be reasonable to proceed with mastectomy, SLN biopsy and reconstruction and wait until the final pathology report to decide on the relative pros and cons of radiating the reconstructed breast. However, in some cases it may be preferable to take the patient to the operating room for a SLN biopsy alone. Frozen section should be planned on, with ALND performed if the SLN positive. Often this procedure can be combined with a ligation of the inferior epigastric vessels if a pedicled TRAM flap is planned. If the nodes are negative, the patient returns to the operating room for a mastectomy and reconstruction with minimal risk of needing postmastectomy with external beam radiation therapy. If the nodes are positive, a discussion can be held with the patient and reconstruction potentially delayed.

Oncoplastic Approaches to Lumpectomy

The ultimate goal of breast conservation therapy is to both remove the cancer with an adequate surgical margin *and* maintain the breast's shape and appearance. This can be difficult depending on the tumor size and location. When a tumor is too large to accomplish this goal, the surgeon typically has two options. The first is to perform a mastectomy with reconstruction, and the second is to give neoadjuvant chemotherapy in hopes of downstaging the primary tumor to allow a more cosmetic lumpectomy. For situations in which neither option is desirable, a third possibility is using oncoplastic techniques for the lumpectomy. The term *oncoplastic surgery* refers to a host of volume displacement operations in which the defect created by a large lumpectomy is filled in using a breast-flap mastopexy closure; advancing breast tissue along the chest wall to help fill in the defect, using a full-thickness segment of breast fibroglandular tissue.

With a typical lumpectomy, the resulting defect is spherical or oblong in shape and left to fill in with seroma fluid and then reabsorb at radiation. If this defect is large, leaving redundant skin over the defect, infolding can occur so that the skin adheres to the chest wall and the nipple deviates toward the lumpectomy site. Oncoplastic approaches to lumpectomy use full thickness lumpectomies, with an overlying skin island removed with the lumpectomy and the fibroglandular tissue resected down to the chest wall. The goal is that there is no direct contact between the skin and the chest wall to prevent this indenting. After the lumpectomy, the breast gland is lifted off of the pectoralis muscle with preservation of the fascia over the muscle. This is advanced over the chest wall and the defect is then closed. If advancement of the tissue seems as though it will displace the nipple-areolar complex, this can be avoided by widely undermining the nipple-areolar complex at the level of the pectoralis fascia, which allows the tissues to shift to an anatomically natural position.

When doing so, the vascular perforators between the pectoralis and breast must be kept in mind. However, the extensive collateral circulation of the breast allows much flexibility for oncoplastic techniques. Once the fibroglandular tissue is mobilized, the breast defect is closed at full thickness. The deep margin of the advanced breast tissue is sutured at the deepest and most superficial edges, and the skin is reapproximated. This decreases the size of the seroma cavity and prevents the skin from adhering to the chest wall, resulting in a better cosmetic outcome.

The removal of a skin island will often cause a distortion of the breast. In some cases, excision of a large amount of skin will cause upward displacement of the nipple-areolar complex, which can be quite awkward looking. In this situation, it is better to use a linear incision in the skin and not remove any skin island. When a skin island is to be resected with the specimen, the ideal defect has superior and inferior margins that are equal in length. A useful design is a rounded parallelogram (Fig 14–20). The two skin incisions are tapered at the corners so that the two incision lines can approach each other easily at the corners, diminishing the V angle at the corner and minimizing any dog ear. Full thickness excision is performed with advancement of the fibroglandular tissue.

A useful approach for cancers underneath the nipple-areolar complex is the batwing mastopexy (Fig 14–21). Two closely similar half-circle incisions are made with angled wings to each side of the areola. Full thickness excision is performed with advancement of the fibroglandular tissue. This will minimize the defect and maintain the natural shape of the breast, however, it will cause lifting of the nipple, resulting in asymmetry. A contralateral lift will be necessary to alleviate the asymmetry.

For large tumors in the lateral or upper portions of the breast, the donut mastopexy lumpectomy can be used. A donut of skin is excised around the nipple-areolar complex

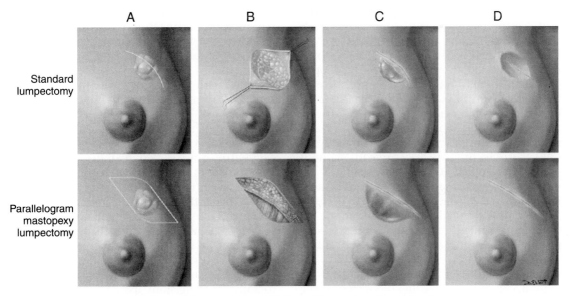

Figure 14–20. The rounded parallelogram is useful when skin needs to be excised.

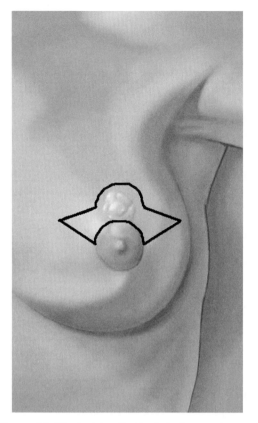

Figure 14–21. Incision for the batwing mastopexy.

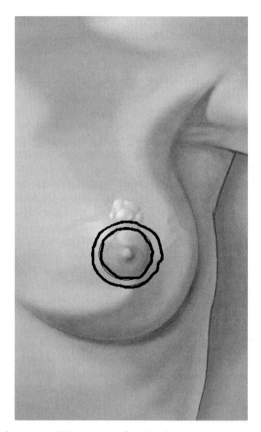

Figure 14–22. Incision for the donut mastopexy.

(Fig 14–22). This tissue ring is removed to allow adequate access to the breast tissue. A generous lumpectomy is performed down to the chest wall and the remaining fibroglandular tissue is advanced and sutured at both the deep and superficial margins. The skin is reapproximated with a purse-string closure. Cancer in the lower part of the breast is difficult because retraction of the lumpectomy cavity will cause downturning of the nipple. For large lesions in the lower hemisphere of the breast, the approach used for breast reduction can also be used to perform a lumpectomy (Fig 14–23). The donut mastopexy and reduction mastopexy are more challenging oncoplastic techniques and surgeons without specific training should be cautious.

There are several issues that need to be kept in mind when the decision is made to perform an oncoplastic resection. Positive margins are often more difficult to deal with after an oncoplastic lumpectomy than with a standard lumpectomy. Knowing the exact extent of the cancer before and during the operation is helpful, so preoperative magnetic resonance imaging (MRI) and intraoperative ultrasound may facilitate achieving negative margins on the first excision. Taking additional margins at the time of the lumpectomy will help minimize the likelihood of positive margins, especially considering that the close or positive margin is often the result of ink running down cracks in the fibroglandular tissue (especially after wire localized specimens are imaged). As with standard lumpectomy, specimens should be inked with the six-color system so that the surgeon knows which margin is positive. Some surgeons ink their own specimens for optimum confidence. Using multiple colors allows the surgeon to reenter the biopsy cavity and excise the one or two margins of concern. When a donut mastopexy or reduction mastopexy is used, reexcision may not be possible, and a mastectomy is indicated for positive margins. One advantage of the donut mastopexy is that the periareolar incision still allows for a skin-sparing mastectomy.

Another concern with oncoplastic lumpectomy is the planning of the adjuvant radiation therapy. The incisions used may confuse the

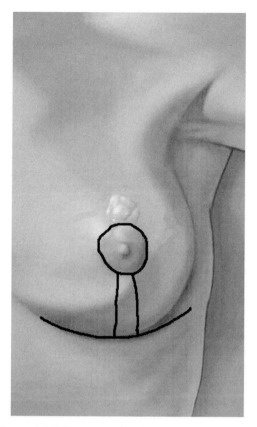

Figure 14-23. Incision for the reduction mastopexy.

radiation oncologist as to the location of the lumpectomy cavity. The placement of multiple clips around the cavity will help, however, these have to be placed carefully to truly represent the extent of the cancer because the advancement of fibroglandular tissue will distort the true cavity. Oncoplastic techniques may also not be compatible with partial breast irradiation (PBI), in which knowledge of the cavity is essential to success. However, oncoplastic surgery is typically reserved for big tumors and PBI is typically not recommended for larger tumors.

Finally, oncoplastic techniques will often maintain the natural shape of the breast and avoid large indentations, but will often decrease the volume of the breast. Many of these patients will require contralateral breast reduction. This can be done at the same time as the lumpectomy, which helps avoid a second surgery or can be done at a later date. Delaying the breast reduction until it is known that mastectomy will not be necessary and the radiation is completed is beneficial so that the contralateral breast can be perfectly matched to the final result.

Suggested Readings

1. Alderman AK, Wilkins E, Kim M, et al. Complications in post-mastectomy breast reconstruction: two year results of the Michigan breast reconstruction outcome study. Plast Reconstr Surg 2002; 109:2265–2274.
2. Alderman AK, Kuhn LE, Lowery JC, et al. Does patient satisfaction with breast reconstruction change over time? Two-year results of the Michigan Breast Reconstruction Outcomes Study. J Am Coll Surg 2007;204(1):7–12.
3. Alderman AK, Wilkins EG, Kim HM, et al. Complications in postmastectomy breast reconstruction: two-year results of the Michigan Breast Reconstruction Outcome Study. Plast Reconstr Surg 2002; 109(7):2265–2274.
4. Anderson BO, Masetti R, Silverstein MJ. Oncoplastic approaches to partial mastectomy: an overview of volume-displacement techniques. Lancet Oncol 2005;6:145–157.
5. Asgeirsson KS, Rasheed T, McCulley SJ, et al. Oncological and cosmetic outcomes of oncoplastic breast conserving surgery. Eur J Surg Oncol 2005;31(8): 817–823.
6. Chawla A, Kachnic L, Taghian A, et al. Radiotherapy and breast reconstruction: complications and cosmesis with TRAM versus tissue expander/implant. Int J Radiat Oncol Biol Phys 2002;54(2):520–526.
7. Cunnick GH, Mokbel K. Skin-sparing mastectomy. Am J Surg 2004;188(1):78–84.
8. Garvey PB, Buchel EW, Pockaj BA, et al. DIEP and pedicled TRAM flaps: a comparison of outcomes. Plast Reconstr Surg 2006;117(6):1711–1719.
9. Harcourt D, Rumsey N, Amber NR, et al. The psychological effect of mastectomy with or without breast reconstruction: A prospective multicenter study. Plast Reconstr Surg 2003;111:1060–1068.
10. Helvie MA, Bailey JE, Roubidoux MA, et al. Mammographic screening of TRAM flap breast reconstructions for detection of nonpalpable recurrent cancer. Radiology 2002;224(1):211–216.
11. Javaid M, Song F, Leinster S, et al. Radiation effects on the cosmetic outcomes of immediate and delayed autologous breast reconstruction: An argument about timing. J Plast Reconstr Aesthet Surg 2006;59:16–26.
12. Jones G. The pedicled TRAM flap in breast reconstruction. Clin Plast Surg 2007;34(1):83–104.
13. Jugenburg M, Disa JJ, Pusic AL, et al. Impact of radiotherapy on breast reconstruction. Clin Plast Surg 2006;x(x):29–37.
14. Masetti R, Di Leone A, Franceschini G, et al. Oncoplastic techniques in the conservative surgical treatment of breast cancer: an overview. Breast J 2006; 12(5 Suppl 2):S174–S180.
15. Nahabedian MY, Momen B, Galdino G, et al. Breast reconstruction with the free TRAM or DIEP flap: patient selection, choice of flap, and outcome. Plast Reconstr Surg 2002;110(2):466–475.
16. Nahabedian MY. Nipple reconstructon. Clin Plast Surg 2007;34(1):131–137.
17. Rainsbury RM. Skin-sparing mastectomy. Br J Surg 2006;93(3):276–281.
18. Rainsbury RM. Surgery insight: Oncoplastic breast-conserving reconstruction—indications, benefits, choices and outcomes. Nat Clin Pract Oncol 2007; 4(11):657–664.

19. Senkus-Konefka E, Welnicka-Jaskeiwicz M, Jaskeiwicz J, et al. Radiotherapy for breast cancer in patients undergoing breast reconstruction or augmentation. Cancer Treat Rev 2004;30:671–682.

20. U.S. Department of Labor. Your rights after a mastectomy ... Women's Health & Cancer Rights Act of 1998. Available at www.dol.gov/ebsa/publications/whcra.

21. Wilkins E. University of Michigan Breast Reconstruction Handbook. Available at www.med.umich.edu/surgery/plastic/clinical/breast/index.shtml.

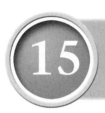

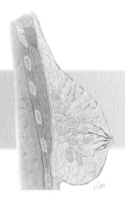

15

Principles of Radiation Therapy for Primary Breast Cancer

INTRODUCTION

HOW DOES RADIATION KILL CANCER?

BENEFIT OF RADIATION THERAPY IN BREAST CANCER
Breast Conservation Therapy
Postmastectomy Radiation

DELIVERY OF RADIATION TO THE BREAST AND CHEST WALL

COMPLICATIONS OF BREAST AND CHEST WALL RADIATION

PARTIAL BREAST IRRADIATION
Interstitial Brachytherapy
Balloon-Catheter Brachytherapy
External Beam Radiation
Intraoperative Radiation
    Therapy

Principles of Radiation Therapy for Primary Breast Cancer: Key Points

- Describe how radiation kills cells and the concept of sublethal damage repair.
- Be familiar with the prospective randomized data comparing lumpectomy alone to lumpectomy and radiation therapy.
- Understand how reducing local recurrence risk may improve overall survival.
- Describe the indications for postmastectomy radiation.
- Understand how radiation is delivered to the breast and chest wall.
- Appreciate the complications of radiation therapy and their management.
- Know the methods and potential for partial breast irradiation and the unanswered questions and possible risks.

Introduction

Shortly after the discovery of x-rays by Wilhelm Roentgen in 1895 and of radium by Marie Curie in 1898, it was realized that ionizing radiation could be used against breast cancer. In 1905, the first radiologic textbooks proposed the use of radiation therapy for unresectable primary tumors, including breast cancer. In 1937, Sir Geoffrey Keynes, a surgeon in England, proposed the notion of radium needle insertion into operable breast cancer as an alternative to mastectomy. He reported 5-year local recurrence rates and survivals similar to what was being obtained with radical mastectomy. Similar results were obtained from the Curie Foundation in Paris and other European investigators.

These results, combined with improved methods of delivering radiation, eventually led to the recognition and implementation of using radiation to eradicate cancer cell aggregates remaining after surgical excision. This of course depended on the size of the aggregates and the dose of radiation used. Although radiation doses of 45 to 50 grays (Gy) are capable of eliminating subclinical deposits of cancer 90% to 95% of the time, larger tumor masses require substantially larger doses. Masses greater than a few centimeters require doses greater than the radiation tolerance of the surrounding normal tissue. Therefore, the optimum use of radiation is when it must contend only with microscopic disease. Radiation is used in all stages of breast cancer, from the adjuvant therapy of ductal carcinoma in situ (DCIS) to the palliative treatment of metastases. This chapter will primarily review the most common use of radiation therapy in the management of breast cancer, that is, as an adjuvant to surgical therapy.

How Does Radiation Kill Cancer?

Understanding the way radiation therapy is incorporated into the treatment of breast cancer requires a basic understanding of how ionizing radiation kills cancer cells. Ionizing radiation is defined as energy with sufficient strength to cause the ejection of an orbital electron from an atom when the radiation is absorbed. When this occurs in biologic tissue, the ejected electrons can indirectly or directly lead to irreparable double-stranded DNA breaks. When the cell next enters mitosis, it cannot divide and cell death occurs (reproductive cell death).

Ionizing radiation can take either an electromagnetic form, as high-energy photons, or particulate forms, such as electrons, protons, neutrons, alpha particles, or other particles. Most radiation is delivered through either electrons or photons. Electrons interact directly with tissue causing ionization, in contrast to photons, which affect tissues by the electrons that they eject. Electron beams deliver a high-skin dose and exhibit a rapid fall-off after only a few centimeters, so they are typically only used to treat superficial targets such as skin cancers or lymph nodes within a few centimeters of the surface of the body. Irradiation with photons can penetrate deeper into tissues. Photons can cause the ejection of electrons by a variety of methods (Fig. 15–1), but the most important is the *Compton Effect*, in which a photon collides with an electron, transferring some of its energy to the electron and scattering both the photon and the electron in various directions. The photon can then undergo additional interactions (with a subsequently lower energy), while the electron begins to ionize with the energy it gained from the photon.

The electrons either interact directly with the target molecules within the cell, or they interact indirectly with water to produce free radicals (such as hydroxyl radicals) that

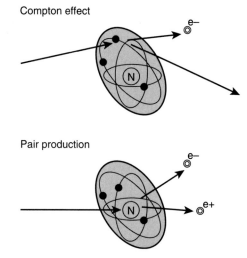

Figure 15–1. Photons can release electrons (which react directly with tissue) by a number of methods. In the Compton Effect, a photon collides with an electron, transferring energy to the electron and scattering both. The photon can go on to have additional interactions, albeit with a lower energy. In pair production, the photon interacts with the nucleus that absorbs the energy and releases a pair of electrons, one positively charged (positron) and one negatively charged.

subsequently interact with target molecules. During their brief life span, electrons and free radicals interact with molecules in a random fashion. If they interact with molecules that are not crucial to cell survival, the effect of the radiation will be harmless. If they react with biologically important molecules, the effect will be detrimental. Molecular oxygen prolongs the life of reactive radicals, increasing the likelihood that it will have a detrimental effect. This is why tumor hypoxia tends to increase resistance to radiation. Antioxidants reduce the life span of free radicals by combining with them, thereby also increasing cellular resistance to radiation.

Although ionizing radiation may damage many molecules with the cell, the most critical injury with respect to cell death appears to be DNA damage in the form of single- or double-strand breaks (Fig. 15–2). Cells have relatively efficient repair mechanisms for single-strand breaks in DNA because there is an intact template on which to replicate a repair patch. However, repair errors may occur resulting in mutations, and ultimately may lead to

the increased incidence of secondary malignancies that occur in between 1 in 500 and 1 in 1000 patients who have had radiation.

Double-strand breaks in DNA are much more difficult for cells to repair because the integrity of the molecule is compromised with the creation of two free ends that separate from one another in space, leaving no template on which to repair the break. Cellular mechanisms for double-strand break repair do exist, however, their efficiency is variable and repair may not be sufficient before cells trigger pathways leading to programmed cell death (apoptosis) or enter into mitosis with damaged DNA, leading to mitotic catastrophe and cell death. Therefore, the ability of ionizing radiation to kill cells is dependent not only on the generation of enough DNA double-strand breaks to overwhelm repair pathways, but also on the time the cell has to repair those breaks before the next mitotic cell division.

This explains the phenomenon known as *sublethal damage repair* in which increased cell survival is observed if a dose of radiation is divided into two fractions separated by a time

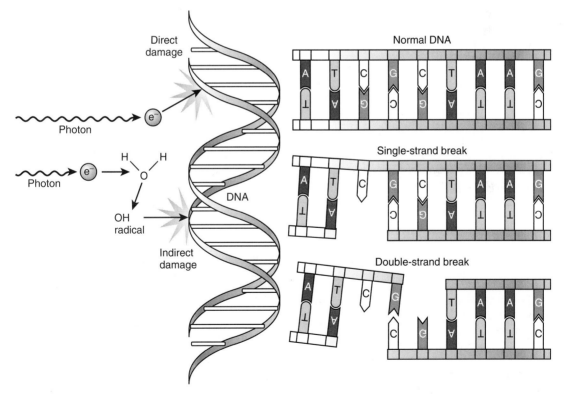

Figure 15–2. Whether directly or indirectly, the electrons lead to DNA damage. This occurs when the "backbone" of the molecule is broken. Single-strand breaks can be easily restored by DNA repair mechanisms within the cell, whereas double-strand breaks are more damaging because they are more difficult to repair by cellular mechanisms. (From Sabel M, Sondak V, Sussman J. Essentials of Surgical Oncology. Philadelphia: Elsevier, 2006.)

interval. As the time interval between the fractions increases, the surviving fraction of the cells also increases because the cells are able to repair double-strand DNA breaks. Furthermore, if the time interval is sufficiently long, the cells will once again begin to proliferate in a process known as repopulation.

Of course, in clinical radiation therapy, the goal is to kill the cancer cells but spare the normal cells. Delivering a single large dose of radiation will have a high rate of killing tumor cells, but the concordant killing of the normal tissue cells may limit the clinical use because of normal tissue toxicity. Fractionation of radiation (delivering a fraction of the dose daily) spares normal tissues because of their greater ability to repair sublethal damage between dose fractions and repopulate with cells if the overall time is sufficiently long. Although tumors may also repair sublethal damage and repopulate, there is increased damage to the tumor because dividing a dose into a number of fractions allows reoxygenation of hypoxic regions within the tumor and reassortment of tumor cells into radiosensitive phases of the cell cycle between dose fractions.

Benefit of Radiation Therapy in Breast Cancer

Radiation has been used for the treatment of locally advanced or inoperable breast cancer for almost a century, beginning shortly after the discovery of radiation's effects on human tissue. After British surgeon Keynes reported how treating operable breast tumors with radium needle insertion alone had both local recurrence rates and survival rates similar to that of radical mastectomy, several European trials of radiation with and without surgery for operable breast cancers began and laid the foundation for breast-conserving therapy (BCT). Today radiation therapy has multiple uses in the management of breast cancer, such as the treatment of chest wall recurrences or palliation of bone metastases, but the primary use of radiation is in the management of early therapy as either a component of BCT, or chest wall irradiation following mastectomy. The optimal local management of breast cancer requires coordination between the surgeon, the plastic surgeon, and the radiation oncologist.

Radiation therapy clearly reduces local recurrence rates. However, does the addition of radiation to surgery improve survival? Several of the randomized trials that established the efficacy of breast conservation included arms in which women underwent lumpectomy alone, without radiation (Table 15–1). These studies demonstrated no significant survival difference between those two groups despite a significant increase in local recurrence. Unfortunately, this led to the incorrect conclusion that "preventing local recurrence has no impact on survival." For this reason, some physicians became willing to offer local therapies that carried a high local recurrence rate under the impression that if patients do recur and undergo salvage mastectomy, their survival remained unchanged. There was little evidence that preventing the local recurrence would have prevented the distant disease. However, the original randomized trials that demonstrated no difference in survival between lumpectomy alone and lumpectomy with radiation did not have the power to detect a small survival advantage from the addition of radiation therapy. In addition, the morbidity and mortality associated with radiation therapy negated some survival advantage, particularly with older methods for delivering radiation. More recent data clearly demonstrates

TABLE 15–1 • Randomized Trials of Lumpectomy Versus Lumpectomy and External Beam Radiation Therapy				Local Recurrence	
Study	N	Follow-Up (Years)	Maximum Tumor Size (cm)	Surgery (%)	Surgery + External Beam Therapy (%)
Milan III	567	4.3	2.5	8.8	0.3
NSABP B-06	1262	12	4	35	10
Ontario	837	7.6	3	35	11
Scottish	585	5.7	4	24.5	5
Upsalla-Orebro	381	10	2	24	8.5
NSABP B-21	1009	6	1	12	5.6

BOX 15-1 CONTRAINDICATIONS TO BREAST-CONSERVING THERAPY

Multicentric disease
Previous radiation
Diffuse malignant-appearing
  microcalcifications on mammography
First or second trimester of pregnancy
Collagen vascular disease
Unable to achieve negative margins

that improved local control does impact survival and establishes that radiation is a critical component of BCT.

Breast Conservation Therapy

The emergence of BCT as an alternative to mastectomy is discussed in detail in Chapter 12 (Box 15–1). The benefits of adding radiation to lumpectomy are clear when one examines the trials comparing lumpectomy to lumpectomy and radiation therapy (see Table 15–1). However, these trials also showed no significant difference in overall survival between these groups. The conclusion was that radiation reduced in-breast recurrence but had minimal impact on the overall survival of the patient.

Subsequent to this, several series noted that patients who underwent lumpectomy and radiation therapy and experienced a local recurrence had a lower survival than their counterparts who did not have a local recurrence. However, it was not able in these retrospective series to determine whether the local recurrence led to the distant metastases. It is also possible (and likely) that patients with more aggressive tumors were more likely to experience both local and distant recurrences, and that preventing the local recurrence would not have improved survival (Fig. 15–3). The strongest evidence for this latter argument was the absence of a survival difference between lumpectomy and lumpectomy with radiation in the randomized trials, despite large differences in recurrence.

Although many patients who experience local recurrence may have harbored distant micrometastases at the time of their initial surgery, is there a fraction of patients whose local recurrence led to their distant disease? The corollary to this is that preventing local recurrence would improve survival. Unfortunately, the individual randomized trials were all underpowered to detect a small difference in survival. In addition, the cardiac toxicity of radiation therapy, and the negative impact it has on survival, may have masked any survival benefit of local control. This is particularly true of the older techniques for delivering radiation.

The improved local control rate achieved with radiation therapy is impressive. The most recent update of the Early Breast Cancer Trialists Collaborative Group (ECGTCG) meta-analysis

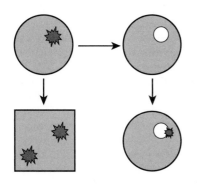

Aggressive tumor biology leads to both local recurrence and distant recurrence. Preventing local recurrence has no impact on
A survival.

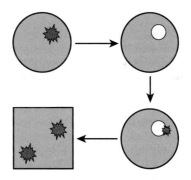

Distant disease did not exist at the time of surgery, but the local recurrence metastasized. Preventing local recurrence does
B impact survival.

Figure 15-3. Impact of local recurrence on distant recurrence. **A,** An aggressive tumor biology leads to both the local recurrence and the distant metastases. Thus, preventing local recurrence has no impact on survival because the micrometastases exist before therapy. **B,** There was no distant disease at the time of definitive surgery, but inadequate local therapy led to a local recurrence, which subsequently developed the ability to metastasize. In this scenario, preventing local recurrence would impact survival. Although it was for a long time accepted that scenario A was most relevant to breast cancer, recent evidence has shown that scenario B is more significant than previously believed.

demonstrated a 5-year local recurrence rate of 7% for breast conservation with radiation therapy and 26% when radiation therapy was excluded. The most recent update of the ECGTCG meta-analysis demonstrates that the 15-year breast cancer mortality risks were also significantly lower in the patients who received radiation therapy (30.5 versus 35.9, $p = 0.002$).

A pooled analysis of mortality data from 13 randomized trials also showed a worse survival in women who did not receive radiation therapy, with an 8.6% excess mortality. This data clearly demonstrates that improved local control does impact survival, and women with an exceedingly high risk of in-breast recurrence with BCT compared to mastectomy may be better served by the latter. It also establishes that radiation is a critical component of breast conservation therapy.

Lumpectomy without Radiation

The benefits of adding radiation are clear, but this is certainly not without cost. Radiation to the breast has both acute and late complications, and although radiation will reduce local recurrence, many patients treated with lumpectomy alone will not recur. Therefore, there has been significant interest in whether there exist subsets of patients for whom the in-breast recurrence risk is low enough that the toxicity of radiation therapy may not be justified. Overall, attempts to identify such a subset of patients who have a low enough risk of local recurrence to justify surgery alone have not been overly successful. Several of the randomized trials sought to identify subsets that may not require radiation therapy. In the Uppsala-Orebro trial, in women over 55 with tumors less than 2 cm (excluding comedo or lobular histologies), the local recurrence rate was 6% with radiation, but only 11% without radiation. The authors suggest that radiation may not be of benefit in this subset because 20 women need to be treated to prevent just one breast recurrence. In contrast to this, the Ontario group could identify no such group. Even among women over 50 with tumors less than 1 cm, the local recurrence rate was 18% without radiation therapy.

Other trials specifically attempted to stratify or select patients to answer whether radiation was needed in all patients. The Scottish trial was designed to specifically look at the impact of radiation therapy in the setting of appropriate systemic therapy. Patients with estrogen receptor (ER)-positive tumors who received tamoxifen had a drop in local recurrence from 14% to 3% with the addition of radiation. Patients who received adjuvant therapy had a decrease from 38.5% to 9%. The conclusion was that adjuvant systemic therapy was not a substitute for breast irradiation. Another study of the need for radiation in the face of adjuvant therapy was NSABP B-21. This trial included 1009 women undergoing lumpectomy for invasive breast cancer equal to 1 cm in size and found that women treated by lumpectomy with tamoxifen had a 16.5% local recurrence rate compared to 2.8% for lumpectomy, radiation, and tamoxifen (and 9.3% for lumpectomy and radiation therapy without tamoxifen). This demonstrates that even with the use of systemic therapy, radiation therapy significantly decreases local recurrence in patients with small tumors. Finally, a prospective trial of women with the most favorable features (tumor size 2 cm, histologically negative axillary nodes, absence of angiolymphatic invasion, or extensive intraductal component [EIC] and margins >1 cm) who underwent surgery alone, the trial needed to be stopped early because of the high local recurrence rate (20%).

One subset of patients for whom the avoidance of radiation seems possible is older women with hormone receptor positive tumors. Several retrospective series of conservative surgery alone in older women have shown varying rates of local recurrence, but similar distant recurrence and survival rates. Two randomized trials have shown comparable results. In a Canadian trial randomizing women over the age of 50 undergoing lumpectomy with adjuvant tamoxifen to radiation or none, radiation therapy significantly decreased the risk of local recurrence (17.6% versus 3.5% at 8 years), but did not appear to impact rates of distant metastases, overall survival, and the number of deaths as a result of breast cancer. However, given what we now appreciate about local control and overall survival, this local recurrence rate seems uncomfortably high. A Cancer and Leukemia Group B (CALGB) trial of women over the age of 70 also showed a difference in the risk of local recurrence in women treated with tamoxifen with or without radiation therapy (4% versus 1%), but no impact on overall survival (86% versus 87% at 5 years). Rates of mastectomy for local failure were also similar. Although the Canadian trial included tumors up to 5 cm, the CALGB trial was limited to tumors less than 2 cm. Thus, in selected women over the age of

70 with small ER-positive breast cancer, treatment with lumpectomy and tamoxifen alone may be a reasonable option.

Postmastectomy Radiation

It is often presented to patients that one of the advantages of mastectomy over BCT is that radiation therapy will not be necessary. However, chest wall recurrence after mastectomy alone is not an infrequent event. The risk of local-regional failure after mastectomy increases with both increasing tumor size and increasing numbers of involved axillary nodes. Trials of postmastectomy radiation, accruing patients in the 60s and 70s, demonstrated that postmastectomy radiation could decrease chest wall recurrences. Similar to the experience with BCT, however, these trials did not demonstrate any significant effect on overall survival. In fact, there was even the suggestion of a decreased survival. But as before, these trials were underpowered to detect a small survival benefit, and they mostly involved radiation techniques that had increased morbidity and mortality compared to today's approaches.

Meta-analysis of these trials, with long-term follow-up and cause-specific mortality recorded, present a different picture. These demonstrate that mortality from late cardiac effects were responsible for canceling out any survival advantage to radiation therapy, something not present to the same degree today using modern radiotherapy techniques. The most recent meta-analysis by the ECGTCG, including 46 randomized trials involving over 23,000 patients, found that postmastectomy radiation therapy was associated with a significant reduction in both local recurrence (5.8% versus 22.8% at 5 years) and in breast cancer mortality for women who are node positive (54.7% versus 60.1%, $p = 0.0002$).

Several trials using more modern radiotherapy and adjuvant systemic therapy have further demonstrated the impact of postmastectomy radiation. The first Danish Breast Cancer Cooperative Group trial included 1708 premenopausal women with either positive nodes or T3 or T4 tumors to undergo mastectomy, axillary sampling, and postoperative chemotherapy and then be randomized to receive chest wall and regional nodal irradiation or not. With a median follow-up of about 10 years, postmastectomy radiotherapy was associated with a significant improvement in locoregional failure (32% versus 9%), disease-free survival (48% versus 34%), and overall survival (54% versus 45%). However, this trial required only axillary sampling, not a complete dissection, and the majority of recurrences were in the axilla, a relatively rare occurrence in patients who had a level I and II dissection. It is unclear what the results of this trial would have been had the patients had a complete axillary lymph node dissection (ALND), as is done routinely in the United States.

In the British Columbia trial, 318 premenopausal women with node-positive breast cancer undergoing modified radical mastectomy (MRM) were randomly assigned to cyclophosphamide, methotrexate, and fluorouracil (CMF) plus chest wall radiotherapy versus CMF alone. Improvements in local-regional recurrence and disease-free survival (DFS) were again seen, with a trend toward improved survival. With 20-year follow-up, the overall survival benefit was statistically significant (overall survival 47% versus 37%, hazard ratio [HR] 0.73 95% confidence interval [CI] 0.55 to 0.98). A third trial, also from the Danish Breast Cancer Cooperative Group, randomized 1375 postmenopausal women with stage II or III breast cancer to adjuvant tamoxifen (30 mg/day for 1 year) alone or with postoperative chest wall irradiation. Once again, significant improvements were seen with postmastectomy radiation therapy in regard to local-regional recurrence (8% versus 35%), 10-year DFS (36% versus 24%), and overall survival (45% versus 36%, $p = 0.03$).

Based on these studies, postmastectomy radiation is recommended for several subsets of patients. Patients with four or more positive lymph nodes clearly benefit from postmastectomy radiation therapy. The data is less clear for patients with one to three positive nodes. Although the impact of treatment on survival might be similar, the risk of recurrence and death is less, and given the questions regarding the surgery used in the Danish trials, it is difficult to translate these findings to the U.S. practice of axillary clearance. For now, there is insufficient evidence to recommend routine chest wall radiation therapy for women with one to three axillary nodes, but these women should have the relative pros and cons of postmastectomy radiation presented to them. Other patients who should undergo postmastectomy radiation therapy include women with T3 and T4 tumors, those with positive margins after mastectomy, patients with advanced nodal disease (N2 or N3), or with gross extranodal extension.

It is important to keep in mind that if post-mastectomy radiation is to be used, this may impact the timing and method of reconstruction. The cosmetic outcome of immediate breast reconstruction will be affected by radiation (Chapter 14). This is particularly true if tissue expanders and implants are used, but radiation can also negatively affect autologous reconstructions. Another less-recognized problem is that the reconstruction can negatively impact the delivery of radiation. One option is to simply delay reconstruction until all treatment is completed. However, if immediate reconstruction is desired, there are options to minimize the likelihood of radiating a reconstructed breast. The simplest option is to perform the sentinel lymph node (SLN) biopsy as a separate procedure before mastectomy. This can be combined with ligation of the inferior epigastric vessels when indicated for reconstruction purposes. If the SLN is negative, the next step is mastectomy and reconstruction. If the patient is node positive, reconstruction can be delayed, especially if tissue expanders were planned.

Delivery of Radiation to the Breast and Chest Wall

When adjuvant chemotherapy is necessary, radiation will follow the chemotherapy. If negative margins were not achieved and the initiation of chemotherapy is being delayed by the need for reexcision, it is reasonable to proceed with the chemotherapy and return to surgery between chemotherapy and radiation therapy. Either way, negative margins must be obtained before beginning radiation. Concomitant chemoradiotherapy may minimize the time necessary to complete therapy, but it also limits the doses of chemotherapeutic agents secondary to increased myelosuppression, increases side effects, and negatively impacts cosmesis. Its use in this setting is strongly discouraged.

When chemotherapy is not used, radiation should follow surgery once adequate time for healing has been allowed (typically 4 weeks). Sometimes this may be delayed because of the formation of a seroma. Repeated aspirations of the seroma during therapy will cause fluctuations in the breast contour and the skin marks. Thus, the need to aspirate the seroma must be balanced against when radiation will commence or conclude and the patient's symptoms. Radiation may also be delayed by the patient's inability to abduct and maintain the arm in

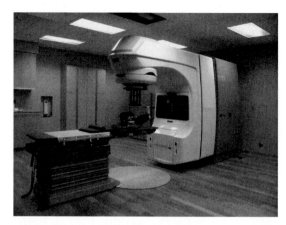

Figure 15–4. Linear accelerator.

the treatment position, as may be seen after an ALND or MRM. A small delay is reasonable; however, a delay in the initiation of radiation therapy beyond 12 to 16 weeks has been associated with increased rates of relapse.

The hallmark of the modern era of radiotherapy is the delivery of radiation in the megavoltage range. This minimized many of the undesirable effects resulting from lower-energy radiation (such as orthovoltage, 150 to 500 kV, or supervoltage, 500 to 1000 kV). The most common machines providing megavoltage radiation therapy are linear accelerators (Fig. 15–4). These have several advantages over the older approaches that have greatly limited toxicity and ultimately allowed the survival advantages of local control to surpass the morbidity of radiation (Box 15–2).

Delivering radiation begins with simulation. Most simulation today is accomplished

BOX 15–2 ADVANTAGES OF THE LINEAR ACCELERATOR

- A higher-energy x-ray beam that treats deeper lesions with greater skin sparing
- In addition to the x-ray beam, it can deliver a high-energy electron beam for more superficial lesions
- Sharper beam edges for more accurate shaping to match the desired target and minimize radiation to surrounding structures
- Greater dose rate, allowing treatment to be accomplished faster
- No exposure to personnel
- No need to change the radioactive material because of isotope delay

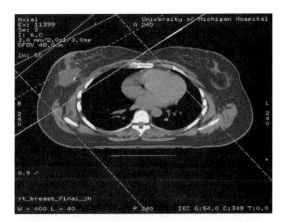

Figure 15–5. Computed tomography simulation allows for better visualization of the breast, chest wall, heart, and lungs. Medial and lateral tangent fields are arranged to minimize damage to normal tissues.

using computed tomography (CT) scanning (Figure 15–5). With modern CT technology, virtual simulation allows for better visualization of the breast, chest wall, and most importantly the relation to the lung and heart, thus minimizing damage to normal tissues. Minimizing toxicity to the underlying heart and lung must be carefully considered in the treatment plan. The patient is scanned with the breast in an immobilization device so that the patient position is reproducible from day to day. Typically this is in the supine position, but the prone position can be used for the patient with a pendulous breast, provided adequate coverage of the tumor is achieved. The scanned information is then brought up on the treatment planning console and the treatment plan is created. The target volume for whole breast radiation therapy extends medially to the middle of the sternum, and laterally to the midaxillary line. The inferior edge of the field is approximately 1 cm below the inframammary fold in the intact breast or the contralateral inframammary fold when treating the chest wall. Superiorly, the field typically ends at the base of the head of the clavicle.

For the initial whole-breast irradiation, 6-MV photon therapy generated by a linear accelerator is generally used. This provides an optimal balance between skin sparing and treatment of the entire breast. Electron beams can be used for postmastectomy irradiation but are unable to penetrate deeper into the breast for whole-breast irradiation.

Once the treatment plan has been formulated, small tattoos are placed to mark the field for daily radiation and treatment is initiated. The radiation will be administered through a medial and lateral tangent field arrangement that parallels the arc of the chest wall. Although they may vary, typical whole breast irradiation doses are 45 to 50 Gy, using daily fractions of 1.8 or 2.0 Gy. Treatments are delivered daily, 5 days per week, Monday through Friday. This takes 5 to 6½ weeks to complete. Several questions need to be addressed when planning whole-breast irradiation as a component of breast conservation therapy.

- Fractionation schedules—In countries where availability to radiation is limited, there is interest in shortening the time it takes to complete therapy. A Canadian trial demonstrated no difference in 5-year local-recurrence free survival, DFS, overall survival, and cosmetic outcome between node-negative patients receiving 50 Gy in 25 fractions (taking 35 days) and those receiving 42.5 Gy in 16 fractions (taking 22 days). Although more information is needed, for selected patients this may be an alternative to the 5 1/2 weeks presently needed.
- Boost—A boost of radiation, often using electrons, can be delivered to the primary tumor site, increasing the total dose delivered to 60 to 66 Gy. Three randomized trials have been performed, two showing that adding a boost can reduce the rate of local failure. The larger trial, performed by the European Organization for Research and Treatment of Cancer (EORTC), stratified patients by resection margins (negative or positive). Local recurrence was significantly lower (4.3% versus 7.3%) in women with negative resection margins who received a boost, without a drop-off in cosmetic outcome. The placement of surgical clips around the cavity at the time of surgery greatly assists the radiation oncologist in planning the boost and should be a standard component of a lumpectomy.
- Regional lymph nodes—Another decision is whether to include the regional lymph nodes in the field. There is no indication to treat the axilla when surgical staging has demonstrated the axillary nodes to be pathologically negative. In addition, it is not recommended when a complete ALND has been performed because the combination of surgery and radiation results in a high rate of lymphedema. Radiation to the axilla can be considered when the axilla has not been

surgically staged. For the patient with a positive axillary SLN, axillary radiation has been proposed as an alternative to completion dissection.

The benefit of irradiating the internal mammary nodes (IMNs) is more controversial. Some recommend a routine inclusion of the IMNs, and some recommend a selective use when either the axillary lymph nodes are involved or the primary tumor is located in the inner quadrant. Today, some use the lymphoscintigraphy obtained for the SLN biopsy to determine whether there is internal mammary drainage. Arguments against internal mammary radiation include the increased incidence of cardiac toxicity and the fact that clinical recurrence in this region is uncommon. In addition, a survival benefit for resecting these nodes (as was done with the extended radical mastectomy) has not been shown, suggesting radiation would not benefit survival. Proponents argue that detection of internal mammary recurrences is difficult, so their incidence may be underreported. With modern CT planning, the IMNs can be irradiated with minimal cardiac toxicity and pathologic involvement of the IMNs can be as high as 37% in patients with node-positive cancers in the inner or central breast.

There are no completed randomized trials evaluating internal mammary radiation; however, a phase II trial of high-risk patients who received postmastectomy irradiation provides some indirect evidence. Although all patients were intended to receive internal mammary radiation, for technical reasons, only 67 of 100 patients received it. At a median follow-up of 77 months, DFS was significantly improved in women who received IM irradiation (73% versus 52%). Two ongoing randomized trials will hopefully provide better answers to this question.

After the initial planning, patients typically spend only 15 to 20 minutes in the treatment room, most of which is spent positioning the patient identical to how she was during the simulation. Once in position, the linear accelerator is rotated to the predetermined treatment angles and the light field aligned with the skin tattoos. The personnel leave the room and treatment is initiated. Patients feel nothing during treatment other than hearing the machine noises. Throughout the course of therapy, interval images are obtained to confirm that the treated field matches the simulated field, and the accuracy verified by computer-based quality assurance. The key to optimal radiation therapy is the meticulous technique reviews by the radiation oncologists, physicists, dosimetrists, technologists, and remainder of the treatment team.

Complications of Breast and Chest Wall Radiation

Because surgeons are typically the first to discuss treatment options for women with breast cancer, they need to be aware of the potential complications of adding radiation to the treatment protocol. Overall, the incidence and severity of long-term treatment complications after radiation therapy for BCT are low. This partly depends on the region that is irradiated; long-term sequelae will increase when nodal radiation is added to breast or chest wall irradiation.

Fatigue—Fatigue is one of the most common side effects of radiation, and the exact reasons that radiation induces fatigue are not fully known. Fatigue often peaks toward the end of therapy. Ten days to 2 weeks after completion, patients start to improve. Most patients will have complete resolution by 6 weeks after completion of therapy.

Skin Changes—Skin changes are the other common complication of breast external beam radiation therapy and include erythema, edema, hyperpigmentation, pruritus, breast discomfort, and desquamation. If the axilla is included, hyperpigmentation, epilation of axillary hair, and desquamation of the axillary skin fold can occur. Moist desquamation is the most frustrating complication of radiation for patients. If it does occur, it is usually at the end of therapy and persists for 1 to 2 weeks. It most commonly occurs in the moist inframammary fold and can be minimized or avoided by continuous aeration, avoiding the use of a bra and cornstarch to absorb moisture. When it does occur, it is treated topically with Xeroform gauze or silver sulfadiazine (Silvadene) ointment.

Some mild skin changes will be long term. Most patients will have some degree of residual hyperpigmentation. There will be some change in the size, shape, and texture of the breast compared to the nontreated side. The breast may be smaller or larger than the opposite breast, may feel heavy (because of breast edema), or feel firmer.

Upper Extremity Lymphedema—Combining regional radiation therapy with axillary surgery will increase the risk of lymphedema; however, this will depend on the extent of both. Full axillary radiation after a complete axillary dissection will result in the highest risk of lymphedema and should be discouraged. When patients undergo breast surgery along with an ALND without radiation, they have a 2% to 10% rate of moderate to severe arm edema. When radiation therapy is added, just to the breast, the rate increases to 4% to 13% of patients. This number jumps to 25% to 30% with nodal irradiation. The incidence also increases with obesity and chemotherapy. It is important to note that patients who had an SLN biopsy also have a risk of lymphedema, between 5% and 7%.

Brachial Plexopathy—Permanent plexopathy is primarily seen in women who receive regional nodal radiation. Women will present with the new onset of numbness, pain, or weakness in the affected arm. Most women will have complete resolution of their symptoms by 1 to 2 years; however, 0.25% will have permanent brachial plexopathy.

Pneumonitis—Approximately 1% to 5% of women receiving breast or chest wall radiation will have transient lung inflammation and symptomatic pneumonitis. The risk will increase with increasing lung volume in the tangent fields. Increased lung irradiation (and an increased risk of pneumonitis) will occur when fields are extended to include the supraclavicular, axillary, and internal mammary lymph nodes. In addition, concurrent chemotherapy will increase the risk of pneumonitis. The incidence of radiation pneumonitis will increase to 8% to 20% for women receiving nodal radiation and adjuvant chemotherapy. Women typically present with cough, low-grade fever, and dyspnea beginning about 2 to 3 months after radiation and persisting for several weeks. In most women these symptoms will be self-limiting, although in rare cases steroids may be necessary. Chest x-ray will show changes confined to the radiation therapy field. Pulmonary fibrosis typically follows in the affected portion.

Rib fracture—Rib fracture is rare after standard radiation. The incidence is approximately 1%, and most rib fractures are seen about 1 year after radiation. Treatment is simple, primarily supportive until healing is completed, however, it is important to differentiate between a rib fracture and a bone metastasis. In patients with preexisting collagen vascular disease, they may develop severe soft tissue ulceration or bone necrosis, and this is one reason why this is a contraindication to radiation.

Cardiovascular morbidity—The risk of late cardiovascular events is dependent on tumor location, technique, and dose. The excess mortality observed in early trials of radiation therapy was largely the result of cardiovascular toxicity; however, more modern techniques have minimized this effect. Women with left-sided breast cancers are at increased risk as they have more myocardium included in the treatment field.

Secondary malignancies—Potential treatment-induced secondary malignancies following locoregional radiation include contralateral breast cancers, sarcomas, lung cancers, and leukemias, all of which are rare.

Sarcoma—Angiosarcoma, a relatively rare tumor, can occur in the breast or chest wall after irradiation. These tumors usually present as multiple reddish, bluish, and purple nodules or areas of skin discoloration (see Chapter 23).

Lung cancer—Radiation therapy for breast cancer has been described as a risk factor for the development of lung cancer, with relative risks between two and three. This is dependent on the volume of lung in the irradiated field. This risk is also increased by smoking, so women undergoing breast or chest wall irradiation should be strongly encouraged to quit smoking.

Acute leukemia—In women undergoing chest wall radiation therapy, the risk of acute nonlymphocytic leukemias (ANLL) appears to be increased. This is related to the volume of bone marrow in the field, the total radiation therapy dose, and the concomitant use of chemotherapy. Though increased compared to controls, the absolute risk is quite low, especially with limited bone marrow in the radiation therapy field.

Contralateral breast cancer—Limited data suggest a slight excess of contralateral breast cancers following breast or chest wall radiation therapy. The risk may be higher with younger age at treatment. Although the risk of radiation-associated contralateral breast cancer is extremely low, measures to reduce scatter to the opposite breast are encouraged.

Finally, there is clearly an impact of both radiation therapy and surgery on cosmetic outcome. Although cosmesis takes a backseat to oncologic principles and patient safety, clearly it cannot be completely overlooked as the driving force for breast conservation therapy is in part cosmetic. Overall, the overwhelming majority of patients and their doctors rate the cosmetic outcome as good to excellent, although both groups are slightly biased. However, there are several factors that will impact the cosmetic outcome.

Most factors contributing to cosmetic outcome are predetermined and include the size of the tumor, the location of the tumor and the preoperative breast size. Tumors in the upper inner quadrant will leave more noticeable defects than the upper outer quadrant, where there is more tissue. The use of chemotherapy and the dose and treatment plan of the radiation therapy will also impact cosmesis, but these are driven by oncologic principles. Other factors, such as the amount of tissue that must be removed to achieve negative margins, the size of the scar, and the location of the scar are controllable by the surgeon, but not at the cost of inadequate surgery. It is believed that the higher local recurrence rate seen among younger women is not the result of biology but rather surgeons compromising their oncologic operation in the name of cosmetic outcome. The surgeon has some maneuverability as to where the incision is placed, but excessive tunneling to remove a cancer is discouraged, and the trade-off for scar location is the excess tissue that needs to be removed. If possible, incisions in the cleavage line should be avoided. Excessively large lumpectomies or quadrantectomies will compromise cosmetic outcome and are not necessary for most tumors. Lesions inferior to the nipple-areolar complex can cause disparity between the two breasts and lead to excessive downturning of the nipple. Radial incisions may help avoid this. Other oncoplastic techniques can further optimize the cosmetic outcome after radiation therapy (Chapter 14). Finally placing radio opaque clips will help the radiation oncologist accurately plan the boost, minimizing its amount.

Partial Breast Irradiation

Although whole breast irradiation after lumpectomy has well-documented, excellent results, it can often add additional inconvenience and cost to both the patient and the health care system. Not every patient lives in close proximity to a radiation oncology center, so the time and travel involved in coming every Monday through Friday for 5 to 6 weeks can be overwhelming for some women. For this reason, some women who are candidates for BCT may opt for mastectomy to avoid not only the inconvenience, but also the toxicity of whole-breast irradiation. This has fueled significant interest in methods to decrease the time needed for treatment. One such approach is the use of more rapid fractionation schedules. A randomized trial from Canada demonstrated that a shorter schedule, in this case 42.5 Gy over 22 days, was equivalent to the standard 45 to 50 Gy over 35 days. But more significant changes in the radiation component of breast conservation may be around the corner.

The argument for using whole-breast irradiation after lumpectomy is based on pathologic studies of mastectomy specimens showing tumor cells located 2 to 3 cm away from the primary tumor. However, clinical observations demonstrate that the overwhelming majority of local recurrences occur close to the site of the tumor bed. This is the reason that many radiation oncologists recommend a boost to the tumor bed to follow whole-breast irradiation, but it raises the question as to whether radiation of the entire breast is necessary. It is feasible that patients may receive the same benefit from irradiating only the tumor bed, sparing the remainder of the breast. This may not only improve the cosmetic outcome, but also would shorten the costs associated with treatment and the time necessary to complete therapy. Several techniques for delivering accelerated partial breast irradiation (APBI) have been evaluated in appropriately selected patients (Table 15–2, Box 15–3).

Interstitial Brachytherapy

The concept of irradiating only the region of the breast near the tumor is not new. Multicatheter, interstitial brachytherapy has been around for some time. This involves the placement of multiple hollow catheters within the breast tissue around the lumpectomy cavity.

TABLE 15–2 • *Relative Advantages and Disadvantages of Methods to Deliver Accelerated Partial Breast Irradiation*

	Advantages	Disadvantages
Multi-catheter interstitial brachytherapy	Well tolerated Short treatment time More clinical experience than other modalities Can be used for any size, shape, or location of cavity	Catheter placement and dosimetry can be technically complex May require hospitalization (low-dose rate) Limited number of clinicians who are familiar with this technique Multiple (10 to 25) catheters are disturbing to patients
Balloon-catheter brachytherapy	Technically simple Well tolerated by patients	Limited by shape of lumpectomy and distance to skin
External beam radiation	Uses technology most facilities already have	May need to radiate larger area than other methods
Intraoperative radiation	Greatly decreases the time needed for therapy	Requires special equipment in the operating room Skin and chest wall complications

A radioactive source is then placed within the catheters. It is somewhat ironic that the first use of radiation to avoid mastectomy, by English surgeon Keynes in the 1920s, used interstitial radium needles to treat the primary tumor, with or without surgery, so APBI is not so much a new approach as much as the field of breast radiation oncology coming full circle.

There are two approaches for delivering the radiation, which is typically done by automated technology to limit the potential radiation exposure of health care providers. Low-dose rate (LDR) brachytherapy involves a continuous exposure to a low dose of radiation (45 to 50 Gy at a rate of about 30 to 70 cGy/h). This typically takes 96 hours, so one drawback to LDR brachytherapy is that this requires admission to hospital rooms specifically designed to shield radiation. The other approach is high-dose rate (HDR) brachytherapy. A total dose of 34 Gy is delivered in twice daily fractions of 3.4 Gy. This can be performed on an outpatient basis and can be completed over 5 days.

BOX 15–3 CRITERIA OFTEN USED TO SELECT PATIENTS FOR PARTIAL BREAST IRRADIATION

Patient age	>45
Tumor size	<2.0 cm
Nodal status	Node negative
Distance from cavity to skin	>5 to 7 mm

Balloon-Catheter Brachytherapy

A significant drawback to interstitial brachytherapy is the complexity of placing the 10 to 25 catheters. In addition, many patients are dissuaded away from multi-catheter brachytherapy when they see pictures of patients with the multiple catheters in place, which can be quite intimidating. This has limited the use of brachytherapy and generated interest in alternate methods for delivering radiation directly to within the lumpectomy cavity. The MammoSite (MammoSite RTS; Proxima Therapeutics, Alpharetta, GA) is a balloon catheter device that greatly simplifies brachytherapy. A catheter sits centrally in a distally located balloon, resembling a Foley catheter. This is placed in the lumpectomy cavity, either at the time of surgery or as a second procedure, and inflated. This catheter is pliable so it can easily be worn within a bra. Treatment is then delivered with a single, centralized HDR.

The MammoSite does have some drawbacks. An adequate distance between the lumpectomy cavity and the skin is needed or skin injury can result. It is also possible that a large (50 ml or more) or irregularly shaped lumpectomy cavity can negatively impact the effectiveness of the MammoSite, limiting the number of patients who would be ideal candidates. However, early results with MammoSite, though highly selective, have been promising.

External Beam Radiation

As opposed to brachytherapy, external beam radiation can be used to deliver PBI. Recent technologic advances in CT-based planning have allowed the introduction of three-dimensional conformal external beam APBI. This allows for improved dose homogeneity within the target volume and does not require additional technology beyond what most radiation facilities already have. One disadvantage is that a larger area of normal breast tissue may need to be irradiated than with other PBI techniques because the breast is a moving target. One way to improve on this is the use of intensity-modulated radiation therapy (IMRT), which delivers radiation using a variable-intensity pattern that is determined with the aid of a computerized optimization algorithm (Figure 15–6). Although more costly and labor-intensive than three-dimensional conformal APBI, IMRT delivers a more uniform and standardized radiation dose without excessive treatment of the surrounding tissue.

Intraoperative Radiation Therapy

The most efficient method of limiting the time necessary to deliver the radiation is to do so in the operating room following lumpectomy. Initially intraoperative radiation therapy (IORT) was proposed as an adjunct to whole-breast irradiation, as a more accurate method of delivering the boost. More recently, it has been examined as a sole method of radiation treatment. Several methods exist for delivering the radiation intraoperatively. One method uses a portable, dedicated linear accelerator. After completion of the lumpectomy, the skin is dissected off of the surrounding breast parenchyma around the cavity, and the parenchyma is dissected off of the pectoralis major muscle. This allows adequate retraction of the skin and the placement of an aluminum-lead disk to protect the chest wall. Once this is completed, 21 Gy are delivered. An alternative approach uses electrons generated by a mobile linear accelerator.

All of these technologies seem promising, but clinical experience is limited and long-term follow-up is not available for the newer approaches (see Table 15–2). In addition, these trials are highly selective, and for the most part, from single institutions. Participation is limited to a patient population with an expected excellent cosmetic outcome and low risk of recurrence with whole-breast irradiation (older patients, node-negative, smaller tumors). PBI is presently being directly compared to whole-breast irradiation in a randomized trial, which will hopefully secure the role of PBI in breast conservation therapy.

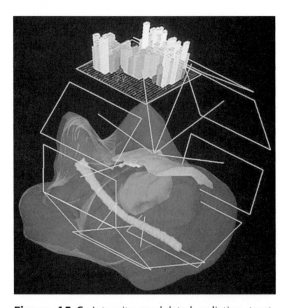

Figure 15–6. Intensity modulated radiation treatment (IMRT) delivers radiation using a variable-intensity pattern that is determined with the aid of a computerized optimization algorithm. IMRT delivers a more uniform and standardized radiation dose without excessive treatment of the surrounding tissue.

Suggested Readings

1. Arriagada R, Lê MG, Rochard F, et al. Conservative treatment versus mastectomy in early breast cancer: patterns of failure with 15 years of follow-up data. Institut Gustave-Roussy Breast Cancer Group. J Clin Oncol 1996;14:1558–1564.
2. Blichert-Toft M, Rose C, Andersen JA, et al. Danish randomized trial comparing breast conservation therapy with mastectomy: six years of life-table analysis. Danish Breast Cancer Cooperative Group. J Natl Cancer Inst Monogr 1992;11:19–25.
3. Buchholz TA, Strom EA, Perkins GH, et al. Controversies regarding the use of radiation after mastectomy in breast cancer. Oncologist 2002;7:539–546.
4. Fearmonti RM, Vicini FA, Pawlik TM, et al. Integrating partial breast irradiation into surgical practice and clinical trials. Surg Clin of N Am 2007;87(2):485–498.
5. Fisher B, Anderson S, Bryant J, et al. Twenty year follow-up of a randomized trial comparing total mastectomy, lumpectomy, and lumpectomy plus irradiation for the treatment of invasive breast cancer. N Engl J Med 2002;347(16):1233–1241.
6. Fisher B, Redmond C, Poisson R, et al. Eight-year results of a randomized clinical trial comparing total mastectomy and lumpectomy with or without irradiation in the treatment of breast cancer. N Engl J Med 1989;320(13):822–828.
7. Fyles AW, McCready DR, Manchul LA, et al. Tamoxifen with or without breast irradiation in women 50 years of age or older with early breast cancer. N Engl J Med 2004;351:963–970.

8. Jacobson JA, Danforth DN, Cowan KH, et al. Ten-year results of a comparison of conservation with mastectomy in the treatment of stage I and II breast cancer. N Engl J Med 1995;332(14):907–911.

9. Kantorowitz DA, Poulter CA, Sischy B, et al. Treatment of breast cancer among elderly women with segmental mastectomy or segmental mastectomy plus postoperative radiotherapy. Int J Radiat Oncol Biol Phys 1988;15:263–270.

10. Morris MM, Powell SN. Irradiation in the setting of collagen vascular disease: acute and late complications. J Clin Orthod 1997;15:2728–2735.

11. Poggi MM, Danforth DN, Sciuto LC, et al. Eighteen year results in the treatment of early breast carcinoma with mastectomy versus breast conservation therapy: the National Cancer Institute Randomized Trial. Cancer 2003;98:697–702.

12. Recht A, Edge SB, Solin LJ, et al. Postmastectomy radiotherapy: clinical practice guidelines of the American Society of Clinical Onology. J Clin Orthod 2001;19:1539–1569.

13. Sanders ME, Scroggins T, Ampil FL, et al. Accelerated partial breast irradiation in early-stage breast cancer. J Clin Orthod 2007;25(8):996–1002.

14. Schnitt SJ, Hayman JA, Gelman RS, et al. A prospective study of conservative surgery alone in the treatment of selected patients with stage I breast cancer. Cancer 1996;77:1094–1100.

15. Taghian A, Jeong JH, Mamounas E, et al. Patterns of locoregional failure in patients with operable breast cancer treated by mastectomy and adjuvant chemotherapy with or without tamoxifen and without radiotherapy: results from five National Surgical Adjuvant Breast and Bowel Project randomized clinical trials. J Clin Orthod 2004;22:4247–4254.

16. Van Dongen JA, Voogd AC, Fentiman IS, et al. Long-term results of a randomized trial comparing breast conserving therapy with mastectomy: European Organization for Research and Treatment of Cancer 10801 Trial. J Natl Cancer Inst 2000; 92:1143–1150.

17. Veronesi U, Cascinelli N, Mariani L, et al. Twenty year follow-up of a randomized study comparing breast-conserving surgery with radical mastectomy for early breast cancer. N Engl J Med 2002; 347(16):1227–1232.

18. Whelan TJ, Julian J, Wright J, et al. Does locoregional radiation therapy improve survival in breast cancer? A meta-analysis. J Clin Orthod 2000;18:1220–1229.

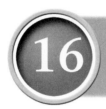

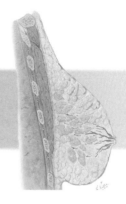

Principles of Adjuvant Chemotherapy for Breast Cancer

Principles of Adjuvant Chemotherapy for Breast Cancer: Key Points

- Be familiar with the principles of how cytotoxic chemotherapy kills cancer cells.
- Describe the benefits of adjuvant chemotherapy after surgery and the data from the EBCTCG.
- Understand the important factors in determining the benefits of adjuvant chemotherapy and the present guidelines clinicians use to guide these decisions.
- Know how to use Adjuvant Online to assess the benefit of adjuvant chemotherapy for the individual patient.

- Understand the potential benefit and unanswered questions of using microarray analysis for making decisions regarding adjuvant therapy.
- Be familiar with the various agents used in breast cancer chemotherapy and the possible side effects.
- Understand the mechanism of action and potential benefit of Herceptin in the adjuvant setting.
- Appreciate the future potential of targeted therapies in the systemic treatment of breast cancer.

Introduction

Breast cancer can essentially be thought of as two simultaneous problems. The first is the locoregional disease, the known cancer within the breast and regional lymph nodes. This is directly addressed through the use of surgery and radiation therapy. The second disease is the possible presence of micrometastatic disease elsewhere in the body. These cells will be unaffected by local therapies, and so the only way to eradicate them (and prevent recurrence) is through the use of adjuvant systemic therapies. These two problems are obviously not mutually exclusive. Systemic therapies will have an impact not only on distant recurrence, but locoregional recurrence as well. Likewise, adequate local control will help minimize the secondary spread of micrometastases and decrease distant recurrence.

Adjuvant systemic therapy refers to the administration of chemotherapy or hormonal therapy following primary surgery for early stage breast cancer to eliminate or delay the subsequent appearance of clinically occult micrometastatic disease. Two observations in the late 1800s led to the concept of using systemic therapy after surgery. The first was the realization that even with aggressive surgical therapy, 20% of patients who were node negative would recur within 5 years, as would 70% of patients with positive nodes. The second was the observation of blood-borne tumor cells post mortem. These led to the awareness that the only way to improve the outcome for patients with breast cancer would be control of the distant micrometastases with systemic therapies.

The first adjuvant therapy for breast cancer was hormonal therapy, which will be discussed in the next chapter. The first clinical trial investigating chemotherapy began in 1958 and was conducted by the National Surgical Adjuvant Breast and Bowel Project (NSABP).

Adjuvant chemotherapy trials in the late 1960s and early 1970s focused on single agents in patients with axillary nodal metastases. With a clear demonstration of improved survival, trials of adjuvant chemotherapy have continued to try to build on these results, examining combination chemotherapy, different treatment durations and schedules, and new agents as they are discovered. This chapter will focus on the use of systemic chemotherapy following surgery.

Principles of Adjuvant Chemotherapy

Chemotherapeutic agents inhibit cell growth and cause apoptosis through interference with normal cellular functions, primarily progression through the cell cycle (Box 16–1). As such, they tend to be more effective in treating rapidly dividing cells. A considerably smaller proportion of cells in a slowly growing tumor are progressing through the cell cycle when chemotherapy is given. Unfortunately, while aggressive,

BOX 16–1 PRINCIPLES OF ADJUVANT CHEMOTHERAPY

- Chemotherapy kills a constant fraction of tumor cells (first-order kinetics) rather than a constant number of cells (log kill hypothesis). Thus, repetitive cycles of therapy are necessary.
- Combination therapy is superior to single-agent therapy by overcoming drug resistance. This will, however, increase toxicity.
- A dose-response effect exists, thus requiring adequate doses of drug.
- Outcome is dependent on the number of malignant cells present when therapy is initiated. Even a single metastatic cancer cell, left alive, can lead to death.

rapidly growing tumors may have more cells in the cell cycle, they are also more likely to acquire resistance to chemotherapy. Chemotherapy not only kills cancer cells, but normal cells progressing through the cell cycle are susceptible, and this is what leads to the significant toxicity associated with adjuvant chemotherapy.

The principles of adjuvant chemotherapy follow several principles that led to the present dosing regimens used. The first is that chemotherapy works by first-order kinetics. This means that the drugs kill a fixed fraction of cells with each cycle and not a fixed number of cells (referred to as log kill hypothesis). If the latter were true, then a large enough single dose could potentially be effective (if tolerated). However, because the drugs kill only a fraction of cells, repetitive cycles are necessary. The effectiveness of adjuvant therapy is therefore related to how efficacious the drug is (how large is that fraction of cells killed), how many cells are there to begin with, how many cycles are used, and how quickly the remaining cells grow between cycles.

There are several other barriers to the efficacy of adjuvant chemotherapy. The first is resistance. Some cancer cells are inherently resistant to particular agents; others will gain resistance via mutation. To some degree, resistance is countered through the use of combination chemotherapy rather than single agents. In general, using agents in combination is more effective and the more common approach when there is a curative intent, as in the adjuvant setting. The best combinations include agents that act synergistically, which are most likely to occur when they have different mechanisms of action and resistance. When combining chemotherapy, however, one must also consider the potential overlapping side effects to avoid excessive toxicity.

When discussing adjuvant chemotherapy, there are several endpoints that are relevant (Box 16–2). Two of the most important endpoints are disease-free survival (DFS) and overall survival (OS). DFS is the time from treatment to the first evidence of recurrence or death, whichever comes first. OS is defined as the time from treatment to death, regardless of disease recurrence. Although this is relatively straightforward, there are several points that bear mentioning. DFS and OS are not linked to the degree that one might expect. For a disease where recurrence is strongly linked to inevitable death, then DFS will

> **BOX 16–2** MEASUREMENTS OF SURVIVAL
>
> Disease-free survival (DFS): Time from treatment to first evidence of recurrence or death.
> Overall survival (OS): Time from treatment to death.
> Distant disease-free survival (DDFS): Time from treatment to first evidence of distant recurrence.

parallel OS. However, if local recurrence is common, but highly curable, this would translate to a low DFS but high OS. For this reason, some studies tend to ignore local recurrences and focus only on distant disease-free survival (DDFS).

One might also assume that improving DFS would improve OS, but this is also not necessarily the case. If a new agent decreases recurrence, but makes subsequent recurrences more aggressive and less susceptible to treatment, then an improvement in DFS might have no effect on OS. It is for this reason that some might argue that OS is the only meaningful endpoint. On the other hand, a delay in recurrence, even in the absence of an OS benefit, may be of significant benefit to patients, and justify the use of an adjuvant therapy.

The benefits of adjuvant chemotherapy are often described in terms of reductions in the odds of disease recurrence or death. It is important to understand the concept of absolute versus proportional reductions when discussing the benefits of systemic therapy. A proportional reduction of 25% is described as an odds reduction of 25%, an odds ratio of 0.75, or a hazard ratio of 0.75. But the absolute benefit of the therapy depends on what the risk of recurrence or death was without treatment. Therefore, let us say that without adjuvant therapy, the likelihood of death was 40% (an overall survival of 60%). If you start with 100 patients, 60 will live regardless of adjuvant treatment. Of the other 40, a 25% proportional reduction would mean that 10 will now survive and 30 will die. Thus, the absolute benefit was 10%. If the risk of death decreases, the proportional benefit stays the same, but the absolute benefit decreases. If the likelihood of death is only 20%, the proportional benefit stays the same at 25%, but the absolute benefit drops to 5%.

Benefits of Adjuvant Chemotherapy in Breast Cancer

A lengthy discussion of the early trials and multiple studies examining adjuvant chemotherapy is well beyond the scope of this book. The impact of adjuvant chemotherapy on breast cancer is best demonstrated in the Early Breast Cancer Trialists' Collaborative Group (EBCTCG) data. The EBCTCG is an international group that meets every 5 years to review the collective data on breast cancer trials. The 1995 overview analysis summarized the results of randomized chemotherapy trials beginning before 1990. The analysis involved 18,000 women participating in 47 trials of adjuvant chemotherapy and revealed several key points regarding the efficacy of adjuvant chemotherapy in breast cancer.

1. Compared to no adjuvant therapy, polychemotherapy significantly improved OS. The proportional risk reductions are shown in Table 16–1 and broken down by age. Overall, combination chemotherapy reduces the risk of recurrence by 23.5% and the risk of death by 15.3%. This translated to an overall 7% to 11% absolute increase in 10 year OS in women under age 50, and a 2% to 3% absolute increase in women aged 50 to 69. There was no significant difference in either recurrence or survival for women 70 years of age or older, however, it should be mentioned that only a small percentage of women in the randomized trials were older than 70.

2. The benefits are true for patients who are both node negative and node positive.

When first introduced into clinical practice, adjuvant chemotherapy was limited to patients who were node positive (hence the importance of the axillary lymph node dissection [ALND] even in the absence of a direct survival benefit, as described in Chapter 13). However, the Oxford overview clearly shows that the proportional reductions in recurrence and death are similar for patients who are node negative and those who are node positive. What changes are the risks of recurrence and death, so that although the proportional benefit stays the same, the absolute benefit changes. Thus, the selection of appropriate patients for adjuvant chemotherapy is based on a more complex calculation of the patient's risk of recurrence rather than node positive versus node negative.

3. Anthracycline-based chemotherapy is superior to non-anthracycline based regimens. Initially, one of the most common regimens used was cyclophosphamide, methotrexate, and fluorouracil (CMF). In the Oxford Overview, they identified 11 trials (over 6900 patients) in which CMF was compared with regimens containing doxorubicin (such as FAC or AC) or epirubicin (such as FEC). There was a 12% reduction in the odds of recurrence and an 11% reduction in the odds of death with the use of an anthracycline regimen. These benefits were seen in patients who were both node positive and node negative. Anthracycline-based regimens are now the most common regimens in the adjuvant setting, although CMF is still a reasonable option for some women.

TABLE 16–1 • *Proportional Risk Reductions Associated with Adjuvant Chemotherapy in the 1995 EBCTCG Systematic Review on Polychemotherapy*		
	Proportional Reduction in Recurrence (%)	**Proportional Reduction in Mortality (%)**
Polychemotherapy vs. None- All Ages	23.8	15.2
<40	37	27
40 to 49	34	27
50 to 59	22	14
60 to 69	18	8
70 or older	—	—

Selection of Patients for Adjuvant Chemotherapy

Several factors have been identified that can help select which patients are most likely to benefit from adjuvant therapy. Factors can be categorized as either prognostic or predictive. A prognostic factor correlates with the clinical outcome at the time of diagnosis, independent of therapy. Examples include tumor size and lymph node status. Larger tumor size and the presence of nodal metastases correlate with the likelihood of distant recurrence and death. Prognostic factors are important because they can help determine the absolute benefit of chemotherapy. As stated, if a drug can reduce the chance of dying of breast cancer by 25%, it is important to know what the chance of dying of breast cancer is, based on prognostic factors. If the chance of dying is only 4%, then the absolute benefit of the drug is only 1% (meaning 100 women need to be treated for 1 woman to survive). On the other hand, if the prognostic signs suggest a 40% chance of dying, the absolute benefit is 10% (10 women need to be treated for 1 woman to survive).

A pure prognostic factor, however, does not give information about the likelihood of a treatment working. Predictive factors provide information on the likelihood of a response to a given modality. These factors are usually the target of the therapy or related to the method by which the treatment works.

Many factors may be both predictive and prognostic. One example is the overexpression of human epidermal growth factor receptor 2 (Her-2/neu). Her-2 neu status is clearly predictive. Women who are Her-2/neu positive are likely to benefit from Herceptin, whereas women who are negative will see no benefit. Her-2 neu status may also predict the response to certain chemotherapeutic regimens. However, Her-2 neu status is also prognostic because women with Her-2 neu overexpressing cancers tend to have a worse outcome than patients who are Her-2 neu negative, regardless of treatment.

Although many prognostic and predictive factors have been examined, only a handful are used clinically (Box 16–3). The primary factors presently in use include both those factors that are patient related (age and comorbidities) and those that are tumor related (size, nodal status, grade, histology, angiolymphatic invasion, hormone receptors, and HER2/neu status). Although the standard approach to systemic therapy is the use of these prognostic and predictive factors, it is an interesting time in cancer

BOX 16–3 AMERICAN SOCIETY OF CLINICAL ONCOLOGY TUMOR MARKER GUIDELINES

- ER and PgR expression should be evaluated on every breast cancer to guide the decision to use hormonal therapy.
- Her-2/neu overexpression should be evaluated on every breast cancer to help guide the selection of trastuzumab (Herceptin) for adjuvant therapy.
- The present data is insufficient to recommend the measurement of p53, cathepsin D, cyclin E, ploidy, or DNA content or S phase measurements. There is also insufficient information at this time to recommend the estimation of the proliferative rate, including mitotic rate counts, S-phase fractions, Ki-67, proliferating cell nuclear antigen (PCNA), or argyrophilic nucleolar organizer regions (AgNOR).*

* Although the American Society of Clinical Oncology (ASCO) guidelines do not recommend the assessment of cell proliferation, it is recommended by the College of American Pathologists, and many institutions do routinely measure Ki-67.
ER, xxxx; Her-2/neu, xxxxx; PgR, xxxx; p53, xxx.***

therapy, with a shift away from using tumor, node, and metastasis (TNM) staging for adjuvant therapy decision making and toward using more detailed genetic information from the primary tumor. With the introduction of Onco Type DX, the first foray into more selective targeting of systemic therapy has been seen. As more research is done and validated, this is likely to dramatically change how we approach adjuvant chemotherapy.

Consensus Groups

Adjuvant hormonal therapy, with a favorable risk-benefit ratio, is generally recommended to all hormone receptor positive patients (see Chapter 17). The decision to administer adjuvant systemic therapy must take into account not only the individual patient's risk of relapse, but also the absolute benefits of treatment, the potential short-term and long-term complications, and the patient's comorbidities and life expectancy. This has made the creation of general guidelines for adjuvant chemotherapy use a challenging problem. One method of addressing the complexities has been through groups of experts reviewing the available data and making recommendations.

National Institutes of Health Consensus Conference

The National Institutes of Health (NIH) Consensus Panel concluded that several months of poly-chemotherapy appear to provide benefit in reducing the risk for recurrence and death and that anthracycline-containing regimens offer a small but significant improvement in survival compared with non-anthracycline regimens. In regard to selecting the most appropriate patients for chemotherapy, this consensus group acknowledged the difficulty in identifying specific patient groups that might not require adjuvant chemotherapy. They agreed on the need to individualize recommendations for node-negative cancers smaller than 1 cm and state that the retrospective data indicate that the use of chemotherapy, in the absence of other worrisome features, does not appear warranted. They also emphasize the need for studies designed to look at women 70 years of age and older and boosting accrual of these patients to trials because there is limited evidence regarding adjuvant chemotherapy in this group (see Chapter 22).

National Comprehensive Cancer Network

The National Comprehensive Cancer Network (NCCN) gathers experts in various fields of oncology to create practice guidelines in oncology, which are available to all practitioners in both published form and on the Internet. Treatment algorithms are presented in flowchart formats based on categories of consensus among the NCCN committee members (Box 16–4), and they are available on the Internet at www. NCCN.org. A sample page from the NCCN guidelines for the adjuvant therapy of breast cancer is shown in Figure 16–1. The guidelines recommend adjuvant chemotherapy for patients with lymph node involvement, for those with hormone receptor negative breast cancer and tumor size greater than 1 cm, and for those with hormone receptor and Her-2/neu positive disease and tumor size greater than 1 cm. They also recommend consideration of chemotherapy for patients with tumor size 0.6 to 1.0 cm regardless of hormone receptor status, and those with hormone receptor positive and Her-2/neu negative disease and tumor size greater than 1 cm.

St. Gallen International Consensus Panel

The St. Gallen International Consensus Conference gathers a worldwide group of breast cancer experts on a regular basis to discuss

BOX 16–4 NATIONAL COMPREHENSIVE CANCER NETWORK CATEGORIES OF CONSENSUS

Category 1: Uniform national comprehensive cancer network (NCCN) consensus based on high-level evidence that the recommendation is appropriate.
Category 2A: There is uniform NCCN consensus, based on lower-level evidence including clinical experience, that the recommendation is appropriate.
Category 2B: There is nonuniform NCCN consensus (but no major disagreement), based on lower-level evidence including clinical experience, that the recommendation is appropriate.
Category 3: There is major NCCN disagreement that the recommendation is appropriate.

the latest research in breast cancer and provide updates on adjuvant therapy recommendations based on low, intermediate, and high risk (Table 16–2). They have defined the features necessary to assess adjuvant therapy needs as the size of the primary tumor, nodal status, estrogen receptor (ER) and progesterone receptor (PR) expression, and Her-2/neu overexpression (Box 16–5). Additional features that may influence the decision would be grade, lymphovascular invasion, and certain histologies. They recommend adjuvant chemotherapy for patients with hormone receptor positive, high-risk disease, or hormone receptor negative, intermediate- or high-risk disease. They also recommend consideration of chemotherapy for patients with hormone receptor positive, intermediate-risk disease. High-risk disease is defined as four or more nodes positive with any Her-2 status, or one to three nodes positive and Her-2 overexpressed. Low-risk is considered age greater than 35, tumor size less than or equal to 2 cm, grade 1, no angiolymphatic invasion, and Her-2 negative.

The St. Gallen guidelines differ slightly from the NCCN recommendations, being slightly more conservative. For example, a woman with a 1.5-cm, node-negative, grade 1 tumor, ER positive, Her-2 negative has an approximate 15% 10-year risk of recurrence without systemic therapy. The NCCN guidelines would recommend considering adjuvant chemotherapy in addition to hormonal therapy, whereas the St. Gallen guidelines would recommend hormonal therapy only. One can see how this may lead to confusion for both clinicians and patients.

SYSTEMIC ADJUVANT TREATMENT – HORMONE RECEPTOR POSITIVE – HER-2 NEGATIVE DISEASE[b]

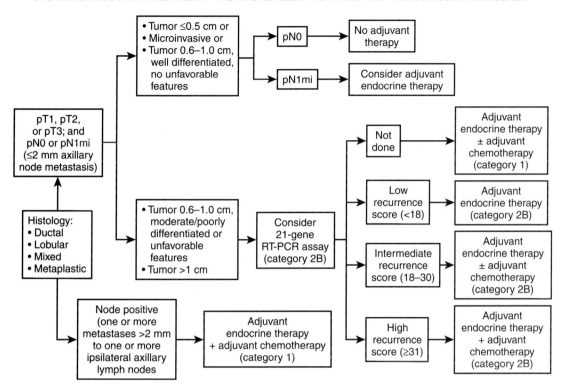

Figure 16–1. A sample page from the National Comprehensive Cancer Network Guidelines for Adjuvant Therapy in Breast Cancer. Available at www.nccn.org/professionals/physician_gls.

TABLE 16–2 • *St. Gallen Systemic Adjuvant Therapy Recommendations*		
Risk Category	**Associated Features**	**Adjuvant Therapy Options**
Low risk	Node-negative, ER/PR positive, T ≤ 1 cm, grade 1, no LVI, Her-2/neu negative, age ≥ 35	1. None 2. Endocrine only 3. Consider Oncotype DX
Intermediate risk	Node-negative and at least one of the following: T > 2 cm, grade >1, LVI, age < 35, Her-2/neu positive Node-positive (one to three nodes) and Her/2-neu negative	1. Endocrine only (ER/PR+) 2. CTX followed by endocrine (ER/PR+) 3. Consider Oncotype (if node negative and ER/PR+) 4. CTX (ER/PR-)
High risk	Node positive (one to three nodes) and Her-2/neu positive Node positive (≥ four nodes)	1. CTX followed by endocrine (ER/PR+) 2. CTX

CTX, chemotherapy; ER, estrogen receptor; LVI, lymphovascular invasion; PR, progesterone receptor; T, tumor size.

Adjuvant Online

To make it easier for physicians to apply guidelines to individual patients and help patients understand the decision they are making, there are several computer programs that are now available to assess the risks of recurrence and death from breast cancer and the relative and absolute benefits of adjuvant therapy. These are particularly helpful in discussing adjuvant therapy decisions with

BOX 16–5 ST. GALLEN INTERNATIONAL CONSENSUS CONFERENCE FEATURES IMPORTANT IN ADJUVANT THERAPY DECISIONS

Necessary

Tumor size (invasive component)
Nodal status
Hormone receptor expression
Her-2/neu overexpression

Additional

Histologic grade
Angiolymphatic invasion
Primary histology (metaplastic changes carry increased risk)

patients. The most popular program is Adjuvant! Online (Adjuvant! Inc.), which is easily accessible to all practitioners via the Internet at www.adjuvantonline.com. Taking survival

information derived mainly from surveillance, epidemiology, and end results (SEER) data combined with the benefits of adjuvant therapy based on the Oxford overview, this program uses a Bayesian method to make estimates for individual patients based on their demographic and staging information. After entering the patient age, comorbidities, menopausal status, tumor size, nodal involvement, grade, and ER status, baseline prognostic estimates are shown. In addition, estimates for the efficacy of endocrine therapy, systemic chemotherapy, and the combination (for both relapse and death) are shown in both numerical and graphical forms (Figure 16–2). The user can examine several chemotherapy regimens and print out graphs that help patients visualize the information. Recently, Adjuvant Online has been updated to include the Oncotype DX assay in assessing the benefit of adjuvant therapy.

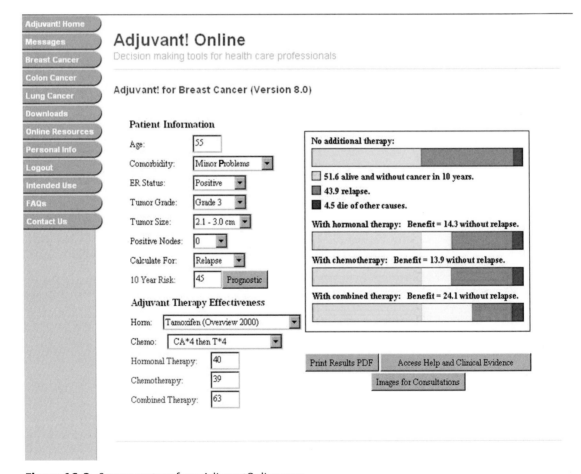

Figure 16–2. Screen capture from AdjuvantOnline.com.

Microarray Analysis and the Oncotype DX Assay

The present methods for selecting patients for adjuvant chemotherapy are based on rather crude measures of the cancer's likelihood of returning; tumor size, nodal metastases, tumor grade, angiolymphatic invasion, etc. The end result of this is that although chemotherapy clearly improves overall survival when one looks at a population of patients with breast cancer, for the individual patient the chance that the chemotherapy is extending their life may be quite small. For any group of patients with similar-appearing tumors (similar size, grade, nodal status), some patients would never have the cancer return after surgery and radiation, regardless of whether they take chemotherapy. However, because we can not differentiate these patients from those patients likely to recur, we must offer chemotherapy to the entire group, to realize the benefit in only a few.

The optimal management of breast cancer would be to use alternate factors that could predict the likelihood of cancer recurring regardless of the size or grade of the tumor. This would not only identify those patients with small, seemingly nonaggressive cancers who might benefit from chemotherapy, but also spare women with tumors unlikely to recur from the morbidity of treatment. For some time, researchers have used immunohistochemical staining to identify individual tumor markers expressed on breast cancer cells that may provide additional prognostic information. Although some of these do correlate with outcome, few provide information above and beyond size, grade, and nodal status, and thus do not help to select patients for chemotherapy.

That has changed significantly with microarray analysis. Microarray analysis allows for the measurement of thousands of genes in a single RNA sample. Although there are a variety of microarray platforms that have been developed to accomplish this, the basic idea is the same. Microarray analysis involves spotting up to 25,000 genes in an ordered "array" on a glass slide. These genes are then hybridized to RNA from a tumor sample (labeled with a red fluorophore) or from a reference sample (labeled with a green fluorophore). For each gene, if the tumor sample expresses levels of a particular RNA that are higher than those of the reference sample (the gene is up regulated by the tumor), the spot will fluoresce red. If the reference sample expresses more RNA than the tumor (the tumor down regulates the gene), the spot will fluoresce green. If the tumor and reference sample express a particular transcript at an equal level, the spot will be yellow (Figure 16–3). The fluorescent array is scanned, digitized, and analyzed by computer programs that provide researchers with a readout of which genes are down regulated and up regulated in the tumor sample.

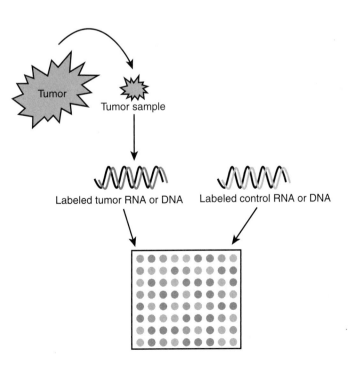

Figure 16–3. Microarray analysis involves spotting genes in an ordered "array" on a glass slide. These genes are then hybridized to RNA or DNA from a tumor sample (labeled with a red fluorophore) or from a reference sample (labeled with a green fluorophore). For each gene, if the tumor sample expresses levels of a particular RNA that are higher than those of the reference sample (overexpressed), the spot will fluoresce red. If the reference sample expresses more RNA than the tumor (underexpressed), the spot will fluoresce green. If the tumor and reference sample are equal, the spot will be yellow.

Tumor

Tumor sample

Labeled tumor RNA or DNA

Labeled control RNA or DNA

DNA microarrays have been used to analyze thousands of genes from fresh frozen tissue obtained from patients with breast cancer. Comparing the over- and underexpression of certain genes with follow-up information on these patients, researchers can identify the genes that most strongly correlate with outcome and create molecular "signatures." Several reports now demonstrate how gene expression profiling can be used to predict clinical outcome in patients with breast cancer, above and beyond standard clinical and pathologic prognostic features. For example, tissues from almost 300 patients in the Netherlands (all young women with stage I or II breast cancer) were classified according to a 70-gene prognosis profile. The patients with a "good" molecular signature had a 10-year overall survival of 95%, whereas the women with a "bad" signature had a 55% survival. In multivariate analysis, the molecular signature of the tumor was a more powerful predictor than any clinical or histologic criteria. Unfortunately, efforts to validate these findings have not been as impressive. Prospective studies are presently under way. Other drawbacks to microarray analysis are the cost, and the fact that fresh tissue is required, so the decision to use the test must be made at the time of surgery.

A more clinically feasible method to use genetic information to select women for chemotherapy is now available to clinicians. The Oncotype DX assay is a reverse-transcriptase polymerase chain reaction (RT-PCR) based assay that measures the expression of several genes that appear to be important in predicting outcome. The advantage of using RT-PCR is that the test can be performed on paraffin-embedded tissue. This not only allows the test to be studied and verified using tissue from completed adjuvant therapy trials, but allows the test to be ordered on patients after surgery, after it has been determined that they are appropriate candidates.

The Oncotype DX assay measures the expression of 21 genes in patients with node-negative, ER-positive breast cancer. Using tumor blocks from patients that were treated on NSABP B14, an algorithm was constructed to predict a recurrence score. This score is based on the expression of 16 genes relative to 5 reference genes. Based on this score, patients could be stratified into three groups based on their likelihood of recurrence (low, intermediate, or high risk). In the NSABP B14 data, about half of the patients were low risk, with a 10-year recurrence rate of 6.8%. One quarter of the patients were intermediate risk with a 10-year recurrence rate of 14.3%, and the remaining quarter were high risk, with a 30.5% chance of recurrence. It is important to remember that because this information was verified on the patients in NSABP B14, which was limited to node-negative, ER-positive patients, the results would only be accurate in this patient population. Oncotype DX cannot be used to make chemotherapy decisions in patients who are node positive or patients who are ER negative.

The Oncotype DX assay was then evaluated for its ability to predict which patients would benefit from adjuvant chemotherapy in addition to tamoxifen. Using data from both NSABP B14 and NSABP B20, the benefit of chemotherapy was assessed for low-, intermediate-, and high-risk patients. The results suggested that chemotherapy adds little to tamoxifen alone for patients with low or intermediate scores, but significantly improves survival among high-risk patients. This was independent of tumor size or grade.

Thus, the Oncotype DX assay is available to help women with node-negative, ER-positive breast cancer decide whether they should be treated with tamoxifen alone or whether they should receive adjuvant chemotherapy in addition to tamoxifen. Women in the low-risk group would see little added benefit to chemotherapy, and hormonal therapy alone should be sufficient. On the other hand, women in the high-risk group should receive chemotherapy in addition to hormonal therapy. The recommendation for women in the intermediate group is slightly more controversial. The data suggests that these women see little benefit to adjuvant chemotherapy, and hormonal therapy alone should suffice. However, some medical oncologists feel that appropriate recommendations cannot be made for these women based on the assay. A randomized trial to help answer this question is underway.

The Oncotype DX assay should only be ordered in women who are appropriate candidates (node negative, ER positive) and are unsure as to whether they would take chemotherapy. If a woman was low risk, but would take the chemotherapy anyway for a less than 3% benefit over 10 years, there is no need to order the test. Likewise, if a woman is not interested in chemotherapy regardless of her risk, the test is also not indicated.

Other gene assays are moving toward clinical use. The MammaPrint assay was recently cleared for marketing by the U.S. Food and

Drug Administration (FDA) for women under the age of 61 with node-negative tumors less than 5 cm in size. This is a 70-gene signature developed at the Netherlands Cancer Institute based on the data previously described. Although this assay can provide additional prognostic information, there is less data regarding the ability of the MammaPrint assay to improve patient outcome. This assay is presently being studied in a randomized trial. Another molecular signature is being developed in conjunction with Veridex LLC (San Diego, CA). However, as previously stated, these latter two assays use fresh frozen tissue for DNA microarrays, which may be more difficult to use in the United States, where immediate fixation of tumor specimens is more common.

Chemotherapeutic Agents Used in Breast Cancer

Table 16–3 and Box 16–6 highlight some of the more common agents used in breast cancer treatment.

Anthracycline-Based Regimens

Several different regimens exist for the adjuvant treatment of breast cancer. Trials in the 1970s and 1980s demonstrated the efficacy of cyclophosphamide, alone or in combination, in reducing breast cancer recurrence rates. Cyclophosphamide is an alkylating agent. This class of agents was one of the first chemotherapies and includes the nitrogen mustards first used in the 1940s. All alkylating agents contain an alkyl group ($-CH_2C$) which covalently binds DNA. Agents with a single alkyl group damage DNA bases or cause single-stranded DNA breaks. Agents with two alkyl groups form DNA crosslinks, which lead to interference with DNA synthesis and transcription and double stranded DNA breaks. Side effects include myelosuppression, nausea and vomiting, alopecia, infertility, hemorrhagic cystitis, and syndrome of inappropriate antidiuretic hormone (SIADH).

Ultimately, two combination regimens involving cyclophosphamide gained acceptance, both delivered in 3-week cycles. One was CMF. Both methotrexate and fluorouracil fall into the category of antimetabolites. Antimetabolites are structural analogues to a variety of cellular substrates. 5-Fluorouracil (5-FU) is metabolized to FdUMP, which inhibits the enzyme thymidylate synthase, necessary for thymidine synthesis. It is also misincorporated into RNA, leading to aberrant RNA processing. FdUMP and another metabolite, FdUTP, are both misincorporated into DNA, inhibiting further DNA synthesis. Methotrexate is a folate analogue that binds to dihydrofolate reductase (DHFR) and inhibits its ability to reduce folate, which is necessary for the synthesis of thymidylate, purines, serine, and methionine.

The other popular regimen was cyclophosphamide, doxorubicin, and fluorouracil (CAF). Doxorubicin falls into the class of drugs known as antitumor antibiotics. Most of these are derived from the *Streptomyces* species of fungus. These drugs work by intercalating into DNA and inhibiting its synthesis and transcription. Doxorubicin also inhibits topoisomerase II and causes DNA breaks through the formation of free radicals. Although doxorubicin is the most commonly used anthracycline in the United States and Canada, epirubicin (4′-epidoxorubicin) is commonly used elsewhere. This is the semisynthetic L-arabino derivative of doxorubicin in which the amino sugar daunosamine is replaced with acosamine. It appears to have a better safety profile than doxorubicin on a milligram per milligram basis, with less nausea and cardiotoxicity when given at roughly equal myelosuppressive doses and with similar response rates. The FDA did recently approve the use of epirubicin for adjuvant therapy in breast cancer. There is little data to support using one over the other.

The dose-limiting toxicity of all anthracyclines is myelosuppression. Neutrophil nadirs typically occur 10 to 14 days after treatment. Other common toxicities include alopecia, nausea and vomiting, diarrhea, and mucositis. The most concerning toxicity of the anthracyclines is the cardiac toxicity. An acute pericarditis/myocarditis syndrome with fever, chest pain, and congestive heart failure can occur, but it is quite rare. Chronic cardiac toxicity is dose dependent, and rarely occurs when a cumulative dose of less than or equal to 450 mg/m^2 is given. If it does occur, however, it can lead to irreversible congestive heart failure. The risk increases with advanced age, diabetes, a history of cardiomyopathy, and chest wall radiation, particularly for left-sided breast cancers.

As previously described, one of the findings of the Oxford Overview, in reviewing over 6900 patients from 11 trials in which CMF was compared with regimens containing doxorubicin (such as FAC or AC) or epirubicin (such as FEC), was that there was an improvement with the doxorubicin- or epirubicin-based regimens

TABLE 16–3 • *Chemotherapeutic Agents Used in Breast Cancer*

Agent	Type of Agent	Side Effects	Precautions
Cyclophosphamide	Alkylating agent	Myelosuppression Nausea/vomiting Alopecia Infertility Hemorrhagic cystitis Syndrome of inappropriate antidiuretic hormone (SIADH) Second-degree malignancies	-Encourage oral fluids (2–3 L/day) to prevent hemorrhagic cystitis -May increase the effects of anticoagulation
Thiotepa	Alkylating agent	Myelosuppression Nausea/vomiting Mucositis Hypersensitivity Rash Hemorrhagic cystitis Second-degree malignancies	-Have resuscitation supplies nearby during administration for hypersensitivity reactions
Paclitaxel	Antimicrotubule	Myelosuppression Hypersensitivity Neurotoxicity Alopecia Mucositis Diarrhea Cardiac arrhythmia Hepatotoxicity	-Dexamethasone, antihistamines, and histamine-2 blockers should be administered before treatment to avoid hypersensitivity -Resuscitation supplies should be available during administration -Activity reduced by phenytoin and carbamazepine
Docetaxel	Antimicrotubule	Myelosuppression Hypersensitivity Fluid retention Neurotoxicity Alopecia Arthralgias Myalgias Mucositis Diarrhea Rash	-Administer dexamethasone before and after treatment to prevent hypersensitivity and fluid retention -Resuscitation supplies should be available during administration -Activity reduced by phenytoin and carbamazepine
5-Fluorouracil	Antimetabolite	Myelosuppression Blepharitis Cardiac ischemia	-Severe toxicity in patients with DPD deficiency -May increase toxicity of antiepileptic medications
Capecitabine	Antimetabolite	Mucositis Hand-foot syndrome Diarrhea Nausea/vomiting Hepatotoxicity Blepharitis Cardiac ischemia	-Severe toxicity in patients with DPD deficiency -May increase the effects of Coumadin
Methotrexate	Antimetabolite	Myelosuppression Mucositis Hepatotoxicity Renal failure Pneumonitis Arachnoiditis (when given intrathecally)	-Accumulates in third space fluid and should not be given to patients with ascites, pleural effusions, etc. -May increase the effects of Coumadin -Ineffective if given with folate -Activity reduced by phenytoin and carbamazepine -May decrease activity of phenytoin or valproic acid
Gemcitabine	Antimetabolite	Myelosuppression Nausea/vomiting Flulike syndrome Hepatotoxicity Dyspnea Rash Hemolytic-uremic syndrome	

(Continued)

TABLE 16–3 *Chemotherapeutic Agents Used in Breast Cancer*

Agent	Type of Agent	Side Effects	Precautions
Doxorubicin	Antitumor antibiotics	Myelosuppression Nausea/vomiting Cardiotoxicity Alopecia Mucositis Diarrhea Rash (radiation recall)	-Infuse through a central venous catheter as a result of vesicant properties -Obtain baseline left ventricular ejection fraction (LVEF) and monitor for cardiotoxicity -May decrease activity of valproic acid or carbamazepine
Mitomycin-C	Antitumor antibiotic	Myelosuppression Nausea/vomiting Mucositis Pulmonary toxicity/ARDS Renal failure Hemolytic-uremic syndrome Cystitis (intravesicular treatment)	-Avoid FiO2 > 50% that may worsen pulmonary toxicity

ARDS, adult respiratory distress syndrome; DPD, dihydropyrimidine dehydrogenase.

(12% reduction in the odds of recurrence, 11% reduction in the odds of death). These benefits were seen in patients who were both node positive and node negative, and so anthracycline-based regimens are now the most recommended regimens in the adjuvant setting. CMF is still a reasonable option, especially if there is concern regarding the cardiac risk associated with the anthracycline.

For many years, anthracycline-based regimens dominated the adjuvant breast cancer landscape. In the late 1990s, three advances occurred that dramatically changed the choices for adjuvant therapy. The first of these was the emergence of the taxanes as a highly effective agent against breast cancer. The second was the development of tolerable bone marrow supportive therapy in the form of granulocyte colony-stimulating factors, allowing dose-dense regimens (higher doses within shorter time frames) without the risks of severe neutropenia. Finally, the development of trastuzumab, a monoclonal antibody that targets the Her-2/neu marker, and proven to be effective in the metastatic setting, was recently shown to be extremely effective in the adjuvant setting as well.

Taxanes

Mechanism of Action

The taxanes (paclitaxel and docetaxel) are known as antitubulins and bind to dimeric tubulin, disrupting the microtubule network by inhibiting tubule disassembly, leading to stable microtubule bundles to accumulate in the cell. These cells are incapable of forming normal mitotic spindles and become blocked in the G2 and M phases of the cell cycle. The dysfunctional microtubules can also lead to cell death by interfering with normal microtubule dynamics. Paclitaxel (Taxol) and docetaxel (Taxotere) bind to the same site and have a similar mechanism of action, although there are some small differences in the pharmacologic characteristics. Paclitaxel was first identified as the active component of a bark extract from the Pacific yew *Taxus brevifolia*. Docetaxel

BOX 16–6 COMMON ADJUVANT CHEMOTHERAPY REGIMENS

FAC/CAF	Fluorouracil/doxorubicin/cyclophosphamide
FEC/CEF	Cyclophosphamide/epirubicin/fluorouracil
AC	Doxorubicin/cyclophosphamide
CMF	Cyclophosphamide/methotrexate/fluorouracil
ACx4+Tx4	Doxorubicin/cyclophosphamide then paclitaxel
TAC	Docetaxel/doxorubicin/cyclophosphamide
TC	Docetaxel/cyclophosphamide
AC→T+H	Doxorubicin/cyclophosphamide then paclitaxel plus trastuzumab

is a semisynthetic product derived from the European yew *Taxus bacata*. Docetaxel has a longer plasma half-life and longer intracellular retention. Both taxanes have potent radiosensitizing effects, can induce apoptosis, and have antiangiogenic properties.

The major dose-limiting toxicity of taxanes is profound myelosuppression. Another significant side effect is the hypersensitivity reaction (HSR). Within a few minutes of the first or second dose of paclitaxel, patients may experience hypotension, hives, rash, or shortness of breath. This typically resolves after the taxane is discontinued, and antihistamines, steroids, and sometimes vasopressors are administered. With pretreatment dexamethasone, diphenhydramine and cimetidine, the incidence of HSR is only 1% to 3%. Another difficult side effect of the taxanes is a peripheral neuropathy characterized by numbness and paresthesias in a stocking-and-glove distribution. Like other cytotoxic agents, the taxanes induce a reversible alopecia. Urticaria, dermatitis, and reactive erythema can also occur.

Taxanes in the Adjuvant Setting

With the antitumor activity demonstrated in studies of metastatic breast cancer, taxanes were examined in the adjuvant setting. The first study to demonstrate results was CALGB 9344, which randomized patients with node-positive breast cancer to Adriamycin/cytoxan (three dose levels of Adriamycin) followed by randomization to paclitaxel or no paclitaxel. Preliminary results at a median follow-up of 21 months showed significant reductions in both recurrence (22%) and mortality (26%). Based on these results, paclitaxel was approved by the FDA for adjuvant therapy in node-positive breast cancer. After 5 years of follow-up, results show a 17% reduction in recurrence (DFS 70% versus 65%) and approximately 4% OS advantage (OS 80% versus 77%) with the addition of taxanes. A retrospective subset analysis of CALGB 9344 suggests the benefit to DFS and OS are primarily among the patients who were ER negative, with little benefit seen in patients who were ER positive. NSABP B-28 also evaluated adjuvant taxanes in patients who were node positive. Over 3000 patients were randomized to AC with or without paclitaxel. Early results demonstrated no benefit to DFS or OS,

although as with the CALGB 9344 trial, subset analysis suggested a trend toward benefit for patients who were ER negative. However, the data was updated in 2003 and the addition of paclitaxel to AC resulted in a significant improvement in DFS (relative risk [RR] 0.83, $p = 0.008$). There was still no benefit to OS (RR 0.94, $p = 0.46$). This magnitude of benefit is approximately similar to that seen in CALGB 9344.

A third trial, a single institution trial from MD Anderson, randomized patients to eight cycles of FAC versus four cycles of FAC and four cycles of paclitaxel. After 4 years, the paclitaxel group had a nonsignificant 3% absolute improvement in DFS (86% versus 83%), but no better OS.

The Breast Cancer International Research Group (BCIRG) study 001 randomly assigned 1491 women with node-positive breast cancer to six cycles of 5-FU, doxorubicin, and cyclophosphamide (FAC) or six cycles of docetaxel, doxorubicin, and cyclophosphamide (TAC). After a median follow-up of 5 years, the TAC group had a reduction in both the risk of recurrence (DFS 75% versus 68% and death (OS 87% versus 81%). Based on these results, docetaxel was approved by the FDA for the adjuvant treatment of node-positive breast cancer in combination with AC.

Herceptin

The epidermal growth factor receptor (EGFR) family of tyrosine kinases regulates a complex signaling cascade that controls the proliferation, survival, adhesion, migration, and differentiation of cells. This pathway is tightly regulated in normal cells because when there is dysregulation of EGFR signaling, the result can be abnormal cell proliferation and other tumor-promoting activities.

There are four distinct receptors in the EGFR family: EGFR (ErbB-1), Her-2 (Her-2/neu or ErbB-2), Her-3 (ErbB-3), and Her-4 (ErbB-4). Each of these receptors consists of an extracellular binding domain, a transmembrane lipophilic segment, and (with the exception of Her-3), a functional intracellular tyrosine kinase domain. When ligand binding occurs, the tyrosine kinase domains are activated by homo- and heterodimerization. Abnormalities of these receptors can be associated with several types of human cancer. In contrast to the other receptors, Her-2 can adopt a fixed conformation resembling a ligand-activated state, permitting it to dimerize in the absence of a ligand. In addition, overexpression or mutation can induce dimerization. Overexpression of Her-2 is found in approximately one third of breast cancers and is associated with a poor prognosis in breast cancer. Overexpression of Her-2 is associated with increased proliferation, increased properties of metastases (invasion, angiogenesis), and resistance to therapeutic agents (chemotherapy and hormonal therapy).

Because the overexpression of Her-2 correlates with prognosis in breast cancer, it is an important therapeutic target. The first therapy to specifically target Her-2 is trastuzumab (Herceptin), a recombinant humanized monoclonal antibody to the extracellular domain of Her-2. Herceptin binds to Her-2 and disrupts the downstream signaling (Figure 16–4 and Box 16–7).

Trastuzumab is an immunoglobulin G (IgG) antibody that consists of two antigen-specific sites that bind to the juxta-membrane portion of the extracellular domain of the Her-2 receptor. This prevents the activation of its intracellular tyrosine kinase. This may occur through prevention of dimerization, endocytic destruction of the receptor, or inhibition of shedding of the extracellular domain. The IgG does have a conserved Fc portion, so it can trigger immune recognition. Although most investigators consider trastuzumab a "targeted therapy," it may also

BOX 16–7 POTENTIAL MECHANISMS FOR TRASTUZUMAB

Inhibition of tumor cell proliferation
Reduces signaling through cell-proliferative pathways (MAPK)
Promotes apoptosis
Reduces signaling through cell survival pathways (Pt3K/Akt)
Inhibits angiogenesis
Induces G1 arrest
Induces p27 cell cycle inhibitor
Reduces cyclin D1 levels
Initiates ADCC

ADCC, xxxx; G1, xxxx; Pt2K/Akt, xxx; p27, xxx.***

be a form of "immunotherapy" because it is possible that immune activation plays a role in the mechanism of action of trastuzumab. There is some evidence for antibody-dependent cytotoxicity, including increased tumor infiltration by lymphoid cells and a loss of function in mice deficient in immune-cell activating Fc receptors. Whether trastuzumab may be combined with other vaccines or immunotherapies is being investigated.

After several studies demonstrating the efficacy and safety of trastuzumab in the management of stage IV disease, studies in the adjuvant setting were initiated. Four large, multicenter, randomized trials (and some smaller studies) reported a significant benefit

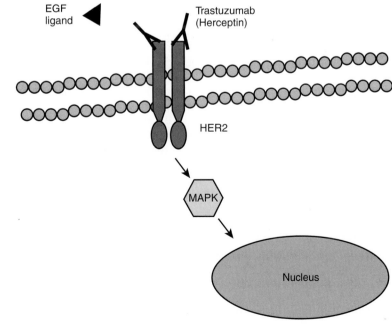

Figure 16–4. Herceptin binding.

from the addition of trastuzumab to adjuvant and neoadjuvant therapy. The use of adjuvant trastuzumab should be considered for women with Her-2-positive breast cancer who are either node positive or have worrisome features despite being node negative. The benefits to patients with small, hormone-responsive tumors who are node negative appear quite modest, so it is unclear whether trastuzumab is indicated in this situation, even if patients are Her-2 positive. One key to the successful use of trastuzumab is the Her-2 testing. In the trials of trastuzumab, response was seen only in patients with 3+ staining or gene amplification on fluorescence in situ hybridization (FISH). No response was seen in patients with 2+ staining unless gene amplification was present. Therefore, all patients who are 2+ should undergo FISH testing.

Trastuzumab alone is relatively safe. About 10% of patients may have a hypersensitivity-like reaction, but this is preventable with antihistamines, antiinflammatories, and corticosteroids. Myelosuppression and nausea and vomiting are rare, and alopecia does not occur. The most concerning side effect of trastuzumab is congestive heart failure, particularly when used in combination with anthracyclines. It is not completely understood how trastuzumab is related to cardiotoxicity, but it appears to be less severe and more readily reversible than the cardiac dysfunction associated with anthracyclines. There appear to be few trastuzumab-related cardiac deaths; however, patients on trastuzumab must be carefully monitored and appropriate actions taken in patients with developing congestive heart failure.

Dose-Dense Chemotherapy

Dose density refers to a shortened interval between treatments under the assumption that more frequent administration may be more effective. The concept is based on experimental models that a dose of chemotherapy kills a certain fraction (rather than number) of exponentially growing cells and tumor regrowth is faster when the number of viable cells is lowest. By giving the next dose faster, there is less time for the cells to regrow. The problem with this approach had been the severe neutropenia triggered by dose-dense chemotherapy. With the introduction of filgrastim, however, neutropenia can be avoided during dose-dense regimens. Filgrastim is an analog of granulocyte-colony stimulating factor (G-CSF) which stimulates the bone marrow to increase the production of neutrophils.

Evidence for the benefit of dose-dense regimens came from CALGB 9741, a trial of adjuvant chemotherapy in 2000 patients with node-positive breast cancer. This study used a 2-by-2 design, randomizing women between sequential doxorubicin, paclitaxel, and cyclophosphamide, and AC for four cycles followed by paclitaxel for four cycles. They were also randomized to an every 3-week regimen versus an every 2-week regimen with filgrastim. At a median follow-up of 36 months, dose-dense treatment significantly improved DFS (RR 0.74, $p = 0.01$) and overall survival (RR 0.69, $p = 0.013$). Further follow-up suggests that although the DFS remains improved, the OS may have lost statistical significance. Longer follow-up is needed. There were no differences between the concurrent and sequential regimens. Although this study provides evidence as to the benefit of dose-dense schedules, there are still many questions regarding the appropriate dosing and scheduling of Adriamycin- and taxane-based regimens in the adjuvant setting. Ongoing clinical trials will continue to change the manner in which systemic chemotherapy is administered (Box 16–8).

High-Dose Chemotherapy with Autologous Stem Cell Support

It was hypothesized that higher doses of chemotherapy, beyond what is in standard clinical use, would improve outcome. In preclinical culture systems, the alkylating agents exhibit a steep dose response in breast cancer, meaning that resistance can be overcome by a fivefold to tenfold higher doses. However, high doses of chemotherapy are limited by the myelosuppression. Because the other side effects of alkylating agents do not reach dose-limiting levels until the dose is many times higher than the myelosuppressive dose, it was felt that if the myelosuppression could be overcome, much higher doses could be given and would result in better outcomes. Thus, extremely high doses were combined with autologous stem cell support. Initial, nonrandomized data seemed promising, and based on public pressure, began to be offered as a choice for high-risk patients before randomized trial data was available. Unfortunately, prospective randomized trials failed to demonstrate a benefit, and this practice has fallen out of favor. A recent meta-analysis suggests that there may be a small benefit to high-dose chemotherapy, although the minimal benefit compared to the significantly increased toxicities do not appear to justify its use.

BOX 16–8 SCHEDULES FOR COMMONLY USED ADJUVANT CHEMOTHERAPY REGIMENS

CMF	Cyclophosphamide 100 mg/m^2 by mouth days 1 to 14 Methotrexate 40 mg/m^2 intravenously days 1 and 8 5-FU 600 mg/m^2 intravenously days 1 and 8 Cycled every 28 days for 6 cycles
AC	Doxorubicin 60 mg/m^2 intravenous day 1 Cyclophosphamide 600 mg/m^2 intravenous day 1 Cycled every 21 days for 4 cycles
CAF	Cyclophosphamide 100 mg/m^2 by mouth day 1 to 14 Doxorubicin 30 mg/m^2 intravenously day 1 and 8 5-FU 500 mg/m^2 intravenously days 1 and 8 Cycled every 28 days for 6 cycles
TC	Docetaxel 75 mg/m^2 intravenously day 1 Cyclophosphamide 600 mg/m^2 intravenously day 1 Cycled every 21 days for 4 cycles.

AC→T	Doxorubicin 60 mg/m^2 intravenously day 1
	Cyclophosphamide 600 mg/m^2 intravenously day 1
	Cycled every 21 days for 4 cycles
	   FOLLOWED BY
	Paclitaxel 175 to 225 mg/m^2 intravenously by 3 hours infusion day 1
	Cycled every 21 days for 4 cycles
	   OR
	Paclitaxel 80 mg/m^2 intravenously by 1 h infusion weekly for 12 weeks

Dose-dense
  AC→T
	Doxorubicin 60 mg/m^2 intravenously day 1
	Cyclophosphamide 600 mg/m^2 intravenously day 1
	Cycled every 14 days for 4 cycles
	   FOLLOWED BY
	Paclitaxel 175 to 225 mg/m^2 intravenously by 3 hours infusion day 1
	Cycled every 21 days for 4 cycles
	All cycles are with filgrastim support.

AC→T+H	Doxorubicin 60 mg/m^2 intravenously day 1
	Cyclophosphamide 600 mg/m^2 intravenously day 1
	Cycled every 21 days for 4 cycles
	Paclitaxel 175 to 225 mg/m^2 intravenously by 3 hours infusion day 1
	Cycled every 21 days for 4 cycles OR paclitaxel 80 mg/m^2 intravenously by 1 hour
	  infusion weekly for 12 weeks
	   WITH
	Trastuzumab 4 mg/kg intravenously with first dose of paclitaxel
	   THEN
	Trastuzumab 2 mg/kg intravenously weekly for 1 year
	   OR
	Trastuzumab 6 mg/kg intravenously every 3 weeks after completion of paclitaxel for 1 year.

Side Effects of Chemotherapy

Short-Term Toxicity

Hair Loss (Alopecia)

The most common side effect of chemotherapy for breast cancer, as well as the most visible and distressing, is hair loss. Alopecia is almost 100% with regimens including an anthracycline or a taxane. Alopecia does not always occur with CMF, with an incidence between 40% and 65% depending on the route and schedule.

Nausea and Vomiting

Nausea and vomiting during chemotherapy are primarily caused by serotonin release from the gastrointestinal mucosa, which leads to stimulation of the emesis center of the medulla. Although severe nausea and vomiting used to be a significant side effect of chemotherapy, the availability of new antiemetic agents has decreased the severity. The prophylactic use of antiemetic medications containing 5-hydroxy-triptamine 3(5-HT3) serotonin antagonists has dramatically improved the tolerability of adjuvant chemotherapy. Dexamethasone may further improve the response to the 5-HT3 serotonin antagonists. Although most women receiving chemotherapy will develop some nausea, less than 5% will have severe nausea and vomiting. Metoclopramide or prochlorperazine may be useful for those cases where nausea occurs several days after treatment.

Myelosuppression

Myelosuppression is a common side effect of chemotherapy, and thus patients are carefully monitored for the development of neutropenia, anemia, or thrombocytopenia. It typically occurs within 5 to 15 days of treatment.

The management of neutropenia depends on the severity. Mild neutropenia, defined as an absolute neutrophil count of less than $1500/mm^3$, but greater than $1000/mm^3$ does not require treatment. It may be prudent to decrease the dose of chemotherapy. Patients with moderate (500 to 1000) or severe (<500) neutropenia are at an increased risk of infection and must be instructed to report any fevers. Fevers should be thoroughly worked up and antibiotics initiated, even if no source is found. Granulocyte colony-stimulating factors should be considered for any patient who had neutropenic fever, with prolonged neutropenia or prophylactically when neutropenia is expected (such as with dose-dense regimens).

Anemia is treated with erythropoietin, or rarely, blood transfusion. Symptomatic patients with hemoglobin counts less than 10 gm/dl are likely to benefit from erythropoietin. Patients with thrombocytopenia may require platelet transfusion.

Neurologic Toxicity

The addition of taxanes (paclitaxel, docetaxel) to adjuvant chemotherapy carries with it several neurologic toxicities. These can take the form of both motor and sensory neuropathies. The severity is dose- and schedule-dependent, and symptoms can be improved by early recognition with subsequent dose reduction. Within 72 hours of receiving paclitaxel, myalgias and arthralgias may develop. These can be relieved by either nonsteroidal antiinflammatory drugs (NSAIDs), or a short course of glucocorticoids.

Weight Gain and Fatigue

As weight loss is commonly associated with cancer, many women are surprised to learn that weight gain is a common side effect of chemotherapy. On average, women gain between 2 and 6 kg, depending on the regimen. The cause for the weight gain is multifactorial.

One of the most common complaints during chemotherapy is fatigue. As with weight loss, the reasons are multifactorial. Anemia should be ruled out, as should other potentially reversible factors, such as sleep disturbance, uncontrolled pain, depression, or poor nutrition. However, in most cases a correctable condition will not be identified. The fatigue should resolve after the cessation of treatment. During therapy, symptomatic relief may be provided by initiating an exercise regimen, changing the diet, or through the use of stimulants or antidepressants.

Long-Term Effects

Adjuvant chemotherapy is given with the goal of improving long-term survival. Therefore, the long-term effects of chemotherapy must be considered in addition to the acute toxicity.

Cognitive Dysfunction

A considerable amount of data is now coming out on the long-term effect of chemotherapy on cognition. As many as one third of patients who receive adjuvant chemotherapy may develop some dysfunction in memory or the ability to concentrate, although for many patients this will eventually return to baseline. There may be a relationship between the intensity of the adjuvant therapy and the incidence of cognitive impairment. Further research is necessary to better clarify the impairment and identify ways to avoid or reverse it.

Ovarian Failure

Premature termination of ovarian function is a significant concern for younger women receiving adjuvant chemotherapy for breast cancer. On one hand, the induction of premature menopause may be beneficial. Removal of estrogen may improve DFS and OS in women with ER+ breast cancer. However, many young women being treated for breast cancer would like to maintain reproductive function, hoping to have children after completing therapy.

Even in women who no longer desire to have children, premature ovarian failure can affect quality of life by heralding menopausal symptoms (hot flashes, vaginal dryness, dyspareunia, depression, sleep disturbance) and result in significant bone loss.

Premature ovarian failure can occur in any woman, but the risks are higher for older women, a longer duration of treatment and for CMF regimens compared to AC. Women receiving taxanes may actually have a lower incidence of ovarian failure. It may be possible to reduce the incidence of ovarian failure by reducing ovarian function during treatment by using gonadotropin-releasing hormone (GnRH) agonists or oral contraceptives. This is presently being studied in a prospective randomized trial. In women who do suffer ovarian failure, supplemental calcium, vitamin D and regular exercise should be used to mitigate bone loss. Bisphosphonates can treat osteoporosis in women with premature menopause.

Cardiac Toxicity

Women treated with anthracyclines or with Herceptin may be at an increased risk of cardiac toxicities. This may be higher in women who receive radiation therapy for left-sided breast cancers. Anthracyclines directly damage the myocardium and can lead to cardiomyopathy. The risk of cardiac failure greatly increases after cumulative doses of doxorubicin greater than 450 mg/m^2. The risk is also higher in older patients and those with a history of cardiac disease.

Leukemia and Myelodysplastic Syndromes

Although chemotherapy can lead to the development of leukemias and myelodysplastic syndromes, the incidence appears low for regimens used to treat breast cancer, less than 1% overall. This may be slightly higher among women who receive radiation therapy or with the administration of G-CSF, although the data is not clear. Two distinct types of treatment-related leukemic syndromes can occur. The first is typically associated with alkylating agents and takes 3 to 7 years to develop, often preceded by a myelodysplastic syndrome. The second is associated with topoisomerase II inhibitors and has a more rapid onset, within 2 to 3 years of therapy. Unfortunately the treatment-related leukemias have a poor prognosis and are more refractory to conventional antileukemic therapies.

On the Horizon

With the success of Herceptin, there is considerable interest in other targeted therapies—agents that exploit certain characteristics of the cancer cells rather than relying on more universal "cytotoxicity" of standard chemotherapy. Many of these targeted therapies are early in their development and evaluation, but several may soon be in clinical use.

Tyrosine kinase inhibitors (TKIs) are small molecules that block the intracellular kinase domain of the transmembrane receptor, preventing its autophosphorylation and subsequent activation. TKIs may be specific for a given receptor type or have more broad effects against multiple tyrosine kinases. The less specific they are, the more side effects they may have. Common side effects include skin rashes, diarrhea, and headaches.

Gefitinib (Iressa) and erlotinib (Tarceva) are TKIs that act by blocking EGFR activation. As single agents, both have been relatively disappointing against breast cancer, although more promising results have been obtained by combining these agents with cytotoxic chemotherapy. Further research is looking into identifying subsets of patients who may benefit from EGFR TKIs as the mere presence of EGFR overexpression does not seem to correlate with response to treatment.

Lapatinib (Tykerb) is a TKI that inhibits both EGFR and Her-2/neu. As Her-2 may play a role in the oncogenic activity of EGFR, blocking both could provide a better response. This agent has been studied alone or in combination with hormonal therapy, chemotherapy, and trastuzumab, and several trials in the adjuvant, neoadjuvant and metastatic settings are ongoing. As previously stated, some TKIs inhibit multiple kinases. One example is sunitinib (Sutent), a multiinhibitor vascular endothelial growth factor (VEGF) receptor; platelet-derived growth factor receptor; stem cell factor receptor, Kit; rearranged during transfection (RET) gene; and fetal liver tyrosine kinase receptor-3 (Flt-3). Phase II and III trials are ongoing or planned in patients with breast cancer.

The family of ras proto-oncogenes has been implicated in the development of breast cancer and so it was hypothesized that blocking this pathway could inhibit tumor growth. Farnesyltransferase inhibitors (FTIs) are agents designed to target ras proteins. One example is tipifarnib (Zarnestra), which inhibits growth of several breast cancer cell lines and has shown some clinical activity as monotherapy in clinical studies, particularly when combined with endocrine therapy. Unfortunately, a large randomized study of tipifarnib plus letrozole versus letrozole alone showed no difference in outcome between the two groups. Ongoing studies are looking at tipifarnib in combination with chemotherapy.

Another important pathway in cell growth and proliferation is the PI3-K/Akt pathway. Akt may promote breast cancer cell survival and play a role in resistance to standard therapies. Temsirolimus (CCI-779) and everolimus (RAD-001) inhibit mTOR, a downstream substrate of Akt, and blocks progression in late G1/S phase of the cell cycle. Both are being examined in the treatment of breast cancer.

Crucial to cancer development and growth is angiogenesis, the formation of new blood vessels for oxygen and nutrient delivery. The most potent stimulator driving tumor angiogenesis is VEGF. Bevacizumab (Avastin) is a recombinant monoclonal antibody that binds directly to VEGF, inhibiting angiogenesis and slowing or stopping tumor growth. It is hoped that the addition of Avastin to standard chemotherapy will increase the response rate and outcome with breast cancer therapy. Randomized trials are ongoing.

Cyclooxygenase-2 (COX-2) is an inducible enzyme that converts arachidonic acid to prostaglandins. Deregulation of COX-2 has been demonstrated in tumorigenesis, and multiple tumors (including breast) have elevated COX-2 levels. COX-2 inhibitors, such as celecoxib (Celebrex), have shown promising results in preclinical studies of breast cancer, although the exact mechanisms of action by which these drugs slow tumor growth is not well understood. They may be anti-angiogenic. COX-2 inhibitors are also presently being studied in combination with chemotherapy and hormonal therapy for breast cancer.

Heat shock proteins (HSP) are proteins responsible for the correct folding of a large number of proteins, which is essential to their functional conformation. Cellular stress leads to an increased production of these proteins, which allow cells to adapt to noxious environments, such as heat or hypoxia, but also chemotherapy or irradiation. HSP-90 is essential for the conformation of several protein kinases and transcription factors involved in cell signaling and proliferation (p53, Erb-B2, Akt-kinase, Raf, etc.). Thus, targeting HSP-90 may have antitumor activity or make cells more susceptible to chemotherapy. Many drugs that bind to HSP-90 are unfortunately too hepatotoxic for clinical use, but newer analogs are under development.

Suggested Readings

1. Adjuvant! On Line. www.adjuvantonline.com
2. Burstein HJ. The distinctive nature of HER2-positive breast cancers. N Engl J Med 2005;353:1652–1654.
3. Citron ML. Dose density in adjuvant chemotherapy for breast cancer. Cancer Invest 2004;22(4):555–568.
4. Early Breast Cancer Trialists' Collaborative Group. Effects of chemotherapy and hormonal therapy for early breast cancer on recurrence and 15-year survival: an overview of the randomized trials. Lancet 2005;365(9472):1687–1717.
5. Early Breast Cancer Trialists' Collaborative Group. Multi-agent chemotherapy for early breast cancer. Cochrane Database Syst Rev 2002;1:CD000487.
6. Effects of adjuvant tamoxifen and of cytotoxic therapy on mortality in early breast cancer. An overview of 61 randomized trials among 28,896 women. Early Breast Cancer Trialists' Collaborative Group. N Engl J Med 1988;319(26):1681–1692.
7. Goldhirsch A, Glick JH, Gelber RD, et al. Meeting highlights: international expert consensus on the primary therapy of early breast cancer 2005. Ann Oncol 2005;16(10):1569–1583.
8. Hudis CA. Trastuzumab—mechanism of action and use in clinical practice. N Engl J Med 2007;357:39–51.
9. Mamounas EP, Bryant J, Lembersky B, et al. Paclitaxel after doxorubicin plus cyclophosphamide as adjuvant chemotherapy for node-positive breast cancer: results from NSABP B-28. J Clin Orthod 2005;23(16):3686–3696.
10. Martin M, Pienkowski T, Mackey J, et al. Adjuvant docetaxel for node-positive breast cancer. N Engl J Med 2004;352(22):2302–2313.
11. Newman LA, Singletary SE. Overview of adjuvant systemic therapy in early stage breast cancer. Surg Clin North Am 2007;87(2):499–509.
12. Paik S, Shak S, Tang G, et al. A multigene assay to predict recurrence of tamoxifen-treated, node-negative breast cancer. N Engl J Med 2004;351(27):2817–2826.
13. Piccart-Gebhart MJ, Proctor M, Leyland-Jones B, et al. Trastuzumab after adjuvant chemotherapy in HER2-positive breast cancer. N Engl J Med 2005;353(16):1659–1672.
14. Polychemotherapy for early breast cancer: an overview of the randomized trials. Early Breast Cancer Trialists' Collaborative Group. Lancet 1998;352 (9132):930–42.
15. Ravdin PM, Siminoff LA, Davis GJ, et al. Computer program to assist in making decisions about adjuvant therapy for women with early breast cancer. J Clin Orthod 2001;19(4):980–991.
16. Romond EH, Perez EA, Bryant J, et al. Trastuzumab plus adjuvant chemotherapy for operable HER2-positive breast cancer. N Engl J Med 2005;353(16):1673–1684.
17. Slamon DJ, Clark GM, Wong SG, et al. Human breast cancer: correlation of relapse and survival with amplification of the Her-2/neu oncogene. Science 1987;235:177–182.

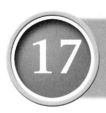 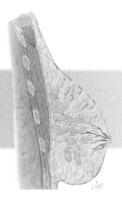

17

Principles of Adjuvant Hormonal Therapy

Principles of Adjuvant Hormonal Therapy: Key Points

- Understand the expression of estrogen receptors and the impact of estrogen on the growth of normal and cancerous breast cells.
- Describe the mechanism of action of selective estrogen receptor modulators.
- Describe the benefits of adjuvant hormonal therapy after surgery and the data from the Early Breast Cancer Trialists Collaborative Group.
- Know the prospective data regarding the use of aromatase inhibitors instead of or after a selective estrogen receptor modulator.
- Describe the side effects of tamoxifen and aromatase inhibitors.
- Understand the potential of ovarian suppression or ablation as hormonal therapy.

In the treatment of most solid tumors, adjuvant systemic therapy typically refers to the use of cytotoxic chemotherapy after surgery to prevent clinically occult micrometastases from becoming distant treatment failures. However, because breast cancer is often stimulated by endogenous estrogen, another form of adjuvant therapy is endocrine or hormonal.

The effects of hormonal therapy on breast cancer were first noted over 100 years ago when Beatson described the regression of advanced breast cancer after oophorectomy. Subsequently, ovarian ablation (typically through irradiation) became a therapy for metastatic breast cancer, and eventually made its way to the adjuvant setting. In the 1960s, hormonal therapy shifted from surgery and radiation for ovarian ablation to pharmacologic methods. This included both suppressing estrogen synthesis (using luteinizing hormone releasing hormone [LHRH] agonists) and blocking the binding of estrogen to the estrogen receptor (ER; using tamoxifen). Since the 1970s, multiple randomized controlled trials have demonstrated its efficacy in reducing relapse rates and death.

The Estrogen Receptor

The steroid hormones estrogen and progesterone are involved in both the development of the normal breast and the changes in the breast seen with the menstrual cycle and pregnancy (see Chapter 1). They influence the molecular processes involved in proliferation, differentiation, and function. They do not act alone, but rather in concert with other steroid hormones (glucocorticoids), peptide hormones (insulin, prolactin, oxytocin, and growth hormones) and peptide growth factors (epidermal growth factor, fibroblast growth factor, insulin like growth factor, and transforming growth factors).

The ER behaves differently than most receptors of the steroid family. The typical steroid receptor is a "translocating receptor." This means that the receptor is distributed in the cytoplasm in the absence of the hormone, moving to the nucleus when the cell is hormone stimulated. The ER works as a "ligand-dependent transcription factor," and is primarily located in the nucleus in the absence or presence of estrogen. Estrogen diffuses through the cell and binds to the ER's ligand-binding domain. This causes a dramatic change in the conformation of the receptor, resulting in the dissociation of the receptor from the heat shock protein 90 (HSP-90) and heterodimerization. These complexes can then bind to DNA sequences, causing the activation or repression of target genes (Fig. 17–1). This can be either the result of direct binding to estrogen response elements (ERE) in the promoter of target genes or to interactions with coactivators at their respective promoter sites.

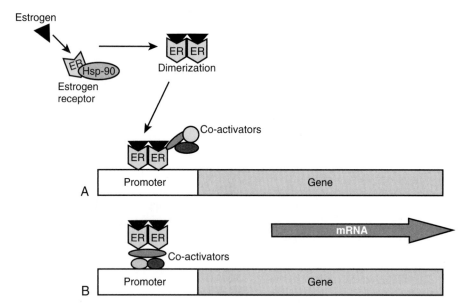

Figure 17–1. Estrogen receptor binding. When estrogen binds to the estrogen receptor, heat shock protein 90 is dissociated, resulting in a change in conformation. This allows the receptors to dimerize. The dimerized hormone receptor molecules then bind to DNA and interact with coactivators to modulate expression of the target gene.

BOX 17–1 EXPRESSION OF α OR β ESTROGEN RECEPTORS BY TISSUE TYPE

Breast	α and β (↑ α in breast cancer)
Uterus	mostly α, some β
Ovary	α and β
Blood vessels	β
Heart	α and β
Bone	α (cortical), β (cancellous)
Brain	α (hypothalamus), β (whole brain)
Gut	β
Immune cells	β
Liver	mostly α, some β

Modified from Fabian CJ, Kimler BF. J Clin Orthod 2005;23:1644-1655.

There are two isoforms of the estrogen receptor; ER-alpha (ERα) and ER-beta. (ERβ) Both have the same basic structure and are made up of six components or "domains," A to F. Estradiol binds to the ligand-binding site in the E domain. This mediates ER dimerization, which is required for DNA binding. Domain D contains a nuclear localization signal. Both isoforms bind estrogens with a similar affinity and activate the expression of genes containing estrogen response elements in an estrogen-dependent manner. They differ in the N terminal A/B (transactivation) domain. These are the regions that promote transcription activation functions, and thus the transcriptional properties of ERα and ERβ are dissimilar. In addition, their distribution is different. ERα is expressed in breast, ovary, uterus, vagina, bone, and hypothalamus. ERβ is found primarily on the ovaries, hypothalamus, cerebral cortex, and in male organs such as the testis and prostate (Box 17–1).

Expression of the ER, and to a lesser degree the progesterone receptor (PR), on breast cancer is crucial for predicting a response to adjuvant hormonal therapy. Estrogen and progesterone receptors can be measured by means of a ligand-binding assay (LBA), which involves the competitive binding of radiolabeled steroid ligand, or by the use of antibodies specific for the receptors through either immunohistochemical staining (IHC) or enzyme immunoassay (EIA).

Estrogen Receptor-Alpha versus Estrogen Receptor-Beta Expression

Although ERα expression is a moderate prognostic sign (meaning that patients who are ER positive will do better than patients who are ER negative in the absence of any treatment; estimated to be about 5% to 10% lower chance of recurrence), it is an extremely strong predictive tool (meaning that patients who are ER positive will respond significantly better to endocrine therapy than those who are ER negative). Whereas 5 years of tamoxifen is associated with a 50% to 60% reduction in the relative risk of relapse and a 25% reduction in the relative risk of death for women with ER-positive breast cancer, there is no significant benefit for women with ER-negative breast cancer. Part of this depends on how one defines ER-negative. The response rates are also related to the quantitative analysis of the receptor. Response rates to endocrine therapy increase with the amount of ER present in the tumors rather than simply the absence or presence of the receptor.

What of ERβ? Although ERβ is present in human breast cancer, its role in the development of breast cancer remains unknown. Some groups have reported that there is a beneficial effect of ERβ, suggesting it may protect against the mitogenic action of estrogen, and may be associated with node-negative and low-grade breast cancers. ERβ-positive tumors may be more likely to respond to hormonal therapy. Other groups have suggested a poor prognostic value of ERβ, and think it may be associated with endocrine resistance. Further research is ongoing, and studies of both ER subtypes may further select subgroups that may benefit from variations in endocrine therapy. Today, however, the routine measurement of ERβ has yet to been shown to be of benefit in the management of breast cancer.

Progesterone Receptor Expression

Although progesterone is necessary for the development of the breast, most research has focused on estrogen and the ER. It is unclear whether the PR has prognostic significance. However, we routinely measure both the ER and PR. How does the PR help with clinical decision making? The presence of PR suggests that the ER is not only present but also functioning, which is crucial for response to hormonal therapy. Therefore the expression of both receptors suggests a better response to endocrine therapy than in ER-positive and PR-negative tumors. Absence or loss of PR over time may be associated with a more aggressive tumor type and decreased responsiveness to hormonal therapy. Although this has been demonstrated for advanced breast cancer, it has not been shown to be true for predicting response to tamoxifen in the adjuvant setting. However, there is that small subset of patients (5%) who will be ER negative but PR positive. These patients will frequently respond to hormonal therapy (possibly because low but critical levels of ER are present, or the ERβreceptor is present and not being measured). So although it may not help predict benefit from adjuvant hormonal therapy in patients who are ER positive, measuring PR is clinically useful for women with both early-stage breast cancer and metastatic disease.

Estrogen and Breast Cancer

Since Beaston's original observation, there has been a preponderance of evidence that indicates exposure to estrogen is an important determinant of the risk of breast cancer. Several studies have shown that women with persistently elevated serum levels of estrogen have an increased risk of breast cancer. Several factors related to estrogen are associated with an increased risk of breast cancer, including an early age of menarche, a late onset of menopause, and obesity (likely related to an increased production of estrogen by aromatase activity in adipose tissue). This evidence suggests that cumulative exposure to estrogen across a woman's life span contributes to the development of breast cancer.

Another piece of evidence comes from the use of hormone replacement therapy. In the United States, hormone replacement therapy typically consists of estrogen alone (conjugated estrone plus various conjugated equine estrogens) or estrogen plus progesterone (medroxyprogesterone acetate). A meta-analysis of data involving more than 160,000 women found that users of hormone replacement therapy for 5 years or longer had a relative risk of 1.35 for the development of breast cancer. An observational study from France showed a similar risk (1.4), although this was limited to women receiving estrogen and progesterone. Another observational study from the United Kingdom showed an even higher risk associated with hormone replacement. The results from these studies suggest that ongoing or recent hormonal replacement therapy is associated with an increased risk of breast cancer. Fortunately, in both the meta-analysis and the United Kingdom study, women who stopped using hormone replacement therapy reduced their risk of cancer, suggesting that this effect may be reversible.

These observational studies prompted a prospective trial—the Women's Health Initiative. Postmenopausal women were randomly assigned to receive placebo or hormone replacement therapy. Women with a uterus received estrogen and progesterone, whereas women who had undergone a hysterectomy received estrogen only. After 5 years, the study was terminated because of the increased incidence of cardiopulmonary events (for which hormone replacement was thought to be protective). Women who received estrogen and progesterone had an increased risk of stroke, coronary heart disease, and pulmonary embolism (PE). These women also had an increased risk of breast cancer. Women receiving estrogen alone had an increased incidence of stroke and PE, but not breast cancer. Why there is a difference between estrogen versus estrogen plus progesterone is unclear, and the contribution to breast cancer of progestin requires additional investigation.

How does estrogen contribute to breast cancer? There are two mechanisms by which this may occur. Metabolism of estrogen involves several cytochrome P-450 enzymes that catalyze the conversion of estrone and estradiol to hydroxycatechols. Several in vitro and animal studies support the hypothesis that oxidative metabolites of estrogen have genotoxic, mutagenic, transforming, and carcinogenic potential (Box 17–2). This has yet to be demonstrated in human breast cancer, however. Another mechanism by which estrogen can contribute to breast cancer is the increased proliferation and inhibition of apoptosis associated with the estrogen receptor signal-transduction pathways (Fig. 17–2).

BOX 17–2 EFFECTS OF ESTROGEN METABOLITES SEEN IN IN VITRO AND ANIMAL STUDIES

- Estrogen 3,4-quinone DNA adducts and depurination
- Oxidative DNA damage
- Gene mutation
- Neoplastic transformation
- Tumor development

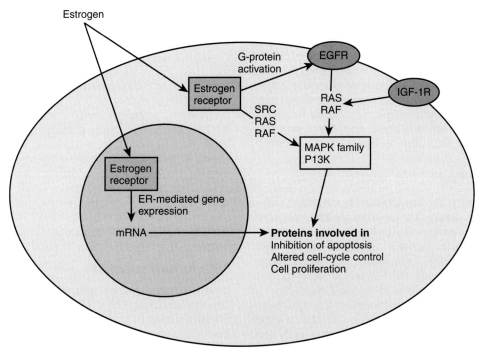

Figure 17–2. Upon binding estrogen, the estrogen receptor interacts with transcription factors to modulate gene transcription for proteins involved in both proliferation and inhibition of apoptosis.

Selective Estrogen Receptor Modulators

Selective estrogen receptor modulators (SERMs) are competitive inhibitors of estrogen binding to estrogen receptors. SERMs include tamoxifen, raloxifene, and related drugs. In the past, these were referred to as "antiestrogens" however this label is misleading because this class of compounds can act as an antagonist in one tissue and an agonist in another. It is this combination of antagonistic and agonistic properties that are responsible for both the effects and the side effects of these drugs. The antagonistic activity can be both beneficial (inhibition of breast cancer cell growth) and detrimental (menopausal symptoms). Likewise, the agonistic effects can be both beneficial (preventing bone demineralization) and detrimental (risk of uterine cancer and thromboembolism).

The process behind how a drug can act positively on one tissue type and negatively on another is just beginning to be understood (Box 17–3). One possibility is that the change in the receptor conformation that follows binding of the ER by a SERM results in variable interactions with cofactors that determine their gene regulation. These nuclear coactivators and corepressors are sensitive to differences between binding of ER to estrogen or a SERM. When estrogen is bound to ER, coactivators promote an interaction between the receptor and the transcriptional apparatus that provides the machinery for gene activation. Corepressors restrain this activity. When ER is bound to a SERM, the ligand-binding domain is distorted, which may result in corepressor binding rather than coactivator binding.

Another variable in the tissue-specific agonist or antagonist activity of SERMs is the relative concentration of ERβ. Tamoxifen, which

BOX 17–3 FACTORS DETERMINING WHETHER A SELECTIVE ESTROGEN RECEPTOR MODULATOR DISPLAYS AGONIST OR ANTAGONIST EFFECTS

Structure of the selective estrogen receptor modulator

Tissue factors

Relative levels of ERα and ERβ
Levels of other growth factors (epidermal growth factor receptor [EGRF]; HER-2, IGFR)
Presence of coactivators or corepressors

Target genes

Promoter site activated by estrogen response element or AP-1

shows agonist activity in some tissues on binding to ERα, has no agonistic activity when it interacts with ERβ. In addition, the partial agonist activity of tamoxifen that is manifest through ERα can be completely abolished on coexpression of ERβ. When coexpressed in tumor cells, ERβ functions as a transdominant inhibitor of ERα transcriptional activity at subsaturating hormone levels and decreases overall cellular sensitivity to estradiol.

Tamoxifen

Tamoxifen is the most studied hormonal therapy for breast cancer and the most widely prescribed anticancer drug in the world (Box 17–4). Tamoxifen is given at a dose of 20 mg/day for 5 years. Trials of higher doses (30 or 40 mg/day) have not demonstrated any increased benefit. Several trials have looked at varying durations. At least four trials have demonstrated a significant improvement in outcome with 5 years as compared to 2 years of tamoxifen therapy. However, taking tamoxifen for longer than 5 years is controversial. Two of three trials, a National Surgical and Adjuvant Breast Project (NSABP) trial and

a Scottish trial, suggest that taking tamoxifen for longer than 5 years may be associated with a worse outcome. The incidence of endometrial cancer appeared to double in women who took tamoxifen for longer than 5 years (2.1% versus 1.1%). One of the three trials, an Eastern Cooperative Oncology Group (ECOG) trial, suggests that prolonged treatment with tamoxifen may improve relapse-free survival and possibly overall survival (OS). Longer-term follow-up is pending; however, recent studies have suggested that the sequential administration of aromatase inhibitors after 5 years of tamoxifen may be optimal therapy.

Benefits of Tamoxifen in the Adjuvant Setting

Relapse and Mortality

As with chemotherapy, it is worth bypassing a lengthy discussion of the individual trials and moving straight to the data from the EBCTCG. The 1998 overview demonstrated a 47% proportional reduction in recurrence and a 27% improvement in mortality rates over a 10-year period (Table 17–1). The 2000 update of the

BOX 17–4 ANTIHORMONAL THERAPIES IN BREAST CANCER

Drug	Mechanism	Setting	Side Effects	Risks
Tamoxifen (Nolvadex)	Selective estrogen receptor modulator	Adjuvant or metastatic	Fatigue, hot flashes, vaginal discharge, mood swings, headache, skin rash, nausea, and fluid retention/weight gain	Thromboembolic events, uterine cancer, and cataracts
Toremifene (Fareston)	Selective estrogen receptor modulator	Metastatic		
Fulvestrant (Faslodex)	Eliminates estrogen receptor	Metastatic	Hot flashes, nausea, or fatigue	
Letrozole (Femara) Anastrozole	Inhibit aromatase and block nonovarian production of estrogen (Arimidex)	Adjuvant or metastatic	Joint stiffness, bone, and joint pain, nausea, headache, and fluid retention/weight gain	Osteoporosis
Exemestane (Aromasin)	Aromatase inactivator			
Goserelin (Zoladex) Leuprolide (Lupron)	Blocks ovarian production of estrogen.	Adjuvant or metastatic	Hot flashes and menopause symptoms.	Osteoporosis
Megestrol acetate (Megace)	Progesterone analog	Metastatic	Headache, nausea, dizziness, SOB, hot flashes, insomnia, and weight gain	Thromboembolic events and allergic reactions

TABLE 17–1 • *Annual Percentage Risk Reduction with 5 Years of Tamoxifen from the Early Breast Cancer Trialists Collaborative Group Overview*		Relapse	Death
Overall		42 ± 3	22 ± 4
Hormonal status	ER positive	50 ± 4	28 ± 5
	ER unknown	37 ± 8	21 ± 9
	ER negative	6 ± 11	−3 ± 11
Lymph nodes	Positive	43 ± 4	28 ± 6
	Negative	49 ± 4	25 ± 5
Chemotherapy		52 ± 8	47 ± 9
Age	<50	45 ± 8	32 ± 10
	50 to 59	37 ± 6	11 ± 8
	60 to 69	54 ± 5	33 ± 6
	>70	54 ± 13	34 ± 13

EBCTCG database now shows that these benefits extend to 15 years.

The studies included trials of 1, 2, and 5 years of tamoxifen and showed a highly significant trend toward greater effect with longer duration of therapy. The EBCTCG was not able to examine duration longer than 5 years, but the data from the aforementioned studies address this issue. The data also included about 8000 patients who were included in these studies but were ER negative or low risk. These patients clearly derive no benefit from adjuvant tamoxifen.

Is there one group that benefits from tamoxifen more than others? No. The relative benefit of tamoxifen was similar for patients who were both node positive and node negative (although the absolute benefit is obviously greater for patients who are node positive) and is irrespective of age, menopausal status, and whether or not tamoxifen is used alone or in conjunction with chemotherapy. The data is clear that hormonal therapy is not indicated in patients who are ER and PR negative; however, one less clear population are those patients who are ER negative but PR positive. The overview suggests a benefit of tamoxifen in these patients, but the numbers are too small to be conclusive.

Beyond the reduction in relapse and death, there are other benefits to adjuvant tamoxifen. Tamoxifen is associated with an increase in bone mineral density in postmenopausal women and may reduce fractures. It is also associated with a reduction in low-density lipoprotein cholesterol. Although it was hypothesized that tamoxifen may reduce the risk for coronary heart disease, and this was suggested by some individual studies, this has not been validated. However, one of the strongest side benefits of tamoxifen is the prevention of new breast cancers. In the 1995 EBCTCG review, tamoxifen reduced the incidence of new contralateral breast cancer by 46%. This is similar to what was seen in the NSABP P-01 prevention trial (see Chapter 8).

Risks of Tamoxifen

Although the risk-to-benefit ratio for tamoxifen is greatly in its favor, the drug is not without risks and side effects. Tamoxifen is associated with an increased incidence of hot flashes, vaginal discharge, and night sweats. Sexual dysfunction is not a common complaint, although it may correlate with vaginal dryness. In addition to menopause symptoms, there is an increased risk of tamoxifen inducing menopause in premenopausal women, although this is restricted to women 45 years or older and is in part related to the normal aging process. Several studies have shown that despite these symptoms, quality of life in women undergoing therapy with tamoxifen is not significantly worse than women receiving placebo. Tamoxifen has also been associated with ocular toxicities, specifically corneal changes and retinopathy. For this reason, it has been recommended that women consider a baseline ophthalmic evaluation during the first year of initiating tamoxifen and have appropriate follow-up.

Thromboembolic disease is a worrisome risk of tamoxifen because these can lead to fatal consequences. This appears to affect less than 1% of patients and is more common in women over the age of 50.

The most significant risk of tamoxifen appears to be that of uterine cancer. Most of these cases consist of adenocarcinoma of the endometrium, although a small percentage of reported cases of uterine cancers consist of uterine sarcoma, a rare and aggressive form of uterine cancer. Half of these cases are mixed mullerian tumors, which have been linked to estrogen use and carry a worse prognosis. In the prevention trial of tamoxifen, the incidence of endometrial adenocarcinoma was 2.2 per 1000 woman-years for women on tamoxifen (and with an intact uterus) compared with 0.71 per 100 woman-years for placebo. For sarcomas, the incidence was 0.17 compared with 0. Routine screening with transvaginal ultrasound or endometrial biopsy is not useful and thus not recommended. Instead, women should be counseled about the need to alert their physician for abnormal vaginal bleeding and undergo regular gynecologic evaluations.

Raloxifene

Raloxifene (Evista) resulted from efforts to design SERMs that have estrogen activity in bone and cardiovascular tissue but not in the reproductive tissues, for the purpose of lowering the risk of osteoporotic fractures. They have been found to have similar effect to tamoxifen on the chemoprevention of breast cancer. This was incidentally discovered in a trial of raloxifene or placebo in over 7700 postmenopausal women with osteoporosis. With 4 years of follow-up, there was an 84% relative reduction in the incidence of ER-positive breast cancer. This data prompted the Study of Tamoxifen and Raloxifene (STAR) trial, which randomized postmenopausal women who are high risk for the development of breast cancer to receive either tamoxifen or raloxifene. The initial results of STAR show that the drug raloxifene is as effective as tamoxifen in reducing the breast cancer risk of the women on the trial. In STAR, both drugs reduced the risk of developing invasive breast cancer by about 50% (see Chapter 8). However, raloxifene has never been studied in the adjuvant setting, and its effect on known breast cancer remains unknown. Thus it is not recommended for the adjuvant therapy of breast cancer in postmenopausal women.

Aromatase Inhibitors

Although tamoxifen has had tremendous success in the treatment of hormone-receptor-positive breast cancer, it is not without problems. As a partial estrogen agonist it has several potentially serious side effects and tamoxifen resistance poses a significant problem for clinicians. The introduction of aromatase inhibitors (AIs) has changed the scope of adjuvant hormonal therapy for postmenopausal women.

AIs act by inhibiting the cytochrome P450 enzyme aromatase, which is responsible for the peripheral aromatization of androgens, converting them to estrogens. In postmenopausal women, aromatase is primarily located in the skeletal muscle and fat and represents the predominant source of estrogen in the body. AIs can either be steroidal inhibitors, (formestane or exemestane) which are irreversible, or nonsteroidal inhibitors (anastrazole, letrozole), which bind to a site distant to the hormone-binding site and are reversible. AIs do not impact the ovaries, and thus they are only effective in postmenopausal women.

Several trials have examined AIs in the adjuvant setting (Table 17–2). Most of these trials compared an AI to tamoxifen or placebo. Little data has emerged comparing one AI to another. One has to be careful in interpreting data interchangeably for anastrozole, letrozole, and exemestane. Likewise, findings from AI trials in early breast cancer can only be applied to the select group of patients in which the trial was conducted. Further trials meant to better define the use of AIs in the adjuvant setting are ongoing, and the recommendations for AI use in the adjuvant setting are likely to continue to change over the next several years.

Anastrozole

The Arimidex, Tamoxifen, Alone or in Combination (ATAC) trial randomized 9366 postmenopausal women to either tamoxifen or anastrozole or the combination of the two. The goal of this study was not only to see

TABLE 17–2 • *Aromatase Inhibitors in the Adjuvant Setting*					
Trial	**Groups**	**N**	**Median Follow-Up**	**Disease-Free Survival**	**Contralateral Tumors**
Arimidex, Tamoxifen, Alone or in Combination	T versus A versus combination	9366	68	DFS: A > T	42% reduction with A
Italian	T versus A after 2–3 years of tamoxifen	426	30	DFS: A > T	Study too small
MA-17	L versus placebo after 5 years of tamoxifen	5187	29	DFS: L > placebo	46% reduction with L
Intergroup Exemestane Study	T versus E after 2–3 years of tamoxifen	4742	31	DFS: E > T	56% reduction with E

A, Arimidex; DFS, disease-free survial; E, exemestane; L, Letrozole; T, tamoxifen.

whether Arimidex was superior to tamoxifen, but also if the combination might be synergistic. In the most recently published results, after a median follow-up of 68 months, anastrazole significantly prolonged disease-free survival (DFS; hazard ratio 0.87, $p = 0.01$). Time to recurrence and number of distant metastases were also significantly improved. It will take considerably more time before any conclusions regarding OS can be made. Anastrozole was also superior to the combination of anastrazole and tamoxifen, and this approach has been abandoned.

Three trials have examined the benefits of switching to Arimidex after 2 or 3 years of tamoxifen, including the Austrian Breast and Colorectal Cancer Study Group (ABCSG) 8 trial, the Arimidex-Nolvadex (ARNO) 95 trial, and the Italian Tamoxifen Anastrazole (ITA) trial. All three showed a benefit to switching to anastrazole.

Finally, the PreOperative Arimidex Compared with Tamoxifen (PROACT) and Immediate Preoperative Arimidex, Tamoxifen or Combined with Tamoxifen (IMPACT) trials compared preoperative treatment with anastrazole with the preoperative treatment of tamoxifen in postmenopausal women with large hormone-receptor-positive breast cancer. In both studies, 3 months of anastrazole appears to increase the likelihood of breast-conserving surgery compared with tamoxifen (43% versus 31%, combined data, $p = 0.019$).

Exemestane

The Intergroup Exemestane Study (IES) randomized 4742 postmenopausal women who had completed 2 or 3 years of tamoxifen to either continue with tamoxifen to a total of 5 years or to switch to exemestane. At 3 years follow-up, switching to exemestane was associated with a significantly improved DFS but no difference in OS. Fewer toxic effects were seen with exemestane.

Letrozole

The MA.17 study performed by the National Cancer Institute of Canada looked at the role of letrozole in women who have completed 5 years of tamoxifen. Over 5000 women were randomized to placebo or letrozole after 5 years of tamoxifen. The 4-year DFS was 93% for patients receiving letrozole and 87% for patients receiving placebo ($p < 0.001$). Unfortunately, without

longer follow-up, it is unclear whether OS or distant DFS is improved or if long-term adverse effects may preclude the benefit.

The BIG 1-98 trial is a four-arm trial comparing 5 years of letrozole, 5 years of tamoxifen, 2 years of letrozole followed by 3 years of tamoxifen, and 2 years of tamoxifen followed by 3 years of letrozole. Mature data are not yet available, although preliminary data suggest that 5 years of letrozole may be better than 5 years of tamoxifen, with an improvement in DFS (0.81, p < 0.001). As with the ATAC trial, an improvement in OS has not yet been seen and will require much longer follow-up.

Toxicity of Aromatase Inhibitors

The AIs have a considerably different side effect profile than SERMs. Because anastrazole, letrozole, and exemestane have different structures and pharmacokinetic profiles, it cannot be assumed they will all have the same safety profiles. However, long-term data (beyond 5 years) is available only for anastrazole and head-to-head comparisons have not been performed.

Gynecological events, a problem for tamoxifen, do not appear to be as much of a problem for AIs. In the ATAC trial, anastrazole was associated with significantly fewer effects on the endometrium, less endometrial cancer, and reductions in hot flashes, vaginal bleeding, and discharge compared with tamoxifen. Similar findings were reported with exemestane and letrozole from those studies, although not all were significant.

Another major concern of tamoxifen is the risk of thromboembolic disease. Again, AIs seem to have a lower risk compared to tamoxifen, as evidenced from both the ATAC trial and BIG 1-98 trial. In the ATAC trial, there was a significant reduction of ischemic cerebrovascular and thromboembolic events with anastrazole.

In contrast, patients on AIs will not receive the estrogen agonist benefits of tamoxifen. This is particularly true for the tamoxifen-induced promotion of bone mass and protective effects on bone. Thus AIs have a higher rate of fracture and joint disorders. These may be minimized by monitoring bone densities and the use of bisphosphonates, where appropriate. Another presumed advantage to tamoxifen is the protection against heart disease by estrogen-induced changes in plasma lipids. However, the data is mixed, and in some cases contradictory, as to whether AIs confer a higher cardiac risk than tamoxifen.

Adjuvant Therapy with Aromatase Inhibitors

With all this recent data about the potential of AIs, how does one incorporate this into clinical practice when treating postmenopausal women? Should postmenopausal women go directly to an AI or should they start with tamoxifen and then switch after 2 or 3 years? Should women already on tamoxifen switch now or finish 5 years and then continue therapy with an AI? Should AIs even be considered in the absence of OS data and long-term safety studies? Several groups, including ASCO, the National Comprehensive Cancer Network (NCCN), and the St. Gallen Expert Consensus Group have concluded that an AI should be included in the adjuvant treatment of postmenopausal women with hormone-receptor-positive breast cancer. The decision should obviously be based partly on the patient's history, including thromboembolic risk, prior hysterectomy, cardiovascular risk factors, osteopenia, and osteoporosis. In the absence of these factors leading one way or the other, only the NCCN has made specific recommendations. They have recommended that anastrazole should be used as initial therapy for women newly diagnosed with breast cancer and beginning adjuvant hormonal therapy; switching treatment from tamoxifen to either anastrazole or exemestane in postmenopausal women 2 to 3 years into tamoxifen therapy, and extending hormonal therapy for an additional 5 years with letrozole in women who have completed 5 years of tamoxifen.

Ovarian Suppression/Ablation

The original hormonal therapy consisted of ovarian ablation, either by surgery, irradiation, or pharmacologic methods. This still remains an option for premenopausal women with hormone-receptor-positive breast cancer (Table 17–3). Ovarian ablation can be achieved through several mechanisms. The first is surgical oophorectomy. The safety of this approach has increased with the introduction of laparoscopic surgery, and there may be additional benefits in regard to prophylaxis against ovarian cancer in high-risk patients, such as those with breast cancer gene 1 and 2 (BRCA 1 and 2) mutations or those with a family history of ovarian cancer. Ovarian irradiation can also be effective at ablating ovarian function. However, there are morbidities associated with both of

these approaches, and they are irreversible, which may be a problem for young patients with breast cancer. An alternative approach is the use of LHRH agonists, a medical form of ovarian ablation. Goserelin acetate is an analogue of LHRH, which suppresses ovarian function, allowing patients to maintain their function after completion of therapy.

The benefits of ovarian ablation/suppression are seen in the meta-analysis conducted by the EBCTCG. A 2000 EBCTCG overview analyzed 4900 women who underwent ovarian suppression with or without chemotherapy. Ovarian suppression was associated with an improvement in OS in women who did not receive chemotherapy, but there was no impact on survival in patients who did receive chemotherapy. The survival benefit of ovarian ablation alone was similar to the survival benefit of chemotherapy alone.

Several individual trials highlight the potential of goserelin as an alternative to chemotherapy in premenopausal women with ER-positive tumors. The Zoladex Early Breast Cancer Research Association (ZEBRA) trial randomized women to either 2 years of goserelin or cyclophosphamide, methotrexate, and fluorouracil (CMF) chemotherapy. Among patients who were ER positive, survival was equal, whereas CMF was significantly better among patients who were ER negative. Importantly, menses returned in the majority of women randomized to goserelin, whereas 77% of women on CMF had ovarian ablation with permanent amenorrhea. Another trial, the ABCSG 05 trial, compared CMF to goserelin plus tamoxifen. Again, no difference in survival was seen, and the authors concluded that goserelin plus tamoxifen is more effective and better tolerated.

The EBCTCG overview found no benefit to ovarian suppression in women receiving adjuvant chemotherapy; however, many women receiving adjuvant chemotherapy will have chemotherapy-induced ovarian ablation. So is there a benefit to ovarian ablation/suppression among women receiving chemotherapy who maintain ovarian function? This has been addressed in several trials without definitive results. The Zoladex in Premenopausal Patients (ZIPP) analysis combined data from four randomized trials initiated by international collaborative groups. Initial results (median follow-up of 4.3 years) suggest that the addition of goserelin to standard chemotherapy will decrease the risk of recurrence, although OS was not improved. Intergroup trial INT-0101 randomized patients

TABLE 17–3 • *Adjuvant Therapy with Ovarian Ablation/Suppression*

Trial	N	Patients	Arms	Results
ZEBRA	1640	Node positive	G × 2 years CMF	No difference in DFS
IBCSG	1063	Node negative	Chemo G × 2 years Chemo + G	No difference in DFS
Scottish Trial	332	Node positive	CMF OA	OS better for OA for ER ≥ 20 but worse for ER < 20
Scandinavian Trial	732	Node positive ER positive	CMF OA	No difference in DFS or OS
TABLE	600	Node positive ER positive	CMF Leuprorelin × 2 years	No difference in DFS or OS
ABCSG	1034	ER positive	CMF G + T	G + T improved DFS
GROCTA	244	ER positive	OA + T CMF	No difference in DFS or OS
France	162	Node positive ER positive	FAC OA + T	No difference in DFS or OS
FACS 06	333	Node positive ER positive	Triptorelin + T FEC	No difference in DFS or OS
ZIPP	2631		G T G + T No further treatment	G improved DFS
INT-0101	1504	Node positive ER positive	CAF CAF + G CAF + G + T	T improved DFS
Vietnam	709		OA + T No further treatment	↑ DFS and OS with OA + T
France	926		Chemo Chemo + OA	No difference in DFS or OS
Mam-1 GOSCI	466	Node positive	Chemo Chemo + G + T	DFS ↑ with G + T
IBCSG	174	Node positive ER positive	Chemo + OA + T OA + T	No difference in DFS or OS

CAF, cyclophosphamide, doxorubicin, fluorouracil; CMF, cyclophosphamide, methotrexate, and fluorouracil; DFS, disease-free survival; ER, estrogen receptor; FAC, fluorouracil, doxorubicin, cyclophosphamide; FEC, fluorouracil, epirubicin, cyclophosphamide; G, Goserelin; Mam-1 OA, ovarian ablation; OS, overall survival; T, tamoxifen; ZEBRA, Zoladex Early Breast Cancer Research Association; ZIPP, Zoladex in Premenopausal Patients.

to chemotherapy, chemotherapy plus goserelin, or chemotherapy plus goserelin plus tamoxifen. The triple therapy arm had an improvement in 5-year DFS, with no improvement in OS. The effect was greatest in women less than 40, which may be as a result of the higher fraction of women who maintained ovarian function. However, there was no chemotherapy plus tamoxifen arm, which is the standard of care, so it is difficult to know how to use this data clinically. Finally, the International Breast Cancer Study Group (IBCSG) trial randomized women to chemotherapy, goserelin, or both (a no adjuvant treatment group was dropped during the course of the trial). No difference in DFS or OS was seen between the three groups.

Further data is necessary to answer whether ovarian suppression added to chemotherapy and tamoxifen is beneficial in patients who are premenopausal and ER positive, particularly if ovarian function is maintained after chemotherapy. An ongoing study of ovarian ablation/suppression will hopefully answer this question. For now, the only conclusion one can make is that ovarian ablation/suppression is a potential alternative to chemotherapy in this subset of patients.

Suggested Readings

1. Arimidex, Tamoxifen, Alone or in Combination (ATAC) Trialists' Group, Forbes JF, Cuzick J, et al. Effect of anastrozole and tamoxifen as adjuvant treatment for early-stage breast cancer: 100-month analysis of the ATAC trial. Lancet Oncology 2008;9(1):45–53.

2. Baum M, Budzar AU, Cuzik J, et al. Anastrozole alone or in combination with tamoxifen versus tamoxifen alone for adjuvant treatment of postmenopausal women with early breast cancer: first results of the ATAC randomized trial. Lancet 2002;359(9324):2131–2139.

3. Buzdar AU. Aromatase inhibitors: Changing the face of endocrine therapy for breast cancer. Breast Disease 2006;24:107–117.

4. Coombes RC, Hall E, Gibson LJ, et al. A randomized trial of exemestane after two to three years of tamoxifen therapy in postmenopausal women with primary breast cancer. N Engl J Med 2004;350(11):1081–1092.

5. Fisher B, Costantino J, Redmond C, et al. A randomized clinical trial evaluating tamoxifen in the treatment of patients with node-negative breast cancer who have estrogen-receptor positive tumors. N Engl J Med 1989;320(8):479–484.

6. Fisher B, Dignam J, Bryant J, , et al. Five versus more than five years of tamoxifen therapy for breast cancer patients with negative lymph nodes and estrogen receptor positive tumors. J Natl Cancer Inst 1996;88(21):1529–1542.

7. Goss PE, Ingle JN, Martino S, et al. A randomized trial of letrozole in postmenopausal women after five years of tamoxifen therapy for early stage breast cancer. N Engl J Med 2003;349(19):1793–1802.

8. Ovarian ablation for early breast cancer. Cochrane Database Syst Rev 2000;3:CD000485.

9. Ovarian ablation for early breast cancer: overview of the randomized trials. Early Breast Cancer Trialists' Collaborative Group. Lancet 1996;348(9036):1189–1196.

10. Tamoxifen for early breast cancer. Cochrane Database Syst Rev 2001;(1):CD000486.

11. Tamoxifen for early breast cancer: an overview of the randomised trials. Early Breast Cancer Trialists' Collaborative Group. Lancet 1998;351:1451.

12. Winer EP, Hudis C, Burstein HJ, et al. American Society of Clinical Oncology technology assessment working group update: use of aromatase inhibitors in the adjuvant setting. J Clin Oncol 2003;21(13):2597–2599.

13. Yager JD, Davidson NE. Estrogen carcinogenesis in breast cancer. N Engl J Med 2006;354:270–282.

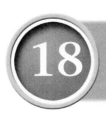

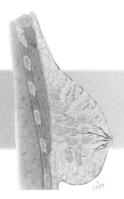

Neoadjuvant Therapy

Neoadjuvant Therapy: Key Points

- Describe the potential benefits of delivering chemotherapy before surgery.
- Know the indications and contraindications to neoadjuvant chemotherapy.
- Be familiar with the implications of neoadjuvant chemotherapy on breast surgery.
- Develop an algorithm for interrogating the sentinel lymph node in patients undergoing neoadjuvant chemotherapy.
- Understand the potential of neoadjuvant hormonal therapy.

Neoadjuvant therapy refers to the delivery of systemic therapy before surgical intervention in an attempt to not only control distant disease, but also to decrease the size of the primary tumor. This allows for the potential resection of an inoperable cancer or the use of breast-conservation therapy (BCT) in a case in which a mastectomy would have been indicated. Neoadjuvant therapy can include preoperative chemotherapy or preoperative hormonal therapy.

Using systemic therapy upfront is considered the standard treatment for patients who present with inoperable breast cancer. This includes patients with locally advanced tumors

(T4 tumors), inflammatory breast cancer, and patients with involvement of the supra or infra-clavicular lymph nodes (N3). This was not always the case because there was concern that the effect of chemotherapy would increase the surgical complication rate or negatively affect overall survival (OS) by delaying the surgery. However, surgery first was associated with dismal results in treating locally advanced breast cancer (LABC), and trials of primary chemotherapy quickly demonstrated the benefits of preoperative downstaging of disease to improve respectability. This will be discussed in more detail in Chapter 19.

The success of primary systemic therapy in inoperable breast cancer led to the suspicion that it may be preferable in operable breast cancer. Today, the phrase *neoadjuvant therapy* typically refers to the use of preoperative chemotherapy as an alternative to postoperative chemotherapy. Based on the experience with LABC, it was thought that giving the chemotherapy before surgery to treat the occult micrometastases at an earlier time may increase survival. However, all the large randomized trials of preoperative chemotherapy demonstrated equivalent disease-free survival (DFS) and OS. What did become apparent was that the rate of breast conservation was significantly increased after neoadjuvant therapy (Table 18–1). The primary indication today for neoadjuvant chemotherapy is the patient with operable breast cancer (good candidates for mastectomy) who desires breast conservation. It may

BOX 18–1 POTENTIAL ADVANTAGES TO NEOADJUVANT CHEMOTHERAPY

- May allow for breast-conservation therapy in a woman who would otherwise require a mastectomy.
- May improve the aesthetic outcome of a lumpectomy by decreasing the volume of tissue needing to be resected.
- Allows for an assessment of the response of the tumor to chemotherapy. This may allow for modifications of therapy based on response. In addition, a demonstrable response may also have a positive effect on the patient's compliance with further treatment and on the patient's willingness to accept some adverse events.
- Allows patients to delay surgery so they have more time to accept the need for mastectomy, consider reconstructive options, or undergo genetic counseling and testing if prophylactic mastectomies are considered.
- Allows women in their second or third trimester of pregnancy to delay the surgery and radiotherapy until after delivery.
- May reduce distant metastases compared with classic adjuvant systemic therapy.

also be considered for patients who could technically undergo a lumpectomy but will receive a better cosmetic outcome if the tumor decreases in size (Box 18–1).

It must be remembered that delivering the chemotherapy preoperatively is an *alternative* to adjuvant chemotherapy. The determinant for the use of chemotherapy is the risk of distant recurrence. Therefore, neoadjuvant chemotherapy should only be offered to patients who, based on clinical staging (tumor size, grade, estrogen receptor/progesterone receptor [ER/PR] status, clinically involved lymph nodes, and possibly genetic profiling), would be candidates for chemotherapy. It should not be used to shrink a primary tumor in a patient who would not otherwise require systemic therapy. For example, a small-breasted woman with a 1.5-cm, intermediate-grade, ER/PR-positive primary tumor, clinically node negative, may benefit from shrinking the tumor, but she might not require adjuvant chemotherapy based on her low risk of distant recurrence. This would be particularly true if her genomic profiling suggested a low risk of recurrence (see Chapter 16). An improved

TABLE 18–1 • Breast Conservation Rates After Neoadjuvant Chemotherapy

Study	Patients	Breast-Conservation Therapy Rate	
		Preoperatively (%)	Postoperatively (%)
Institut Bergonie	272	63.1	0
Institut Curie	414	82	77
Royal Mardson	309	89	78
NSAPB B18	1523	68	60
EORTC	698	37	21
ECTO	892	71	35
ABCSG	423	67	60

ABCSG, Austrian Breast and Colorectal Cancer Study Group; ECTO, European Cooperative Trial; EORTC, European Organization for Research and Treatment of Cancer; NSAPB, National Surgical and Adjuvant Breast Project.

TABLE 18–2 • *Hormonal Therapy in the Neoadjuvant Setting*

Study	Therapy	Breast-Conservation Therapy Rate (%)
IMPACT	anastrazole	46
	tamoxifen	22
	anastrazole + tamoxifen	26
Letrozole 024 Trial	letrozole	45
	tamoxifen	35
St. Petersburg	anastrazole	21
	doxorubicin and paclitaxel X4	37

IMPACT, Immediate Preoperative Arimidex, Tamoxifen or Combined with Tamoxifen.

cosmetic result does not justify the toxicity and sequelae of chemotherapy. In addition, as the primary goal of neoadjuvant chemotherapy is to allow BCT, patients who will still require mastectomy after chemotherapy (Box 18–2), are not ideal candidates, although there are other reasons why neoadjuvant chemotherapy might be considered.

There are other potential and real advantages to neoadjuvant therapy. In addition to allowing more women to proceed with breast conservation, it also allows women who will require mastectomy to come to terms with their diagnosis, think about whether to have reconstruction and what type of reconstruction to have, and possibly undergo genetic counseling and testing and decide whether to undergo bilateral mastectomies. In addition, the patient's response to the chemotherapy provides prognostic information. Patients who have a complete pathological response (pCR) have a better long-term outcome than those who do not. Whether this information can be used to adjust pre- or postsurgical chemotherapy is still an area of investigation. However, clinical trials using neoadjuvant chemotherapy do allow for a more rapid and less expensive means for evaluating the efficacy of new agents and regimens. Adjuvant therapy trials require many patients over many years, whereas neoadjuvant therapy trials can be completed over the course of just a few years. This chapter will address several of these issues.

Neoadjuvant Therapy Regimens

Most of the attention in neoadjuvant therapy has been focused on chemotherapy. However, hormonal therapy plays a crucial role in the management of breast cancer, particularly among women who are post-menopausal and hormone-receptor positive. This patient population often does not require systemic chemotherapy. It should then seem reasonable to believe that these patients could receive the benefits of preoperative therapy without the need for chemotherapy. Neoadjuvant hormonal therapy has been less extensively studied than chemotherapy protocols, but it is a viable option for postmenopausal women who have hormone-receptor-positive disease. Several trials examined the effect of preoperative hormonal therapy. In a direct comparison of hormonal therapy to chemotherapy, the St. Petersburg trial showed that comparable, though not equivalent, rates of both response (75.8% versus 89.8%) and breast conservation (21% versus 37.2%). Other studies demonstrated that neoadjuvant aromatase inhibitors were superior to tamoxifen in the neoadjuvant setting (Table 18–2). The data suggest that primary endocrine therapy is a valid option for postmenopausal patients with hormone-receptor-positive breast cancer who desire breast conservation but for whom cytotoxic chemotherapy is not indicated.

At least 3 to 4 months of neoadjuvant endocrine therapy is generally needed to achieve a significant clinical response, and this may need to be continued for 6 months to see a benefit. As opposed to chemotherapy, the response takes a longer time to become clinically apparent. Often a response is not visible until 2 months into therapy, a point important for surgeons and patients alike, so they do not discontinue therapy and proceed with surgery too quickly. Current data suggests that aromatase inhibitors may offer better clinical responses than tamoxifen and increased rates of breast-conserving

TABLE 18–3 • *Taxanes in the Neoadjuvant Setting*		
Study	**Regimen**	**Breast-Conservation Therapy rate (%)**
Geparduo	APx4 q2W	66
	ACx4 → Tx4	75
Geparduo	TACx6	81
AGO	ETx4	55
	Ex3 → Tx3, q2W	66
NSABP B-27	ACx4	62
	ACx4 → Tx4	64

A, doxorubicin; C, cyclophosphamide; E, epirubicin; P, paclitaxel; T, docetaxel.

surgery. Ongoing prospective clinical trials will better define which aromatase inhibitor (if any) might be best and provide valuable clinical information regarding the clinical use of neoadjuvant hormonal therapy on downstaging tumors. Future trials directly comparing neoadjuvant hormonal therapy to neoadjuvant chemotherapy are planned.

Most neoadjuvant therapy consists of cytotoxic chemotherapy. Anthracycline-based regimens are the most extensively studied, and the typical neoadjuvant approach consists of four to six cycles of Adriamycin and cyclophosphamide. More recent data demonstrate a higher clinical and pathologic response rate with the addition of a taxane, and four cycles of Adriamycin/cyclophosphamide followed by four cycles of taxol have become a common neoadjuvant regimen (Table 18–3). For patients who are human epidermal growth factor receptor 2 (Her-2/neu) positive, even higher response rates may be achieved with the addition of Herceptin. Although a wide variety of timing schedules have been studied, there is no consensus on whether sequential, concurrent, or dose-dense approaches should be considered the standard of care.

Patient Selection for Neoadjuvant Therapy

As stated, the primary indication for delivering chemotherapy in the neoadjuvant setting is to downstage the primary tumor to increase the likelihood of successful breast conservation. Patients who will require mastectomy regardless of response, such as those with multicentric disease, widespread calcifications, or those who cannot undergo radiation therapy,

do not directly benefit from the chemotherapy being delivered before surgery as compared to after surgery, although giving neoadjuvant therapy may give the patient time to consider reconstructive options or contralateral mastectomy, and the tumor response may yield prognostic information. Likewise, patients who would not require adjuvant chemotherapy (based on their risk of distant disease) should not be given neoadjuvant chemotherapy simply to downstage their primary tumor. The indications for chemotherapy should be clear. For example, some patients with large-volume, palpable ductal carcinoma in situ (DCIS) may require a mastectomy based on the size of the tumor, but clearly do not merit chemotherapy, and thus neoadjuvant chemotherapy is contraindicated. It is important, however, to confirm that they have only DCIS or DCIS with microinvasion and not a large invasive component. If this cannot be done with multiple core-needle biopsies, an open, incisional biopsy may be necessary.

Recommendations for neoadjuvant chemotherapy may also be based on the likelihood of downstaging occurring. Hormone receptor status, Her-2/neu status, tumor grade, primary tumor histology, and patient age are factors that may influence this. ER/PR-positive, low-grade tumors are less likely to decrease in size than ER/PR-negative or high-grade tumors. Compared with ductal carcinoma, lobular carcinoma tends to present at a more advanced stage and is less likely to respond to neoadjuvant therapy. These women have lower rates of breast conservation after neoadjuvant therapy than women with ductal carcinoma, and although this should be discussed with the patient with lobular carcinoma, it is not an absolute contraindication to neoadjuvant chemotherapy.

Neoadjuvant Chemotherapy and Surgery

Breast Conservation Rates

The National Surgical Adjuvant Breast and Bowel Project (NSABP) B-18 trial was the first and largest study to compare delivery of chemotherapy before surgery, with postoperative chemotherapy. This trial found that although doxorubicin and cyclophosphamide (four cycles) given preoperatively did not improve survival, there was a 7% higher rate of breast conserving surgery ($p < 0.01$). Other trials confirmed these results, although they varied in the eligibility criteria and the regimen of chemotherapy. Using

Concentric

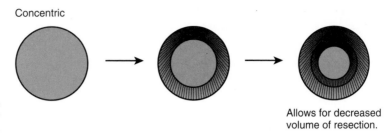

Allows for decreased
volume of resection.

Figure 18-1. As with a lollipop being licked, chemotherapy may shrink the tumor concentrically, toward a smaller central mass but leaving no disease at the periphery. A smaller area of resection is appropriate. However, if the tumor shrinks in a way that leaves microscopic satellite lesions, the same area of resection as before chemotherapy may be needed.

Honeycombed

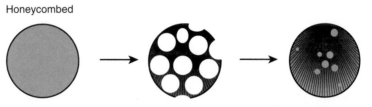

Requires the same
volume of resection as
before chemotherapy

four cycles of fluorouracil, epirubicin and cyclophosphamide (FEC), both the Institute Curie and the European Organization for Research and Treatment of Cancer (EORTC) reported increased rates of breast conservation with preoperative chemotherapy (5% and 16% increases, respectively).

Using improved combinations or sequences of drugs, the breast conservation rate can be further increased. The European Cooperative Trial (ECTO) compared preoperative or postoperative doxorubicin and paclitaxel in combination, followed by four cycles of cyclophosphamide, methotrexate, and fluorouracil (CMF). In this study, the breast-conserving surgery rate increased from 34% to 65%. Subsequent studies confirmed that the response rates and breast-conserving surgery rates could be further improved by adding taxanes to the combination. The NSABP B-18 trial had a pathologic complete response rate of 9.8%. This is substantially higher in studies using taxanes (GEPARDUO-22%; AGO-18%; NSABP B27-26%).

Local Recurrence Rates after Neoadjuvant Chemotherapy

The primary indication for neoadjuvant chemotherapy, outside of a clinical trial, is to downsize the primary breast tumor, facilitating a margin-negative lumpectomy with a smaller volume. However, there are two ways the tumor may shrink (Fig. 18–1), often compared to either a lollipop or a dandelion. As with a lollipop being licked, the tumor may shrink down concentrically, toward a smaller central mass but leaving no disease at the periphery. This would lend itself quite well to a reduced-volume lumpectomy. However, if the tumor shrinks in a way that leaves microscopic satellite lesions, then breast conservation may be compromised. This honeycombed response has been compared to blowing on a dandelion to completely rid it of its seeds. The tumor disappears in a more scattered pattern, leaving microsatellite lesions anywhere within the original tumor volume. After lumpectomy, this would result in a high rate of margin failure and local recurrence rates.

Of the major randomized studies of neoadjuvant chemotherapy, local recurrence rates have been either equivalent or higher in the preoperative chemotherapy arms, but within acceptable limits (Table 18–4). Local recurrence rates varied between 3% and 27% and depend on the duration of follow-up, the type of surgery, and the margins obtained. The largest study, NSABP B-18, randomized over 1500 women with stages I through IIIA breast cancer to preoperative or postoperative chemotherapy. There was a statistically significant increase in breast conservation (68% versus 60%), but with a median follow-up of 72 months, there was no statistically significant difference in local recurrence following BCT

TABLE 18–4 • Local Recurrence Rates After Neoadjuvant Chemotherapy

Study	Patients	Median Follow-Up (Months)	Overall Survival		Local Recurrence	
			Preoperatively (%)	Postoperatively (%)	Preoperatively (%)	Postoperatively (%)
Institut Bergonie	272	124	55	55	23	NA
Institut Curie	414	66	86	78	24	18
Royal Mardson	309	48	80	80	3	4
NSAPB B18	1523	108	69	70	10.7	7.6

NSAPB, National Surgical and Adjuvant Breast Project.

(7.9% versus 5.8%). However, this includes those patients who were candidates for lumpectomy before they received their chemotherapy. If you look at just those patients who would have required mastectomy, but were downstaged to become eligible for BCT, there was a higher local recurrence rate. The rate of local recurrence in patients who had BCT after neoadjuvant chemotherapy instead of mastectomy was 16% compared to the 10% of patients who were considered candidates for BCT before chemotherapy. It is hard to say how significant this increase in local recurrence this was, because most of these were T3 tumors and would have had an increased rate of chest wall recurrence if mastectomy would have been performed.

Primary Surgery after Neoadjuvant Chemotherapy

When neoadjuvant chemotherapy was first proposed, there was some concern that this might increase the rate of surgical complications or radiation side effects. After 30 years of experience, this has not been seen and should not be a concern. Surgery should not be performed until leukocyte counts and hemoglobin and hematocrit levels are back to normal, which typically takes 3 to 4 weeks after the last cycle of chemotherapy (although it may take up to 6 weeks in some patients).

The goal of the chemotherapy is to shrink the primary tumor to allow for breast conservation. Hopefully, the tumor will completely disappear because a complete pathologic response is associated with an improved OS. The surgeon therefore needs to plan on the possibility that at the time of surgery, there will be no way of identifying where the primary tumor was. Therefore, before the initiation of chemotherapy, the

surgeon should assure that precise localization will still be possible when the chemotherapy is completed. Several methods have been proposed for this. One option is to mark on the skin of the patient the exact location and size of the tumor and the proposed surgical skin incision and then photograph this. The boundaries of the tumor can also be marked on the skin with small tattoos, similar to the tattooing done for radiation therapy. The most common method is to place a metal clip or coil in the center of the lesion. In the patient who had a core biopsy of a palpable mass performed in the office, this may require an additional procedure. However, this will be well worth it if there is complete clinical resolution of the mass. With improving chemotherapeutic regimens, a complete clinical response is becoming more frequent.

When the decision is made to use preoperative chemotherapy, it is accepted that surgery is an obligatory part of the multidisciplinary approach to the tumor. However, after a complete clinical response, patients often question why they still need to undergo surgery. It is important to inform patients that even when there is a complete disappearance of the tumor on physical examination, mammography, or ultrasound, there remains uncertainty whether there is microscopic disease still in the region. Therefore, lumpectomy is still required to assess the pathologic response. Although some studies have suggested magnetic resonance imaging (MRI) may be more accurate for assessment of residual disease, it is still not reliable enough to avoid lumpectomy. Likewise, the presence of a residual mass does not always mean that a complete pathologic response has not been achieved because it may not be possible to differentiate chemotherapy-induced fibrosis from tumor.

A careful physical examination should be performed to document the extent of disease in both the breast and regional lymph nodes. This should be accompanied by repeat imaging studies including mammography and ultrasound. MRI should only be used if it was also used preoperatively. The surgeon must decide whether the residual mass may be excised with a satisfactory cosmetic result and negative margins. The geography of the residual mass, the shape and size of the breast, and the presence of microcalcifications will influence this decision. Malignant-appearing calcifications do not always resolve with chemotherapy, and if there remain large areas of calcifications on the postchemotherapy mammogram, these must be incorporated in the lumpectomy. Patients who began with locally advanced cancer should have regression of any skin or chest wall involvement. Patients who began with inflammatory carcinoma should undergo mastectomy regardless of their clinical response.

When the surgeon takes the patient to the operating room, they are faced with a question of how much tissue to remove. Obviously, if the tumor was large enough to warrant a mastectomy, then using the original tumor size to guide the excision would preclude breast conservation and obviate the need for having delivered the chemotherapy upfront. However, there may be no macroscopic evidence of disease to guide the surgeon in how much tissue to remove. What about the patient who was a candidate for a lumpectomy before neoadjuvant chemotherapy? Should the lumpectomy be guided by the size of the present tumor, or should the extent of excision be based on the original size of the tumor? Within the limits of aesthetics, the wider margins the better (with an optimum margin of 1 cm). Reducing the volume of tissue will increase the likelihood of reexcision; however, this can often still successfully clear the margins satisfactorily. The balance between the oncologic resection and the cosmetic outcome is a decision for the surgeon and patient, but should tilt toward the former.

Sentinel Lymph Node Biopsy after Neoadjuvant Chemotherapy

Before the introduction of sentinel lymph node (SLN) biopsy as a method of staging the axilla, there was little impact surgically on whether patients received neoadjuvant chemotherapy or not because either way they would be receiving an axillary lymph node dissection (ALND).

The most significant impact of preoperative therapy was that there were some patients who may have been node positive initially but were node negative after chemotherapy and so their true nodal status remained unknown. This did not alter their surgery, and at the time there was less impact of nodal status in guiding radiation therapy.

This changed dramatically as lymphatic mapping and SLN biopsy became standard in the surgical therapy of breast cancer. Now patients who opted for neoadjuvant chemotherapy to shrink their primary tumor were obligated to undergo ALND as part of their surgery, whereas if they had surgery first, they could opt for an SLN biopsy and avoid ALND if they were node negative. In addition, the nodal status plays a larger role in therapy decisions. Some medical oncologists would reserve the use of taxanes or dose-dense regimens for patients they know to be node positive. The use of postmastectomy radiation for patients who are node positive has become more prevalent. These practices made it more important to know whether the patient was node positive. Thus the question arose of how to best integrate SLN biopsy with neoadjuvant chemotherapy for clinically node-negative breast cancer.

SLN biopsy is only necessary in patients who are clinically node negative. Patients with palpable disease in the lymph nodes can have this confirmed by fine-needle aspiration (FNA) and proceed with neoadjuvant chemotherapy with a planned ALND at the completion of systemic therapy. Patients who are clinically node negative should have an ultrasound of the axilla looking for abnormal lymph nodes. Ultrasound-guided FNA can then document these patients to be node positive before neoadjuvant chemotherapy. For patients who are clinically and ultrasonographically node negative, there are two options for the use of SLN biopsy if they are candidates for neoadjuvant chemotherapy.

The first option is to perform the SLN biopsy before beginning chemotherapy. There are several advantages to this approach. The first is that the true nodal status is known before initiating chemotherapy, which may be important if this will help decide what regimen and schedule to use. Likewise, this will help the radiation oncologist decide whether they would recommend postmastectomy radiation should the patient not be a candidate for BCT. However, there are several factors that go into this decision, including the size of the primary tumor.

BOX 18–3 ADVANTAGES AND DISADVANTAGES OF SENTINEL LYMPH NODE BIOPSY BEFORE OR AFTER NEOADJUVANT CHEMOTHERAPY

	Advantages	Disadvantages
Before chemotherapy	• Higher identification rate • Likely lower false-negative rate • Accurate pretherapy nodal staging	• Requires an additional surgery • Delays the beginning of chemotherapy • May subject patients converted to node negative to an unnecessary axillary lymph node dissection
After chemotherapy	• No need for surgery before chemotherapy • No axillary lymph node dissection performed on patients who become node negative	• Slightly lower identification rate • Higher false-negative rate • Will mislabel some patients who were initially node positive as node negative

If the nodal status would not change either the medical oncologists' or radiation oncologists' recommendations, then knowing the prechemotherapy nodal status becomes less important. This emphasizes the importance of presenting these patients at a tumor board and formulating a treatment plan in a multidisciplinary setting.

Another advantage to performing SLN biopsy before chemotherapy is the confidence in the feasibility and accuracy of the procedure. There has been some concern that the chemotherapy may affect the lymphatic drainage and make identification of the SLN more difficult. In addition, performing SLN biopsy after chemotherapy supposes that if there was disease in the lymph nodes it will either completely disappear from all the nodes, or if not, it will remain in the sentinel node. However, if it is eradicated from the sentinel node, but not the nonsentinel nodes, this will lead to a false-negative finding. Unfortunately, performing SLN biopsy before the onset of chemotherapy means an extra procedure and a delay in the initiation of therapy (Box 18–3).

The second option is to perform the SLN biopsy after completing chemotherapy. This presumes that it is accurate to do so. Several studies of SLN biopsy after neoadjuvant chemotherapy have been performed, and although some have suggested an unacceptably high false-negative rate, overall this seems to be reasonable (Table 18–5). Although a clear disadvantage of this approach is not knowing the true nodal status, if this would not impact the chemotherapy decisions, this is less of a factor. In regard to postmastectomy radiation, some might argue that the nodal status after chemotherapy might serve as a better indicator of whether to offer radiation to the chest wall. Delaying the SLN biopsy to after

chemotherapy also allows the chemotherapy to start immediately and may preclude the need for an additional surgery. The most important advantage to SLN biopsy after chemotherapy is that patients who may have been node positive before chemotherapy, but are now node negative, will be spared from ALND. Approximately 20% of patients may be converted from node positive to node negative, and the use of SLN biopsy before chemotherapy would obligate those patients to undergo ALND. Future clinical trials will

TABLE 18–5 • Success Rates and False-Negative Rates of Sentinel Lymph Node Biopsy After Neoadjuvant Chemotherapy

Author	Patients	Sentinel Lymph Node Identification Rate (%)ate	False-Negative Rate (%)
Breslin	81	85	12
Nason	15	87	33
Haid	33	88	0
Fernandez	40	90	20
Tafra	29	93	0
Stearns	26	88	6
Julian	34	91	0
Miller	35	86	0
Brady	14	93	0
Piato	42	98	17
Balch	32	97	5
Schwartz	21	100	9
Reitsamer	30	87	7
Mamounas	428	85	11
TOTAL		87	9

better define the timing of SLN biopsy with neoadjuvant chemotherapy.

Neoadjuvant Chemotherapy and Outcome

Does Earlier Delivery of Chemotherapy Improve Survival?

The ultimate danger of breast cancer is not the primary tumor, but rather the ability of breast cancer metastases to cause vital organ dysfunction. Therefore, the persistence of distant micrometastases through systemic therapy is ultimately what will determine survival after treatment. The original hypothesis of neoadjuvant chemotherapy was that instead of delaying systemic therapy until after surgery, the earlier initiation might do a better job of eradicating these micrometastases. There are animal studies to suggest that after resection of the primary tumor, an increase in the growth rate of micrometastases is seen. The explanation for this is unclear, possibly related to inhibitory factors released by the primary tumor or an immunosuppressive effect of surgery. However, these studies show that preoperative chemotherapy can prevent this growth spurt. This survival advantage to neoadjuvant chemotherapy for operable breast cancer, however, has not been borne out by any of the randomized trials, all of which had equivalent survivals between preoperative and postoperative chemotherapy.

Can Neoadjuvant Chemotherapy Be Used as a Chemosensitivity Test?

A pCR is defined as the complete absence of residual invasive and in situ disease following neoadjuvant chemotherapy and surgery, although some have defined a complete absence of invasive disease, even in the presence of in situ disease, as a pCR. Although the studies failed to show any difference in OS or DFS between preoperative and postoperative chemotherapy, they did demonstrate a correlation between the response of the tumor to chemotherapy and the outcome. For example, in the NSABP B-18 trial, patients who had a complete clinical response had an overall survival of 78%. This dropped to 67% for patients with a partial clinical response and 65% for patients with no clinical response. The correlation between response and outcome is independent of tumor size, nodal status, or age. A better predictor of outcome than clinical response is pathologic response. At 9 years of follow-up, the OS of patients who achieved a pCR was 85%, compared to 73% for patients with residual cancer.

In addition to downstaging the primary tumor, the status of the regional lymph nodes is also downstaged. Patients who have a pCR in the breast are more likely to have a pCR in the axillary lymph nodes as well, although not always. Kuerer and others, from the MD Anderson Cancer Center, found that of the 16% of patients who had a pCR in the primary tumor, 75% also had a pCR in the axillary nodes. Rouzier and others reported that of patients with documented disease in the regional nodes before chemotherapy, a pCR in the axillary nodes was associated with a significantly better 5-year DFS. The effect in the nodes may be a better marker of outcome than the effect on the primary tumor. In the NSABP B-27 trial, patients who received a pCR in the breast, but still had residual disease in the nodes, had a similar outcome with those patients who did not receive a pCR in the breast. This suggested that the response in the nodes may be the strongest prognostic factor. This makes biologic sense because distant micrometastases (whose ablation ultimately defines overall survival) are probably more similar to nodal metastases than the primary tumor.

Knowing that a pCR in the primary tumor and axillary nodes is associated with a significantly improved outcome, how can this information be used? The potential for research is evident. Without neoadjuvant chemotherapy, the only way to assess a new systemic therapy is to perform a prospective randomized trial comparing the new agent to standard chemotherapy and looking at DFS or OS. This takes many patients and will take several years to provide an answer. In the neoadjuvant setting, new systemic therapies can be delivered before surgery, with pathologic response as the endpoint. This takes considerably less patients and can be concluded in a matter of months. In addition, the use of neoadjuvant therapy, with the ability to obtain tumor specimens before and after chemotherapy, allows for the investigation of molecular markers for prediction of tumor response.

Does this benefit individual patients? In other words, is there a benefit to the patient to assess in vivo their individual response to the chemotherapy? Patients showing a poor response to therapy can have ineffective chemotherapies stopped, avoiding unnecessary toxicity. They can then opt to proceed with surgery or try a different agent.

What about the patient who completes their chemotherapy and undergoes surgery but is found to have only a partial response? As patients with residual disease in either the breast or axillary lymph nodes are known to have a poorer outcome compared with those who have a pCR, does this mean that these patients should receive additional chemotherapy with a new agent after surgery?

Achieving a pCR is clearly associated with better outcome but does the response rate translate into better DFS and OS? In other words, if you can increase the pCR rate (perhaps by changing drugs or treating for more cycles) will this translate into improved outcome? The NSABP B-27 trial hoped to answer this. Patients were randomized into three groups. The first group received preoperative doxorubicin/cyclophosphamide (AC). The second group received preoperative AC, had surgery, and then received postoperative docetaxel. The third group received AC and docetaxel before surgery. As expected, the addition of taxanes increased the pCR rate. Arms 1 and 2, which had AC before surgery, had pCR rates of 12.8% and 14.3%, respectively. Arm 3, which had preoperative AC and docetaxol, had a pCR rate of 26%. In all three groups, a pCR was associated with a significantly improved outcome compared to patients who did not achieve a pCR. However, all three groups had the same OS. Perhaps the increase in pCR rate was not sufficient enough to translate to a statistically significant improvement for the entire group. Unfortunately, without a difference in survival, the trial could not answer whether patients who did not achieve a pCR with AC received any survival benefit to the addition of docetaxel. To date, therefore, no data exist in the literature to guide clinicians, and so decisions about further systemic therapy must be made on an individual patient basis.

If it were demonstrated that patients who do not receive a pCR benefit from additional systemic therapy, then the indication for neoadjuvant chemotherapy as a "chemosensitivity test" would argue for the expanded use of chemotherapy before surgical intervention, even in patients for whom breast conservation is feasible. However, there may be additional markers that can be used besides pCR. The search continues for new molecular markers of response through the use of proteomics, microarray analysis, and immunohistochemical staining. It may be feasible in the future to analyze the tumor during or after chemotherapy to determine whether the regimen should be altered or if additional therapy is needed after surgery.

Suggested Readings

1. Bear HD, Anderson S, Brown A, et al. The effect on tumor response of adding sequential preoperative docetaxel to preoperative doxorubicin and cyclophosphamide: preliminary results from National Surgical Adjuvant Breast and Bowel Project Protocol B-27. J Clin Oncol 2003;21:4165–4174.
2. Beresford M, Padhani AR, Goh V, et al. Imaging breast cancer response during neoadjuvant systemic therapy. Expert Review of Anticancer Therapy 2005;5(5):893–905.
3. Kaufmann M, von Minckwitz G, Smith R, et al. International expert panel on the use of primary (preoperative) systemic treatment of operable breast cancer: review and recommendations. J Clin Oncol 2003;21:2600–2608.
4. Khan A, Sabel MS, Nees A, et al. Comprehensive axillary evaluation in neoadjuvant chemotherapy patients with ultrasonography and sentinel lymph node biopsy. Ann Surg Oncol 2005;12(9):697–704.
5. Kuerer HM, Sahin AA, Hunt KK, et al. Incidence and impact of documented eradication of breast cancer axillary lymph node metastases before surgery in patients treated with neoadjuvant chemotherapy. Ann Surg 1999;230:72–78.
6. von Minckwitz G, Costa SD, Raab G, et al. Dose-dense doxorubicin, docetaxel, and granulocyte colony-stimulating factor support with or without tamoxifen as preoperative therapy in patients with operable carcinoma of the breast: a randomized, controlled, open phase IIb Study. J Clin Oncol 2001;19:3506–3515.
7. Wolmark N, Wang J, Mamounas E, et al. Preoperative chemotherapy in patients with operable breast cancer: nine-year results from National Surgical Adjuvant Breast and Bowel Project B-18. J Natl Cancer Inst Monogr 2001;30:96–102.

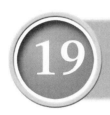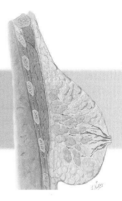

19

Locally Advanced and Inflammatory Breast Cancer

Locally Advanced and Inflammatory Breast Cancer: Key Points

- Define locally advanced breast cancer.
- Describe the workup and staging of the patient presenting with locally advanced breast cancer.
- Know the benefits of induction chemotherapy in the management of locally advanced breast cancer.
- Understand the clinical presentation and diagnosis of inflammatory breast cancer.
- Describe the treatment algorithm for inflammatory breast cancer, including the surgical management.

With the promotion of breast self-examination (BSE) and screening mammograms, the average size at which breast cancer is detected have been steadily decreasing. Some women, unfortunately, will either not be diagnosed or will not seek treatment until the breast cancer is more advanced. This is generally referred to as locally advanced breast cancer (LABC) and continues to represent a significant burden. This is especially true in areas where access to screening and adequate health care is limited. Today, in the United States, approximately 5% of patients that are newly diagnosed with breast cancer have LABC. Worldwide, however, LABC is the most common presentation of breast cancer. For example, in India, the number of patients with breast cancer presenting with LABC may be as high as 50% to 70%.

Locally Advanced Breast Cancer

The definition of LABC has changed over the years. Originally, the term referred to patients who had features associated with a high chance of local recurrence and low chance of cure after radical mastectomy. These included significant skin involvement or satellite nodules in the skin, lymphedema of the arm, internal mammary or supraclavicular metastases, chest wall fixation, or large axillary lymph nodes. These types of observations ultimately led to more formal staging systems based on prognosis.

In general, LABC is defined as either large, bulky primary tumors or extensive adenopathy. Patients with American Joint Commission on Cancer (AJCC) T3 or T4 tumors (associated with chest wall fixation, skin ulceration, or both) are classified as LABC. Also classified as LABC are patients with AJCC N2 or N3 disease (matted axillary nodes, supraclavicular or internal mammary metastases; Table 19–1).

Inflammatory breast cancer (IBC) is distinct from LABC and will be discussed later in the chapter. IBC should be considered separately from LABC because it has a distinct biologic behavior. However, because it is staged as T4d, it has been included in series of LABC cases. Whether to include AJCC T3 tumors (tumors > 5 cm) as LABC has also been controversial because although T4 lesions are generally inoperable, T3 tumors are generally operable, albeit by mastectomy. Finally, ipsilateral infraclavicular or supraclavicular nodal involvement used to be considered metastatic disease, so many older series of LABC would not include these patients. However, the updated AJCC staging system includes these patients as having N3 disease based on the fact that these patients can achieve long disease-free survival (DFS) and potentially be cured. Therefore, more recent series of LABC will include these patients.

However one defines LABC, this group of patients clearly represents a subset of patients with more advanced disease. Whether this is as

TABLE 19–1 • American Joint Committee on Cancer Staging for Locally Advanced Breast Cancer

Stage	Primary Tumor	Regional Lymph Nodes
IIB	T3	N0
IIIA	T0	N2
	T1	N2
	T2	N2
	T3	N1
	T3	N2
IIIB	T4	Any N
	Any T	N3

T3, Tumor more than 5 cm in greatest diameter.
T4a, Extension to chest wall, not including pectoralis muscle.
T4b, Edema or ulceration of skin or satellite nodules confined to same breast.
T4c, Both T4a and T4b.
T4d, Inflammatory carcinoma.
N1, Movable, ipsilateral lymph nodes.
N2, Fixed or matted ipsilateral axillary nodes or clinically apparent ipsilateral internal mammary nodes.
N3, Metastasis in ipsilateral infraclavicular or supraclavicular lymph nodes or in clinical apparent internal mammary nodes *and* clinically evident axillary node metastases.

a result of neglect and delayed diagnosis or a more aggressive tumor biology is not completely understood, nevertheless a more aggressive approach to therapy will be necessary.

Diagnosis and Workup of Locally Advanced Breast Cancer

The diagnosis of LABC is relatively straightforward. By definition, patients present with either a large, firm, fixed palpable mass or large or matted lymph nodes (Fig. 19–1). As with all women with a suspicious breast mass, workup includes diagnostic imaging (mammography, ultrasound and possibly magnetic resonance imaging [MRI]) and tissue biopsy. If there is no palpable adenopathy, an ultrasound of the axilla should be performed, with fine-needle aspiration (FNA) biopsy of any abnormal lymph nodes. If patients present with multiple or matted lymph nodes, but no identifiable mass in the breast on either physical examination or mammogram (and possibly whole-breast ultrasound), an MRI should be obtained to look for an occult breast cancer.

The breast imaging should be carefully reviewed for other abnormal lesions. If present,

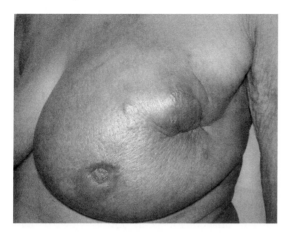

Figure 19–1. Locally advanced breast cancer.

biopsy of these additional lesions is necessary because the identification of multicentric disease would preclude breast conservation therapy (BCT) after chemotherapy. Likewise, the identification of multicentric disease or diffuse calcifications before chemotherapy should prompt a discussion with the patient regarding the need for mastectomy regardless of degree of response to the chemotherapy. In this way, there are no surprises or mixed messages, and the patient has time during the chemotherapy to come to terms with the need for mastectomy. Likewise, there may be time for genetic counseling and testing, and for patients to consider whether they want the contralateral breast removed for prophylaxis.

Core biopsy is the optimal method for diagnosing LABC because this provides adequate tissue for immunohistochemistry (IHC) staining for estrogen receptor (ER), progesterone receptor (PR), and human epidermal growth factor receptor 2 (Her-2/neu), which are imperative to make decisions regarding systemic therapy, which will be the first step. Multiple cores should be taken to confirm the entire mass is invasive because occasionally (although rarely), ductal carcinoma in situ (DCIS) can present as a large bulky mass. If the core biopsy is non-diagnostic, negative, or suggests primarily noninvasive disease, the surgeon should perform an incisional biopsy of the breast for a more definitive diagnosis. If patients have skin involvement, a punch biopsy of the affected skin can also provide the diagnosis.

Because of the high risk of distant disease, all patients with LABC should undergo a thorough search for metastatic disease. The incidence of metastatic disease rises from approximately 2% to 3% for early stage disease to as high as 30% for LABC. The metastatic workup should include laboratory work, bone scan, and computed tomography (CT) scans of the chest, abdomen, and pelvis. Positron emission tomography (PET) scan is being investigated as a staging examination, and although it should not serve as a substitute for these other studies, it may serve as a useful adjunct. MRI of the brain is only indicated when central nervous system symptoms are present. Even with the advanced nature of their primary disease, the majority of patients with LABC will have no evidence of distant disease.

Treatment of Locally Advanced Breast Cancer

History of Treatment for Locally Advanced Breast Cancer

Because breast cancer had always been a surgical disease, surgery was also the primary therapy for LABC, specifically the radical mastectomy. Haagensen and Stout first reported the extremely poor outcomes associated with this approach, with high local recurrence rates and poor survival. It was this experience on which early staging systems for breast cancer were based, identifying poor candidates for surgery as those with extensive breast skin edema, satellitosis, intercostal/parasternal nodules, lymphedema of the arm, supraclavicular metastases, or IBC. Patients with ulceration, limited skin edema, fixation, or bulky adenopathy were not necessarily considered inoperable, but as having a poor prognosis.

Given the limitations of surgery in controlling LABC, the potential of radiation was examined, but likewise yielded poor local control and had minimal impact on survival. A combination of radiation and surgery failed to improve disease control. It was not until the introduction of preoperative chemotherapy that improvements in the outcome of patients with LABC were realized. When first proposed, surgeons were hesitant to deliver chemotherapy before surgery, worried not only about an increase in surgical complications but also a negative impact on survival secondary to delaying the operation. However, several series not only showed that the operative morbidity was not worse, but also showed that it may actually improve tumor downstaging. And in contrast to concerns that preoperative treatment and deferral of surgery may increase rates of unresectability, approximately 80% of patients will have at least 50%

shrinkage of the primary tumor mass, and only 2% to 3% will have signs of progressive disease. More importantly, both local control rates and survival improved significantly with the introduction of preoperative chemotherapy for LABC.

Induction Chemotherapy

Today, the treatment of LABC will be multi-modality, beginning with systemic chemotherapy. Not only will this provide early treatment of the micrometastases that are highly likely to be present, but also downstaging the primary and regional disease will facilitate surgery.

In the setting of LABC, the preoperative chemotherapy is often referred to as induction chemotherapy or neoadjuvant chemotherapy. *Induction chemotherapy* is a better term because it differentiates the mandatory therapy used in LABC from the optional neoadjuvant chemotherapy used when mastectomy is feasible; however, tumor downstaging may allow for breast conservation. The use of the term *neoadjuvant chemotherapy* for both clinical situations sometimes confuses students and residents into thinking the chemotherapy for LABC is optional.

Although there is no standard regimen for the induction chemotherapy in LABC, the most aggressive regimens are typically chosen. Adriamycin, cytoxan, and a taxane is the most common regimen used. Several trials have demonstrated the benefit of adding a taxane, particularly docetaxel, in patients with LABC. If the patient is Her-2/neu positive, Herceptin should be considered, given the increased response rate associated with it.

During chemotherapy, the patient should have periodic assessments of their response, including not only physical examination, but also after one or two cycles, repeat imaging with breast ultrasound or mammogram. Other imaging modalities such as MRI, PET, and sestamibi nuclear medicine studies have been examined as methods of monitoring response to induction chemotherapy, but they are still considered experimental. If no clinical response is noted, repeat biopsies of the lesion may also help determine if there is a pathologic tumor response. If no clinical or pathologic response is noted, or worse, if the disease progresses, a decision should be made to either abandon systemic therapy and move to surgery or switch to a different systemic regimen. This will require a multidisciplinary assessment to determine whether the patient is presently resectable or the likelihood of a different regimen working.

Local Surgery after Induction Chemotherapy

After the completion of induction chemotherapy, the patient will return to the surgeon. Most patients will be ready to undergo surgery approximately 3 weeks after the last chemotherapy treatment, when the absolute neutrophil and platelet counts have normalized (greater than 1500 and 100,000, respectively). For most patients, this means a mastectomy. Breast conservation is an option, but this will depend on the stage of their cancer after chemotherapy. Researchers at the MD Anderson Cancer Center retrospectively studied their LABC population to determine the optimal candidates for BCT. They recommended that patients only be considered for breast conservation if they met certain criteria (Box 19–1). As with all patients with breast cancer, the patients must be desirous of breast conservation, have no contraindications to radiation, and not have multicentric disease or widespread calcifications on mammography. In their series, the pretreatment size was not as strong a predictor of local recurrence as the posttreament size. Patients with clinical N2 or N3 disease before chemotherapy do have higher rates of local failure, but this is true for both BCT and mastectomy and is not a contraindication to lumpectomy.

Many patients are desirous of immediate reconstruction after mastectomy. However,

BOX 19–1 CONTRAINDICATIONS TO BREAST CONSERVATION SURGERY AFTER INDUCTION CHEMOTHERAPY FOR LOCALLY ADVANCED BREAST CANCER

Before Chemotherapy
- Multicentric disease
- Extensive suspicious microcalcifications
- Contraindication to radiation therapy
- Extensive intramammary lymphatic invasion
- Inflammatory breast cancer

After Chemotherapy
- Skin edema has not completely resolved
- Residual tumor >5 cm (or still too large for reasonable cosmetic outcome)

most of these patients will be recommended to undergo postmastectomy radiation. Radiating tissue expanders and implants results in a high rate of complications and is generally discouraged (see Chapter 14). In addition, recent studies have demonstrated excessive rates of cosmetic complications following irradiation of autogenous tissue reconstructions, but occurring in a delayed fashion. The decision to proceed with immediate breast reconstruction in patients with known LABC should be made cautiously, and implant reconstructions should be avoided whenever postmastectomy radiation is planned. Occasionally, patients with LABC will require plastic surgery at the time of mastectomy purely for soft tissue coverage of an extensive chest wall defect. In these cases the latissimus dorsi flap is the most frequently used approach because this flap is a relatively straightforward procedure technically, and it provides durable, radiation-tolerant chest wall coverage.

Regional Surgery after Induction Chemotherapy

The majority of patients with LABC will present with regional metastases. With the routine use of axillary ultrasound and ultrasound guided FNA biopsy, most of these patients will have documented disease in their regional nodes before induction chemotherapy. At the completion of induction chemotherapy, axillary lymph node dissection (ALND) should be performed at the time of either their mastectomy (modified radical mastectomy) or lumpectomy.

With the introduction of sentinel lymph node (SLN) biopsy, several researchers have proposed using SLN biopsy after induction chemotherapy as a method of sparing women who were downstaged to N0 disease from the morbidity of ALND (see Chapter 13). Approximately 20% of patients may be converted from node positive to node negative. This approach presumes that SLN biopsy will work after induction chemotherapy. There have been concerns that lymphatic pathways may have been altered by either the disease or by the chemotherapy, leading to increased false-negative rates. Series of SLN biopsy followed by ALND in patients receiving neoadjuvant chemotherapy have been variable, with some suggesting an unacceptably high false-negative rate, and others suggesting accuracy similar to SLN biopsy in operable breast cancer. Although SLN biopsy after chemotherapy appears to be safe, the

---

BOX 19–2 TREATMENT SUMMARY FOR LOCALLY ADVANCED BREAST CANCER

1. Diagnosis by physical examination, breast imaging, and core biopsy.
2. Complete staging for distant metastases (computed tomography, bone scan).
3. Consider sentinel node biopsy for patients who are clinically node negative.
4. Induction chemotherapy, typically four cycles of doxorubicin and cyclophosphamide (AC) followed by four cycles of a taxane (paclitaxel or docetaxel). Inclusion of Herceptin for patients who are positive for Her-2/neu.
5. Surgery. Lumpectomy and axillary lymph node dissection (ALND) versus modified radical mastectomy. For patients determined to be sentinel lymph node (SLN) negative before chemotherapy, ALND may be omitted. SLN after chemotherapy is controversial.
6. Radiation therapy.
7. Hormone therapy for patients who are hormone-receptor positive.

---

patients in these trials were primarily patients with operable breast cancer undergoing neoadjuvant chemotherapy. There is little data regarding the safety of SLN biopsy specifically after induction chemotherapy for LABC. Further research is necessary before this can be recommended, although it may be an option for selected patients (Box 19–2).

Inflammatory Breast Cancer

A much more aggressive form of LABC is IBC, with 5-year survival rates of only 15%. IBC is a discrete form of breast cancer, and although neglected LABC may develop inflammatory changes, primary IBC is a distinct entity. Although it only accounts for 1% to 5% of breast cancers in the United States, it has a much more significant impact on mortality. The incidence varies with geography and is considerably higher in areas such as the mid-East and northern Africa. The median age at diagnosis is slightly younger than for non-IBC.

Women present with a red discoloration of a large portion of the breast. The involved area is warm to the touch, edematous, and has dimpling of the overlying skin, known as *peau*

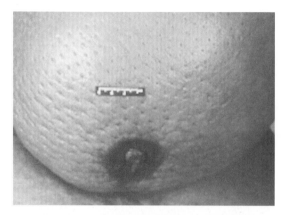

Figure 19–2. Inflammatory breast cancer showing the classic finding of *peau d'orange*. (Image courtesy of Dr. Tara Breslin, Department of Surgery, University of Michigan).

d'orange (orange peel skin; Fig. 19–2). Physical examination often shows palpable adenopathy (approximately in one third of patients, although almost all patients with have pathologic involvement). Often the axillary lymph nodes are matted. The most striking aspect of IBC is that these changes tend to come up rather quickly, over the course of a few weeks. It is not, therefore, difficult to imagine how most physicians who initially see IBC would think these changes were related to infection rather than malignancy.

Diagnosis and Workup

Because mastitis is more common than IBC, it is not unusual for the first physician to see the patient to start the patient on a course of antibiotics. However, in the patient who has the rapid onset of these symptoms without a clear initiating factor for infection (trauma, recent breast-feeding, etc.), a high suspicion of IBC must be entertained and biopsy obtained early. In addition, patients with IBC do not have the fever and elevated white blood cell count that women with mastitis have. Biopsy should also be performed immediately in a patient with inflammatory changes who does not rapidly respond to antibiotics. Antibiotics tend to be of immediate benefit in mastitis. Sometimes in a woman with IBC, a slight decrease in the erythema will be seen with antibiotics, without complete resolution, leading the physician to incorrectly conclude this is infectious and leading to several trials of different antibiotics. Several weeks go by before a biopsy is performed, and this delay in

diagnosis can be devastating for the patient. Sometimes IBC may be confused for skin problems such as atopic dermatitis, psoriasis, eczema, or vasculitis, and steroids are initiated before obtaining a biopsy. Again there may be a minimal response that leads to an incorrect diagnosis, whereas a skin biopsy would confirm the diagnosis and avoid a delay in initiating therapy for IBC.

For any patient suspected to have IBC, a core-needle biopsy should be obtained of any palpable mass; however, there is often no palpable abnormality except for some induration of the involved area. A skin biopsy should also be obtained. The classic histologic finding of IBC is dermal lymphatic invasion by tumor cells. These tumor emboli obstruct lymphatic drainage, leading to the clinical manifestations of IBC. If palpable adenopathy is present, FNA biopsy may also help secure the diagnosis. Dermal lymphatic invasion will be present in about 75% of cases, but its absence does not rule out IBC; the diagnosis can be made on clinical assessment only.

Mammography and directed breast ultrasound should be obtained to document the presence of any underlying abnormalities and provide a baseline to compare to when trying to assess response. However, biopsy should not be delayed until the breast imaging is obtained; it should be done immediately on seeing the physical changes suspicious for IBC. Mammography will often demonstrate a mass or thickening in the breast. In addition there are other signs of inflammation in the breast, such as skin thickening and stromal coarsening (Fig. 19–3).

Once IBC is diagnosed, the patient should have a full staging workup, including a thorough history and physical, CT scan of the chest/abdomen/pelvis, and bone scan. Further imaging studies should be directed by the presence of symptoms.

It should also be mentioned that sometimes a primary breast cancer, treated by lumpectomy and radiation therapy, can recur with inflammatory features. Biopsy of the skin will show widespread invasion of the cancer into the dermis and epidermis. Although this is not true IBC, it does require immediate intervention. Often this inflammatory recurrence is misdiagnosed as a postoperative infection or lymphedema of the breast following radiation therapy. If the condition fails to resolve with antibiotics or other interventions, biopsy should be performed sooner rather than later.

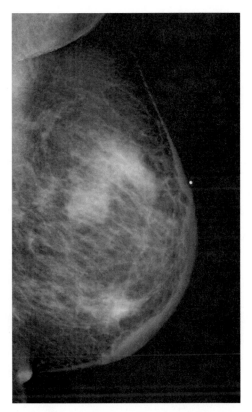

Figure 19–3. Right MLO view demonstrates skin thickening. A 3×2-cm area of focal asymmetry is seen in the superior breast. Core-needle biopsy of breast demonstrated invasive ductal carcinoma. Skin punch biopsy demonstrated tumor in the dermal lymphatics. Findings are consistent with inflammatory breast carcinoma. (Image courtesy of Dr. Alexis Nees, Department of Radiology, University of Michigan).

Treatment of Inflammatory Breast Cancer

The treatment of IBC is multimodality: neoadjuvant chemotherapy followed by surgery (if the patient becomes resectable) followed by radiation therapy (Box 19–3). This is followed by hormonal therapy in patients with hormone-receptor-positive disease, although IBC is more commonly ER/PR negative than non-IBC. Patients treated by all three modalities have significantly improved survival over patients treated with radiation alone, chemotherapy alone, surgery plus radiation, or radiation plus chemotherapy. Several studies have examined whether mastectomy is necessary, looking instead at chemotherapy followed by radiation only. Although some studies found no difference in either disease-free or overall survival, others found a significant benefit to local-regional control with the mastectomy

BOX 19–3 TREATMENT SUMMARY FOR INFLAMMATORY BREAST CANCER

1. Diagnosis by physical examination, breast imaging, core biopsy, and punch biopsy of skin.
2. Complete staging for distant metastases (computed tomography, bone scan).
3. Induction chemotherapy, typically four cycles of doxorubicin and cyclophosphamide (AC) followed by four cycles of a taxane (paclitaxel or docetaxel). Inclusion of Herceptin for patients who are positive for Her-2/neu.
4. Modified radical mastectomy
5. Chest wall radiation.
6. Hormone therapy for patients who are hormone-receptor positive.

and a possible impact on overall survival. Therefore there is no reason to exclude surgery in suitable candidates. In addition, there are other advantages to surgery as part of the multimodality treatment of IBC. Surgery provides important prognostic information regarding the pathologic response to the chemotherapy. The clinical response rate (based on physical examination and mammography) does not accurately reflect the pathologic response rate, and this information is useful in deciding whether additional chemotherapy after radiation therapy may be of use. In addition, surgery provides prompt control of bulky tumor burden and may allow for a lower dose of radiation therapy to be delivered to the chest wall.

Surgery for IBC consists of a modified radical mastectomy. Nodal involvement is present in almost all cases, and the accuracy of SLN biopsy after neoadjuvant chemotherapy for IBC appears poor. Although there have been some reports of using breast conservation in patients who have a complete or nearly complete pathologic response, the body of evidence is minimal compared to that for neoadjuvant chemotherapy for T1 through T3 tumors (or even LABC), and it is difficult to predict what the local recurrence rate would be. Breast conservation is therefore strongly discouraged and should only be considered for highly selected patients in whom a complete pathologic response has been clearly demonstrated. Even then, it is best restricted to research protocols.

Mastectomy should be followed by postmastectomy radiation therapy, even in patients who had a complete pathologic response. Local-regional failures are significantly lower in patients who receive modified radical mastectomy and electron beam therapy compared to electron beam therapy alone. Although the exact impact this has on overall survival is unknown, the benefits of postmastectomy electron beam therapy on overall survival for high-risk breast cancer can be extrapolated to IBC (see Chapter 15). The exact protocol for postmastectomy electron beam therapy for IBC can vary among institutions and with the response to chemotherapy.

Suggested Readings

1. Brito RA, Valero V, Buzdar AU, et al. Long-term results of combined-modality therapy for locally advanced breast cancer with ipsilateral supraclavicular metastases: The University of Texas M.D. Anderson Cancer Center experience. J Clin Oncol 2001;19:628–633.
2. Cancer WG, Carey LA, Calvo BF, et al. Long-term outcome of neoadjuvant therapy for locally advanced breast carcinoma: effective clinical downstaging allows breast preservation and predicts outstanding local control and survival. Ann Surg 2002;236:295–302.
3. Cristofanilli M, Buzdar AU, Hortobagyi GN. Update on the management of inflammatory breast cancer. Oncologist 2003;8(2):141–148.
4. Cristofanilli M, Valero V, Buzdar AU, et al. Inflammatory breast cancer (IBC) and patterns of recurrence: understanding the biology of a unique disease. Cancer 2007;110(7):1436–1444.
5. Gonzalez-Angulo AM, Hennessy BT, Broglio K, et al. Trends for inflammatory breast cancer: is survival improving? Oncologist 2007;12(8):904–912.
6. Lee MC, Newman LA. Management of patients with locally advanced breast cancer. Surg Clin North Am 2007;87(2):379–398, ix.
7. Newman LA. Management of patients with locally advanced breast cancer. Curr Oncol Rep 2004; 6(1):53–61.
8. Singletary SE, McNeese MD, Hortobagyi GN. Feasibility of breast-conservation surgery after induction chemotherapy for locally advanced breast carcinoma. Cancer 1992;69:2849–2852.
9. Waljee JF, Newman LA. Neoadjuvant systemic therapy and the surgical management of breast cancer. Surg Clin North Am 2007;87(2):399–415.
10. Walshe JM, Swain SM. Clinical aspects of inflammatory breast cancer. Breast Disease 2005-2006; 22:35–44.
11. Yang CH, Cristofanilli M. Systemic treatments for inflammatory breast cancer. Breast Disease 2005–2006;22:55–65.

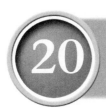
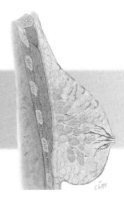

Surveillance of the Patient with Breast Cancer after Treatment

PATTERNS OF RECURRENCE FOR
BREAST CANCER
Local Recurrence
Regional Recurrence
Distant Recurrence
Second Primary Breast
  Cancers
Nonbreast Cancers

TREATMENT-RELATED
TOXICITY

SURVEILLANCE FOR PATIENTS
WITH BREAST CANCER
Recommended Follow-up for
  In Situ Cancer
Recommended Follow-up for
  Invasive Cancer
Not Recommended Follow-up
  Studies

Surveillance of the Patient with Breast Cancer after Treatment: Key Points

- Understand the importance of adequate surveillance after breast cancer treatment.
- Know the common patterns of recurrence of breast cancer.
- Develop a follow-up schedule for patients with breast cancer based on stage of presentation.
- Understand the risks of second primary cancers after successful treatment of breast cancer.
- Know the limitations of surveillance studies and the risks of ordering excessive tests in the surveillance period.
- Know the treatment-related toxicities that must be monitored for after treatment.

BOX 20–1 GOALS OF BREAST CANCER FOLLOW-UP

- Detect and treat recurrence of the cancer
- To diagnose and treat second cancers
- To address complications of therapy
- To gather data for research purposes

Throughout the their lifetime, women treated for breast cancer face a risk of disease recurrence. Following completion of their treatment, patients require surveillance to recognize and treat potentially curable recurrences and identify second primary breast cancers (Box 20–1). Understanding the patterns of breast cancer relapse, and the benefits and down sides of surveillance testing is necessary to establish a cost-effective follow-up strategy.

Breast cancer can recur many years after therapy. Traditionally, the annual frequency of recurrence has been relatively predictable, highest during the first 3 years and gradually declining thereafter. Most recurrences occur within the first 5 years of therapy, and as a result, the greatest emphasis on surveillance is during this time period. Although this is still true, it may be in a state of flux because newer agents and longer periods of systemic therapy (such as the use of aromatase inhibitors [AIs] after 5 years of tamoxifen) may alter these recurrence patterns. A higher percentage of patients are returning with recurrent disease beyond that 5-year window, so lifelong surveillance is necessary.

Who is going to perform this follow-up is still a matter of debate. After completing therapy, patients with breast cancer may now have a team of doctors, including a surgeon, a radiation oncologist, and medical oncologist. It is important to avoid redundancy, so coordination of follow-up among all treating physicians is necessary. The follow-up does not necessarily need to be with an oncologist. The primary care provider may also assume the responsibility to follow the patient after he or she completes therapy. This is not only more cost effective, but several studies have demonstrated that prognosis is no worse with primary care providers following the patient than with cancer specialists. However, most of these studies provided specialized training to the primary care physician in the follow-up of patients with breast cancer, and their participation in the study indicated their interest in following patients with cancer. This may not be true for all primary care physicians.

Patterns of Recurrence for Breast Cancer

Understanding the patterns of recurrence for an individual patient's breast cancer helps focus the surveillance and allows the physician to tailor the appropriate follow-up strategy to each patient. As stated, the majority of breast cancer recurrences occur within the first 5 years after therapy, although they can occur later than this. For this reason, most of the emphasis on surveillance is within the first 5 years. Patients with ductal carcinoma in situ (DCIS) have a low risk of distant recurrence. Therefore, the major risks these women face are of local recurrence or a second primary cancer. Women with large primary tumors or with nodal metastases are at a much higher risk of both loco-regional and distant metastases (in addition to second primary cancers). The surveillance should therefore reflect this.

Local Recurrence

Local recurrence is not only a problem for women who underwent BCT, but chest wall recurrences may also occur after a mastectomy. Local recurrence after breast-conservation therapy (BCT) typically presents in a similar fashion to primary breast cancer, including abnormal mammograms, palpable masses, or other symptoms such as nipple discharge. Local recurrence following a mastectomy most commonly presents as nodularity in or under the skin of the chest wall. This is most often near the mastectomy scar.

The risk of local recurrence will vary depending on the initial stage of the patient and treatment. The risk of a local recurrence after a mastectomy correlates with size of the original tumor, metastases in the regional lymph nodes, the use of adjuvant therapy, and the use of chest wall radiation. Additional factors that have been associated with local recurrence after BCT include positive margins, grossly multifocal disease, high-grade angiolymphatic invasion, and young age. Overall, however, women who undergo BCT or mastectomy have relatively similar rates of local recurrence, approximately 10% to 15% over 10 years. They will differ in their timing. Although most chest wall recurrences are detected within the first

2 to 3 years after surgery, local recurrences are more commonly detected 3 to 4 years after breast conservation, sometimes longer.

After BCT, it is sometimes difficult to differentiate between a true local recurrence and a new ipsilateral primary breast cancer. In either case, the woman will require a mastectomy because radiation cannot be used a second time; however, whether this is a true recurrence or a second primary may impact the decision to use adjuvant therapy. In general, a second primary tumor occurs later than a local recurrence, may be in a different quadrant of the breast, and may have a different histology than the original tumor. Often a careful review of the pathology and estrogen receptor (ER), progesterone receptor (PR) and Her-2/neu expression of both the original primary and the new tumor can help make the diagnosis, but this is not a guarantee. In some cases, a previously ER-positive tumor can recur as an ER-negative tumor. In fact, the opposite can sometimes occur; a previously ER-negative tumor may recur as ER positive.

Although women who underwent BCT and had a local recurrence have a worse prognosis than women who did not have a local recurrence, the majority of these women will be salvaged by mastectomy. The outcome is less optimistic for women who have a chest wall recurrence after a mastectomy. This carries a much worse prognosis because nearly one third of these women will have distant disease at the time of their local recurrence. A chest wall recurrence should be thought of as a harbinger of distant disease, and a staging workup (history and physical, computed tomography [CT] of chest/abdomen/pelvis and bone scan) should be performed before proceeding with salvage therapy. Although it is not imperative, it is not unreasonable to perform a staging work-up in a woman with an in-breast recurrence after BCT.

Regional Recurrence

In addition to local recurrences, recurrences in the regional basins can occur. These include the ipsilateral axillary, infraclavicular, supraclavicular, and internal mammary nodes. Not common, regional recurrences occur in only 1% to 3% of cases.

Although there was some concern that the use of sentinel lymph node (SLN) biopsy may increase this, to date that has not been demonstrated. Axillary, infraclavicular, and supraclavicular recurrences most commonly present as a palpable mass in these regions. In

some cases, axillary recurrence may present as a new-onset lymphedema. Although lymphedema may occur many years after treatment, its onset should prompt the consideration of regional recurrence, especially if no other explanation for its arrival is noted. In other cases, axillary or supraclavicular recurrences may present as pain in the arm and shoulder or increasing sensory or motor loss in the arm or hand. These symptoms are often as a result of brachial plexus involvement (although they may be caused by cervical spine metastases). CT, magnetic resonance imaging (MRI), and bone scan can help make the diagnosis and should be considered in any patient with new onset pain, paralysis, paresthesias, or lymphedema, even in the absence of palpable disease. Internal mammary recurrences often present as a deep, fixed mass in an intercostal space at the ipsilateral sternal border. These often first present with pain and tenderness, without a noticeable mass. It may be difficult to differentiate from a chest wall recurrence or sternal metastasis. Also in the differential of parasternal pain are costochondritis (Tietze syndrome), neuroma, or radiation-induced sarcoma. Persistent pain should prompt a CT, bone scan, or MRI to make the diagnosis.

Sometimes it is not completely clear what type of a recurrence is present. Masses that appear along the sternal border may have originated from the skin flap or chest wall (local recurrence), internal mammary node (regional recurrence), or a sternal metastasis (distant recurrence). Masses inferior to the clavicle could be from the skin flap (local) or infraclavicular nodes (regional). Masses in the pectoralis muscle may be chest wall (local) or from Rotter nodes (regional). The presence of nodal tissue histologically can help make the diagnosis, but the node may be completely replaced. Because of the overlap between local and regional recurrences, they are often reported together as locoregional recurrence (LRR).

Distant Recurrence

The greatest fear for patients with breast cancer and their physicians is that of distant recurrence because this marks a shift from a curable disease to a treatable, but ultimately fatal disease. In the United States, few patients present with metastasis, approximately 6% to 7%. Therefore the overwhelming majority of women with stage IV disease represent distant recurrence among treated patients.

The risk of recurrence is directly related to the size and grade of the primary tumor and the presence of disease in the lymph nodes. Although we commonly talk about 5-year survival, and many women consider reaching that milestone as evidence of cure, over 25% of all metastases occur past 5 years from diagnosis. Much of this is a result of improved systemic therapies and prolonged hormonal therapy, and thus this percentage may even be higher in patients who are hormone-receptor positive. Breast cancer has the potential to return almost anywhere in the body, but the most common initial sites are bone, liver, and lung. Although brain is often mentioned here, fewer than 5% of patients will manifest central nervous system metastases as the first site of metastatic disease.

Second Primary Breast Cancers

One of the most significant risks for the development of breast cancer is a previous history of breast cancer. Thus, breast cancer survivors are at an increased risk of a second primary cancer, particularly if they have a strong family history or known inherited predisposition to breast cancer. Typically, we estimate the risk of a second primary breast cancer as 0.8% per year. This is based on data from Memorial Sloan Kettering of patients followed for a median of 18 years. Thus in the first 5 years after therapy, 4% of women will develop a second primary cancer. By 20 years, this number rises to 16%. However, this risk was age dependent; women under 45 had an average annual rate of 1%, whereas women older than 50 and an average annual rate of 0.5%. For women who were initially ER positive and underwent 5 years of adjuvant hormonal therapy, the risk of a second primary cancer dropped by approximately 50%. For women with a breast cancer gene (BRCA) 1 or 2 mutation, the risk of a second primary cancer is much higher (see Chapter 8). Second primary breast cancers more commonly occur later, past the 5 year mark, necessitating long-term surveillance.

Because of this risk of a second primary cancer, many women may have undergone a prophylactic contralateral mastectomy at the time of their treatment. Although this is an effective strategy, it does not completely eliminate the chance of a second primary tumor. Prophylactic mastectomy will reduce the risk of a new cancer by over 95%, but that still leaves a small chance of a new primary tumor in residual breast tissue. Therefore, surveillance is still mandated in women who have had bilateral mastectomies.

Nonbreast Cancers

Often lost in the conversation is the fact that most women with breast cancer will be successfully treated for their cancer and will go on to have an expected survival no different than had they never been diagnosed. As such, they need to have continued surveillance for new primary nonbreast tumors. Many women and physicians focused on a recurrence of the first cancer, tending to overlook screening guidelines for other cancers such as colon cancer. It is important to make sure women continue their recommended screening programs.

In addition, women who have had breast cancer may be at higher risk of nonbreast cancers either because of common risk factors or as a result of therapy (Box 20–2). Radiation therapy increases the risk of sarcoma; chemotherapy can increase the risk of leukemia; and tamoxifen increases the risk of uterine cancer. Women with breast cancer have an increased risk of ovarian cancer, especially those with a known or suspected BRCA 1 or 2 mutations. An increased risk of melanoma among patients with breast cancer has been suggested, although this is less clear.

Treatment-Related Toxicity

Finally, it is important to remember that breast cancer survivors have several treatment-related toxicities (Table 20–1). Most commonly, this is related to early menopause as a result of chemotherapy-induced ovarian failure or ovarian ablation, or treatment with selective estrogen receptor modulators (SERM).

Many women with breast cancer will have the onset or worsening of hot flashes after therapy. The most effective therapy, estrogen, is contraindicated in breast cancer survivors.

BOX 20–2 OTHER PRIMARY CANCERS AT HIGHER RISK AMONG BREAST CANCER SURVIVORS

- Ovarian cancer
- Endometrial cancer (after treatment with tamoxifen)
- Myeloid leukemia (after treatment with high cumulative doses of alkylating agents or anthracyclines)
- Angiosarcoma (after chest wall irradiation)
- Lymphangiosarcoma (in patients with lymphedema; Stewart-Treves)

TABLE 20-1 • Possible Side Effects of Breast Cancer Treatment

Symptom	Treatment
Hot flashes	Citalopram Fluoxetine Venlafaxine Gabapentin
Sexual dysfunction	Counseling or nonhormonal moisturizing or lubricating formulas (Replens, Astroglide), or intravaginal estradiol preparations
Cognitive dysfunction	Full evaluation to rule out other causes
Depression	Counseling, antidepressants
Weight gain	Counseling, diet, exercise
Fatigue	Full evaluation to rule out other causes
Musculoskeletal pain	Rule out fractures or bone mets, nonsteroidal antiinflammatory drugs or acetaminophen
Osteopenia/ osteoporosis	Screening for high risk women Calcium and vitamin D, exercise, possibly bisphosphonate
Cardiovascular disease	Appropriate medical management
Deep vein thrombosis	Anticoagulation as indicated
Lymphedema	Physical therapy, preferably by a lymphedema specialist

This is particularly true for patients who are ER positive and generally true even for patients who are ER negative. Options for therapy of hot flashes in breast cancer survivors include selective serotonin-reuptake inhibitors (SSRIs), the SSRI and norepinephrine-reuptake inhibitor, venlafaxine, and the anticonvulsant, gabapentin. These may reduce the frequency and severity of hot flashes by 50%. However, paroxetine can interfere with tamoxifen activation and should not be used in women on tamoxifen.

Early menopause can increase the risk of osteopenia, osteoporosis, and fractures among breast cancer survivors, as can the use of AIs. In contrast, postmenopausal women on tamoxifen have a reduced risk. In addition to standard recommendations (calcium and vitamin D, weight-bearing exercise), measurement of bone mineral density is recommended every 1 or 2 years for all breast cancer survivors, particularly those on AIs (bone density scans should

be performed before the initiation of an AI). Bisphosphate therapy should be initiated if osteoporosis is documented and may play a role in the osteopenic patient on an AI.

Another risk of treatment is cardiovascular disease. Radiation therapy to the left chest wall has been associated with an increase of 20% to 30% in the long-term risk of cardiac events, although this is decreasing with newer techniques. Early menopause increases risk, as does chemotherapy with anthracyclines or trastuzumab, whereas tamoxifen may decrease risk. Regardless, all breast cancer survivors should be advised to eat right, exercise, avoid tobacco, and control cholesterol and blood pressure. Although no specific monitoring is recommended, patients showing signs of cardiovascular compromise should be immediately referred to a cardiologist for evaluation.

Surveillance for Patients with Breast Cancer

The appropriate surveillance of patients with cancer is a difficult subject because there are several competing ideologies. Patients are often desirous of frequent and intensive surveillance, using the most advanced technologies. This is understandable, given the anxiety surrounding their diagnosis, and the individual patient would not be expected to focus on issues related to health care economics. Patients, in arguing for more intensive follow-up, would argue that there is an immeasurable psychological benefit to receiving the news that they have no evidence of disease recurrence.

However, there are many negatives to intensive screening, beyond issues related to cost and availability. First and foremost, there are no randomized trials demonstrating a survival benefit to more intensive surveillance beyond history, physical, and mammography. Randomized trials of women with nonmetastatic breast cancer failed to demonstrate any impact on overall mortality compared to more intensive surveillance. Much of this is a result of the fact that the therapies we have available to treat stage IV breast cancer have little impact on extending survival. Instead, they primarily delay or diminish the symptoms associated with metastatic disease. Initiating disease before the onset of symptoms is therefore of minimal benefit. Finding the disease earlier only serves to lengthen the amount of time the patients know they have stage IV disease, and this has a significant negative impact on quality of life.

There is also a negative side to obtaining follow-up chest x-rays, CT scans, or even blood tests. Although there may be that relief in hearing that there is no evidence of distant disease, there is a significant amount of stress experienced in the weeks preceding the test and in the time between when the test is performed and the clinician notifies the patient of the results. More importantly, all of these tests have significant false-negative rates, leading to further increased anxiety, and additional and often more invasive follow-up tests. Detailed and tactful discussions need to be held with the patient explaining why frequent and intensive monitoring is not typically performed Box 20–3).

Many physicians, in an attempt to pacify patients or increase their own level of comfort (treating the physician rather than treating the patient), will still obtain yearly blood tests (complete blood count [CBC], chemistries, tumor markers) and chest x-rays and frequently follow-up with all patients with breast cancer (including those with a low risk of disease recurrence, such as those patients with DCIS only). Although this may make them more popular with their patients, the impact on health care costs is substantial. The estimated cost for this type of screening, compared to the recommended history and physical and yearly mammography can be five times higher. If all physicians used the recommended minimalist approach to surveillance, nearly 1 billion dollars per year could be saved and put toward other aspects of breast cancer care. And this would be accomplished without any compromise of patient outcome. It is therefore imperative that we all practice cost-conscious medicine. With that in mind, the recommended surveillance for patients with breast cancer is detailed next.

Recommended Follow-up for In Situ Cancer

Patients with DCIS are generally treated by lumpectomy with radiation therapy (although the treatment of low-grade DCIS by lumpectomy alone may be considered) or simple mastectomy. Tamoxifen may be used after breast-conserving surgery to further reduce local recurrence. It may also be considered as chemoprevention for contralateral cancers in women treated by mastectomy. This is detailed in Chapter 20.

For the most part, patients with DCIS are at a low risk of developing either regional or distant recurrences. The goal of follow-up in these patients is therefore to look for a recurrent cancer in a conserved breast or a new cancer in either breast. The follow-up for patients with DCIS is limited to history, physical, and mammography. History and physical examination should be performed every 6 months for the first 5 years and then yearly (Box 20–4).

For the patient being treated by breast conservation, an ipsilateral mammogram is recommended after lumpectomy and before radiation when the patient's DCIS was

---

BOX 20–3 DRAWBACKS TO OVERLY AGGRESSIVE FOLLOW-UP STRATEGIES

- Cost to the patient and cost to the health care system.
- Limited options for treatment when asymptomatic distant recurrences are detected.
- No significant improvement in survival (lead-time bias).
- Regularly scheduled physical examinations detect relatively few recurrences.
- Serum markers have a low sensitivity for detecting recurrence.
- Imaging studies may be false-positive, prompting unnecessary worry and additional studies/procedures.

BOX 20–4 NATIONAL COMPREHENSIVE CANCER NETWORK RECOMMENDED FOLLOW-UP AFTER TREATMENT OF BREAST CANCER

- History and physical examination every 4–6 months for invasive cancer and every 6 months for DCIS for 5 years, followed by yearly
- Mammogram every 12 months
- If patient is on tamoxifen:
  - Annual pelvic examination
- If patient is on an aromatase inhibitor or has treatment related ovarian failure
  - Monitoring for bone density loss

diagnosed by microcalcifications. This postlumpectomy mammogram assures that all the calcifications were removed. Occasionally, residual calcifications may be present, even if negative margins were obtained around the DCIS. These should be excised by wire-localized excision as they (1) may represent residual disease and (2) will be suspect for local recurrence at the first surveillance mammogram. Once radiation is completed, the next ipsilateral mammogram should be obtained 6 months later. This will serve as a new baseline mammogram for that side. Any sooner than that is suboptimal because of the radiation induced changes (edema, skin changes, etc.). Six months after that, bilateral mammograms should be obtained and be performed annually. There is no data that more frequent mammograms are of benefit. If treatment was delayed for any reason, it is important to note when the last contralateral mammogram was obtained, so the interval on the contralateral side is not too much longer than 1 year.

For patients treated by mastectomy, contralateral mammography is performed yearly. If the mastectomy was reconstructed by means of a transverse rectus abdominis myocutaneous (TRAM) flap, there are some radiologists who would recommend a TRAMogram-mammography of the reconstructed breast as part of the surveillance imaging. Although this is not a standard recommendation, many cancer centers routinely perform TRAMograms in addition to mammograms of the contralateral breast, particularly for cases of DCIS that required mastectomy. TRAMograms may potentially find calcifications and recurrences before they are detectable on physical examination.

Recommended Follow-up for Invasive Cancer

A history and physical should initially be performed every 3 to 6 months after the completion of therapy. Patients with a higher risk of relapse should be seen every 3 months, whereas low-risk patients can be seen closer to every 6 months. These follow-ups should be coordinated with all of the treating physicians. It does not benefit the patient to be seen three times in 1 month by the surgeon, the medical oncologist, and the radiation oncologist. Follow-up care should be coordinated as not to duplicate effort. In addition, the patient should continue to follow-up with their primary care physician because the oncology team will rarely focus on routine health maintenance. For patients at lower risk, follow-up visits can be alternated between the oncologist and the primary care physician or in some cases left completely to the primary doctor.

As the patient gets further out from their treatment, surveillance visits can be scheduled further apart. The American Society of Clinical Oncology recommends that patient visits should be every 3 to 6 months for the first 3 years after therapy, every 6 to 12 months for the next 2 years, and then annually after 5 years.

History

When seeing a patient with breast cancer for a return visit, the history should start by focusing on signs and symptoms related to local or regional recurrence. Has the patient been performing her recommended monthly BSEs? This is crucial because the majority of local recurrences are discovered by the patient, not by the physician. Has the patient noticed any new masses or changes in the area of the lumpectomy, or in the case of a mastectomy, on the chest wall? In the first few months after surgery and radiation, some posttreatment changes are to be expected. As swelling decreases, seromas resolve, and scar tissue softens, the patient may notice changes in the region. Has the patient noticed any new masses in the contralateral breast? In addition to asking about new lumps in the breasts, the physician should query about lymphadenopathy either under the arm or in the neck. These questions will also serve to remind the patient that they should be performing BSEs of both breasts and lymph node self-examinations. If they are not, time should be taken to review how to perform a self-examination.

The history should then shift toward symptoms consistent with metastatic disease. This should begin with constitutional symptoms; weight loss or gain, changes in appetite or energy levels, fatigue, etc. A full review of symptoms should be performed going by systems. As breast cancer may metastasize to the brain, central nervous system symptoms such as headaches, nausea/vomiting, syncopal episodes, vision changes, or nerve palsies should be reviewed. If patients have symptoms, it is important to ask how long these symptoms have been present. Quite often the patient will report headaches, but her headaches predate the breast cancer by several years.

Breast cancer commonly recurs in the lung and liver; however, the patient has to have rather advanced disease to cause symptoms.

Nonetheless, the patient should be asked about cough, shortness of breast, pain with deep inspiration or pleuritic chest pain, or right upper quadrant pain, melena, or changes in bowel function or habits. Finally, questions regarding constant aching pain may elicit the presence of bone metastases. One of the most challenging aspects of the surveillance examination is differentiating the mild aches and pains that all patients will get as they get older from symptoms that may suggest recurrent disease.

Many patients who are ER positive being seen for surveillance will be on hormonal therapy, such as tamoxifen or Arimidex. It is therefore important to ask about symptoms related to the complications of these therapies. The risk of uterine cancer is significantly increased with tamoxifen, particularly among women over the age of 50. Uterine cancers typically present with abnormal vaginal bleeding. This needs to be asked of patients, and any abnormality worked up because most uterine cancers are highly curable in the early stages. The use of routine endometrial biopsies is not necessary. Tamoxifen also increases the risk of deep venous thrombosis, so patients should be queried on leg or calf pain, swelling, or other signs of thrombotic disease. AIs do not appear to carry the same risk of uterine cancer or thrombotic disease, but they do have an increased risk of bone pain and osteoporosis.

Physical Examination

As with the history, the physical examination should focus on LRR and distant recurrence. The examination should include a thorough examination of the treated breast (or chest wall in the case of a mastectomy) and the opposite breast. An accurate description of the examination in the medical records is important to document postoperative and postradiotherapy changes. These may even include diagrams of the treated breast. This helps the examiner follow these changes over time and recognize new changes. The examination should include a search for axillary, supraclavicular, and cervical adenopathy and should note the presence of lymphedema on the affected side. Not only may this allow for early intervention, but the subsequent development of lymphedema may also represent a regional recurrence.

The remainder of the examination should focus on distant recurrence. Palpation of the spine, sternum, and pelvis for bone tenderness may reveal bony metastases. A heart and lung examination is crucial, not only because of the possibility of pulmonary metastases, but also because several breast cancer therapies may have negative effects on cardiac performance (Adriamycin, radiation, Herceptin). Right upper quadrant tenderness or hepatomegaly may be a sign of liver metastases, and a neurologic examination should be performed to rule out central nervous system metastases. In women on tamoxifen, calf tenderness or a positive Homan sign may be evidence of a deep venous thrombosis. A yearly gynecologic examination is also important in women on tamoxifen who have not undergone hysterectomy. Because it would be unlikely that the breast surgeon would perform this examination, it should be verified with the patient that they are having this done by their gynecologist or primary care physician.

Mammography

Mammography not only detects local recurrences, but also second primary breast cancers, which breast cancer survivors are at an increased risk of developing. A new baseline mammogram of the treated breast should be obtained at 6 months. Bilateral mammography should then be obtained yearly after that. More frequent mammography does not appear to improve outcome and should only be performed when an abnormality is detected on physical examination. It is important to note when the last mammogram was obtained on the contralateral breast because sometimes the focus on the treated breast leads to intervals greater than 1 year between mammograms on the unaffected side.

Referral for Genetic Counseling

Women at high risk of harboring the BRCA 1 or 2 mutation or women at a higher risk of a second primary breast cancer should ideally undergo genetic counseling and possibly genetic testing before their treatment because this might affect their decisions regarding local therapy and prophylactic surgery (Box 20–5). However, some women, overwhelmed by their cancer diagnosis, are not prepared to think about the implications of genetic testing or prophylactic surgery. If this had not been addressed pretreatment, then it should be reassessed in the immediate surveillance period. Even in women who do not desire prophylactic surgery, genetic counseling and testing may alter surveillance strategies and may have implications regarding additional measures (such as oophorectomy).

Not Recommended Follow-up Studies

It seems logical that intensive follow-up should lead to an earlier recognition of distant disease and more successful treatment. However, when one considers the question more closely, taking into account the likelihood of finding disease, the possibility of false-positives, and the impact of initiating therapy earlier in stage IV disease, it becomes apparent that this assumption is false. Thus, in asymptomatic patients, the routine use of blood tests and radiologic imaging to detect distant disease is not recommended. The false-positive rates for these tests can be as high as 50%. False-positives raise anxiety and usually lead to additional studies and possibly invasive biopsies. Two randomized trials compared intensive screening to routine clinical evaluation, and neither found any impact on survival. In fact, one found a significant decrease in quality of life associated with intensive screening.

This is, however, a field that is constantly evolving. Although today there is little evidence that finding metastatic disease earlier does not seem to improve outcome, as systemic therapies and imaging studies improve, this might change.

Blood Tests

Blood chemistries are often recommended as a surveillance tool, but their use is limited. Liver function tests may be elevated in patients with liver metastases, but they are often falsely elevated in patients without metastases and rarely lead to the detection of disease much earlier than the onset of symptoms. Other tests, such as C-reactive protein (CRP) or erythrocyte sedimentation rate (ESR), the acute phase reactants, can also be elevated with metastatic disease, but again are non-specific and not routinely recommended. CBC has little impact on the early recognition of distant disease.

Several tumor-associated antigens can be detected in the serum, such as CA15-3, CA 27.29 and CEA. CA-15-3 and CA-27-29 are glycoproteins secreted by breast cancer cells, whereas CEA belongs to a family of glycoproteins with increased expression on a number of cancers, including breast. Their presence may be predictive of a breast cancer relapse, but they do not have a particularly high sensitivity or specificity. They may fluctuate greatly between tests, making interpretation difficult. These markers are much more useful in monitoring patients with documented advanced disease and to date are not recommended for routine surveillance following treatment.

Chest X-Rays

One of the most commonly used tests for surveillance after cancer treatment is the chest x-ray. Breast cancer can recur not only as lung metastases but in the pleura (resulting in an effusion) or the mediastinum. However, chest x-rays are rarely useful in detecting asymptomatic recurrences and are not necessary for routine surveillance. Less than 5% of patients will present with asymptomatic intrathoracic recurrences detected on chest x-ray. Therefore, the number of yearly chest x-rays needed to find a single recurrence is staggering, certainly not cost effective and not recommended.

Computed Tomography Scans or Positron Emission Tomography Scans

Both CT scans of the chest, abdomen, and pelvis and PET scans have been investigated as follow-up instruments in small, single institution trials with variable results. There are no large prospective trials and the routine use of these tests is not recommended.

Bone Scans

The skeletal system represents the most common site of distant relapse, so it makes sense that bone scans may detect a more significant number of asymptomatic recurrences. However, in a prospective study by the National Surgical and Adjuvant Breast Project (NSABP) of over 2500 women with stage II breast cancer, routine bone scans have minimal benefit, with only 0.6% detecting an asymptomatic recurrence. This and other similar studies failed to provide justification for the routine use of bone scans.

In addition, the overall strategy of intensive surveillance using serial bone scans, liver ultrasounds, chest x-rays, and blood tests has been examined in two prospective randomized studies. Both studies showed that most patients with metastatic disease will present with symptoms rather than on imaging studies and neither study was able to demonstrate a benefit to survival or an improvement in quality of life with intensive screening.

Magnetic Resonance Imaging of the Breast

The use of more sensitive breast-screening techniques such as MRI has been increasing in both the screening and surveillance of breast cancer. MRI has been a double-edged sword, finding cancers not detected by mammography but also finding many benign lesions, lowering the specificity and raising the false-positive rate. The routine use of MRI in the surveillance of breast cancer patients is not recommended. There are, however, some women for whom MRI might be reasonable. These include women with a known BRCA 1 or 2 mutation who opted for breast conservation rather than bilateral mastectomy. Although it may be tempting to use MRI surveillance in women who had a mammographically occult breast cancer, there is no data to suggest that mammography is more likely to miss a second cancer in these women.

Suggested Readings

1. GIVIO Investigators. Impact of follow-up and testing on survival and health-related quality of life in breast cancer patients: a multicenter randomized controlled trial. JAMA 1994;271:1587–1592.
2. Hayes DF. Follow-up of patients with early breast cancer. N Engl J Med 2007;356(24):2505–2513.
3. Khatcheressian JL, Wolff AC, Smith TJ, et al. American Society of Clinical Oncology. American Society of Clinical Oncology 2006 update of the breast cancer follow-up and management guidelines in the adjuvant setting. J Clin Oncol 2006;24(31):5091–5097.
4. Rosselli Del Turco M, Palli D, Cariddi, et al. Intensive diagnostic follow-up after treatment of primary breast cancer: a randomized trial. JAMA 1994;271:1593–1597.
5. Rutgers EJ. Follow-up care in breast cancer. Expert Rev Anticancer Ther 2004;4(2):212–218.

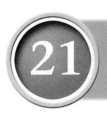

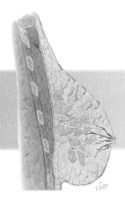

Management of Breast Cancer Recurrence

Management of Recurrence: Key Points

- Know how to look for a local recurrence and diagnostic workup if a recurrence is detected.
- Understand the treatment options for the patient with a local recurrence after breast-conserving therapy or after mastectomy.
- Develop an algorithm for the regional management of the patient with a local recurrence.
- Know the management of the patient with an axillary or supraclavicular recurrence.
- Understand the potential role of surgery for patients with metastatic disease.
- Be familiar with the principles of systemic therapy in the patient with stage IV breast cancer.

BOX 21–1 DEFINITIONS OF LOCOREGIONAL RECURRENCE

Recurrence: Reappearance of a treated cancer in a patient previously considered NED.

Local recurrence: Recurrence in the remaining breast after breast conservation or in the soft tissues of the anterior chest after mastectomy.

In-breast tumor recurrence (IBTR): Local recurrence in the breast after breast-conserving therapy although it is not always possible to differentiate IBTR from a second primary tumor.

Regional recurrence: Recurrence in the ipsilateral axillary, internal mammary, or supraclavicular lymph nodes.

Distant recurrence: Recurrence anywhere outside the ipsilateral breast, chest wall, or regional lymph node basins.

Following surgery for breast cancer, patients can recur in a variety of methods (Box 21–1). A local recurrence may be an in breast recurrence in the case of women treated by breast-conserving therapy (BCT) or a recurrence on the chest wall for patients who underwent a mastectomy. A regional recurrence is defined as recurrent disease in the regional lymph nodes, either the axillary, supraclavicular, infraclavicular, or internal mammary lymph nodes. Finally, a distant recurrence refers to the development of metastatic disease outside of the breast/chest wall and regional nodes. The approach to recurrent disease is multidisciplinary. Surgery plays a major role in the management of locoregional recurrence. The role of surgery in the management of metastatic disease is more limited.

The clinical picture of recurrent breast cancer is changing as the treatment of primary breast cancer changes. The increasing use of neoadjuvant chemotherapy to downsize primary tumors and allow for BCT or the use of post-mastectomy radiation for women at high risk of chest wall recurrence has certainly contributed to this changing picture. So has the use of sentinel lymph node (SLN) biopsies, resulting in a dramatic increase in the number of women who have not had previous axillary lymph node dissection (ALND). Advances in systemic therapy have led to delays in local recurrence rates and possibly an increase in local recurrence as survival from breast cancer increases.

The management of recurrent disease is rarely straightforward, particularly because these changes in management have led to scenarios for which there is little data to guide therapy decisions. As the management of locoregional disease rarely consists of just one specialty, it is recommended that many of these patients be presented at multidisciplinary tumor boards before commencing with a treatment plan. With multimodality treatment, long-term disease control is attainable after a locoregional recurrence, and patients should be approached with curative intent. This chapter will review the management of locoregional recurrence, focusing on the role of surgery. In addition, the role of the surgeon in the treatment of metastatic disease is reviewed.

Local Recurrence

Several factors may ultimately lead to the development of a local recurrence (Box 21–2). The incidence of local recurrence will depend on the stage of the primary cancer and the treatment the woman received. The use of lumpectomy alone, rarely recommended, is associated with a high rate of local recurrence. Women who undergo BCT or mastectomy have relatively similar rates of local recurrence, approximately 10% to 15% over 10 years. There are several differences, however, in the presentation of local recurrences between women who underwent BCT and those who underwent a mastectomy (Table 21–1).

For most women who undergo mastectomy, the presence of recurrent disease is almost always a recurrence of the primary tumor. This, however, depends on the degree of breast tissue that the surgeon left behind at the time of the initial mastectomy. Leaving thick flaps that include significant breast tissue or not taking care to excise the axillary tail of Spence (see Chapter 12) will result in residual breast tissue that can develop second primary tumors. This

BOX 21–2 POTENTIAL EXPLANATIONS FOR LOCAL RECURRENCE

- Incomplete excision of the primary tumor
- Unrecognized multifocal or multicentric disease
- Implantation of tumor cells at the time of surgery
- Entrapment of cells within obstructed lymphatics
- Local implantation of systemically circulating cancer cells

TABLE 21–1 • *Local Recurrence after Breast-Conserving Therapy versus Mastectomy*

	In-Breast Tumor Recurrence After Breast-Conserving Therapy	Chest Wall Recurrence After Mastectomy
True recurrence?	Sometimes a second primary	Rarely a second primary
Median time to recurrence	3 to 4 years	2 to 3 years
Detection	Physical examination or mammography	Almost always physical examination
Surgical approach	Mastectomy	Resection when feasible and radiation
Implications on prognosis	More favorable	Strong association with systemic disease

is particularly true in women with a breast cancer gene (BRCA) 1 or 2 mutation. In contrast, a second tumor in a breast previously treated for breast cancer may represent either an in-breast tumor recurrence (IBTR) or a second primary tumor. In general, a second primary tumor occurs later than an IBTR, may be in a different quadrant of the breast, and may have a different histology than the original tumor. In some cases it is difficult if not impossible to differentiate between the two.

Local recurrences after mastectomy are diagnosed earlier than IBTRs. The median time to recurrence after a mastectomy is 2 to 3 years, compared with 3 to 4 years after BCT. Local recurrences can occur much later than this, however, depending on the use of systemic therapies.

The implications of a local recurrence on prognosis also differ between BCT and mastectomy. Both signal an increased risk of additional disease, but women who have a local recurrence after BCT tend to have a lower rate of simultaneous regional or distant metastases and an improved cancer-specific survival compared to women with a chest wall recurrence. Both forms of recurrence should prompt a thorough search for distant disease, and in the absence of documented metastases, should be approached with a curative intent.

Presentation of Local Recurrences

A local recurrence in an intact breast is usually detected by a change in the physical examination or on surveillance mammography. Physical examination findings may include a palpable mass or increased thickening or retraction at the site of the lumpectomy site. Mammographic findings may include a new mass, architectural changes, or the new appearance of calcifications. However, these changes may not always represent a local recurrence. Both surgery and radiation therapy can lead to changes over time that can be confused with recurrent disease. Likewise, not all IBTRs detected on physical examination will be associated with mammographic change, so a normal mammogram does not rule out a local recurrence.

Postmastectomy recurrences will differ in presentation depending on whether or not women have had breast reconstruction. In patients who have not had reconstruction, postmastectomy recurrences are almost always detected on self-examination or by the physician. These typically present as nodules in the overlying skin of the chest wall or subcutaneous nodules. These may be single or multiple and are often located near the mastectomy scar, although recurrences can occur anywhere in the skin flaps. Suture granulomas, scar, fat necrosis, and even benign breast disease occurring within residual breast tissue are also in the differential diagnosis (Box 21–3). For patients several years past radiation therapy, a radiation-induced sarcoma must also be considered.

If a patient has had reconstruction with an expander/implant, a chest wall recurrence is not typically hidden by the reconstructed breast

BOX 21–3 DIFFERENTIAL DIAGNOSIS OF A LOCAL CHEST WALL RECURRENCE

- Postradiation or postoperative change
- Foreign body cyst around suture material
- Cellulitis
- Fat necrosis
- A bony nodule on a rib or costal cartilage from surgical trauma
- Sarcoma (radiation-induced). These typically appear later, at a median of 10 years posttreatment.

because implants are usually placed submuscular. For patients who have had transverse rectus abdominis myocutaneous (TRAM) reconstruction, recurrences typically occur in the native skin/subcutaneous tissues at the junction between the TRAM tissues and native tissues. Recurrence in the TRAM is extremely rare; masses within the flap are more commonly fat necrosis, although these can mimic recurrent cancer. For patients who have had reconstruction after a mastectomy, mammography is sometimes used for surveillance. Typically this is done in patients who have had a TRAM flap as opposed to implants. Occasionally a TRAMogram-mammography will detect a local recurrence not identifiable on physical examination.

A rare form of local recurrence is an inflammatory recurrence. After breast conservation, an inflammatory recurrence may present as diffuse swelling and erythema of the intact breast, with the associated skin changes associated with inflammatory breast cancer (IBC) such as *peau d'orange*. These can be difficult to differentiate from true breast infections, significant breast lymphedema, or changes related to radiation therapy. Although rare, an inflammatory recurrence must be kept in mind and biopsies performed in any patient not responding to standard therapy. Inflammatory changes can also occur on the chest wall after a mastectomy. Diffuse infiltration of the skin and subcutaneous tissues of the chest wall, resulting in woody induration, ulceration, and nodules, is a distinct form of chest wall recurrence known as "carcinoma en cuirasse." Unfortunately, the tumor has often spread beyond standard surgical or radiation boundaries.

Diagnostic Workup of Local Recurrence

The first step in the workup of a patient suspected of a local recurrence is a biopsy. For palpable lesions, fine-needle aspiration biopsy (FNAB) is a quick, simple, and accurate way of differentiating between scar tissue and recurrent disease. However, false-positive and false-negative results are possible, so the results must be interpreted in light of the clinical suspicion. A negative or inconclusive FNAB of a clinically suspicious lesion mandates a more definitive biopsy. Core-needle or excisional biopsy will provide more definitive results and will provide tissue to assay for estrogen receptor/progesterone receptor (ER/PR) and human epidermal growth factor receptor 2 (HER-2/neu) expressions. These will not only help differentiate between a local recurrence and a second primary tumor, but will also help guide treatment decisions (Table 21-2).

Once the diagnosis of recurrent disease has been established, a complete staging workup is indicated to rule out distant metastases. This is particularly true for a chest wall recurrence after mastectomy, which is often referred to as a "harbinger of distant disease." It is estimated that approximately one third of women who have a chest wall recurrence have distant disease, one third will develop distant disease, and one third have an isolated local recurrence. Although the likelihood of discovering simultaneous distant disease in women with an IBTR is less, a metastatic workup is still indicated. One exception to this would be the woman with an in situ recurrence after BCT.

The staging examination typically includes a thorough history and physical, a computed tomography (CT) scan of the chest, abdomen, and pelvis and a radionuclide bone scan. CT scan or magnetic resonance imaging (MRI) of the head is not necessary in the absence of neurologic symptoms. Positron emission tomography (PET) scans have been increasingly used to restage patients with recurrent disease. PET scans have a higher sensitivity than CT scans and will occasionally detect metastases that would have been missed by CT. However, they have a decreased specificity and a false-positive rate of 10% or higher. A positive finding on a PET scan should prompt dedicated imaging of the region and tissue biopsy to confirm metastatic disease.

Treatment of Local Recurrence after Breast-Conserving Therapy

The standard approach to an IBTR, assuming the metastatic workup shows no evidence of distant disease, is mastectomy, with or without immediate reconstruction. Lumpectomy alone is inadequate, associated with a high risk of a second recurrence, and re-irradiaion is not recommended. Mastectomy can be performed with simultaneous reconstruction, although for patients with a high risk of a second local recurrence, such as those with significant skin involvement, it may be preferable to delay reconstruction. Between 80% and 90% of patients with an IBTR are amenable to a mastectomy. The remaining 10% to 20% recur with either advanced or inflammatory disease and should be treated with systemic therapy first. Many of these patients may respond to systemic therapy allowing for mastectomy.

TABLE 21–2 • *Local Recurrence versus Second Primary Tumor*

	True in-Breast Tumor Recurrence	Second Primary Tumor
Time to occurrence	Shorter	Longer
Histology	Similar to primary	Difference in histology, estrogen receptor/progesterone receptor (ER/PR) expression, human epidermal growth factor receptor 2 (Her-2) overexpression, flow cytometry
Location	Same region as primary tumor	Outside of boost volume
Implications on prognosis	Worse	Better

Unfortunately, some patients will be diagnosed with simultaneous distant metastases. In this situation, the curative potential of a simple mastectomy is limited. However, consideration should be given to a palliative mastectomy to control the locally recurrent disease. The decision to perform a mastectomy in the face of distant disease should take into consideration the volume of distant disease and projected survival, the ER/PR expression of the tumor, chemotherapy history and predicted response to systemic therapy, and the nature of the recurrence in the breast and associated symptoms.

The survival for patients with an IBTR who undergo mastectomy is worse than patients who were treated by BCT and did not experience a recurrence. The risk of distant disease ranges from 20% to 40% at 5 years. There are some factors associated with a significantly worse outcome after mastectomy for an IBTR (Box 21–4).

For the rare patient who was treated by lumpectomy alone, an IBTR can be treated by either mastectomy or lumpectomy followed by radiation. The volume of tissue that needs to be resected and the volume of tissue initially removed need to be taken into account because a second attempt at lumpectomy may result in an unfavorable cosmetic outcome.

Many patients who experience an IBTR after a lumpectomy and radiation are not willing to undergo mastectomy and are desirous of a second lumpectomy. Several series of women undergoing second attempts at breast conservation have been reported. These include patients undergoing lumpectomy alone and excision with reirradiation of the breast. Several of these series demonstrate a high rate of second local recurrences in the breast, and in some series, this is associated with a worse outcome. In addition, the cosmetic outcome may be inferior to that obtained with a mastectomy and reconstruction. In addition, the complication rate of reirradiating a breast is extremely high. Some investigators are examining the use of partial breast irradiation (PBI) as a method of reirradiating women after a lumpectomy for an IBTR, by means of either catheter-based or intracavitary brachytherapy or limited external beam irradiation. Although this may be feasible, this approach should still be considered investigational only.

Treatment of Local Recurrence after Mastectomy

In the patient with a chest wall recurrence and no evidence of distant disease, a multidisciplinary approach is needed for successful management. In this situation, combined modality treatment has the potential to provide long-term disease control. Even in the presence of distant metastases, optimal local treatment can significantly reduce the morbidity of uncontrolled local spread. The approach to therapy will depend on several factors (Box 21–5).

BOX 21–4 FACTORS ASSOCIATED WITH POOR OUTCOME AFTER IN-BREAST TUMOR RECURRENCE

- Inflammatory type of recurrence
- Stage of the primary tumor
- Interval between primary treatment and recurrence (disease-free interval)
- An invasive as compared to noninvasive tumor recurrence
- Large or advanced recurrent tumor, skin, or muscle involvement.
- Multicentric tumor recurrence
- Lack of hormone receptor expression

BOX 21–5 FACTORS TO CONSIDER WHEN PLANNING THERAPY FOR CHEST WALL RECURRENCE

- Extent of local disease (single versus multiple nodules)
- Resectability (need for skin grafts, tissue flaps, or chest wall resection)
- Comorbid conditions of the patient
- Disease-free interval
- History of postmastectomy radiation
- History of systemic therapy
- Present estrogen receptor/progesterone receptor status

The first decision to be made is whether the disease is surgically resectable. If it is, then the wide excision of all gross disease should be the first step. In some cases this will be a rather simple excision of the skin nodules with an adequate margin of normal skin. In other cases, skin grafting or a tissue flap may be necessary to fill in the defect. In rare cases, resection to negative margins may necessitate the resection of muscle or chest wall. Surgical intervention, however, should be planned with the intent of removing all gross disease. Leaving behind gross disease is associated with a high rate of subsequent chest wall failures as compared with patients who undergo complete excision. The potential for radiation therapy to maximize disease control is considerably improved by the excision of all gross disease. In cases in which this can only be accomplished by more extensive surgery needed to control disease, the benefits of surgery (potential for cure or palliation) must be weighed against the risks. Additional factors such as whether or not the patient is a candidate for radiation therapy or systemic therapy should be considered, and these patients are best evaluated within a multidisciplinary setting.

For patients who have had reconstruction, removal of an implant or TRAM flap is not always necessary. If complete surgical removal of the recurrence is possible, it should be undertaken. In patients who did not receive postmastectomy radiation, radiation to the reconstructed breast is also possible. However, it is important to note that in the case of an implant, capsular contracture is frequent, and in the case of a TRAM flap, contraction and shrinkage is possible.

For the patients who were initially treated by mastectomy alone, external beam radiation therapy is recommended after resection of the recurrent disease. The field to treat depends on the patient's previous treatment and extent of disease. Optimal management typically involves treatment to the entire chest wall and draining lymph node basins. This is true even if the local recurrence is isolated to a small area because the risk of subsequent failure in this area is high if radiation is limited to the chest wall. For the patient who has not undergone a previous ALND, treatment should include the chest wall, axillary, supraclavicular, and internal mammary lymph nodes. However, this may be altered by how the axilla is managed surgically.

A more difficult situation is the woman who underwent postmastectomy radiation and presents with a chest wall recurrence. Further radiation is generally frowned on given the significant risks of tissue damage and the low likelihood that it will control the disease. In selected cases, retreatment with limited doses of radiation can be used for palliative purposes, but this is unlikely to contribute to long-term cure. The need for radiation will also be influenced by whether systemic therapy is feasible. These cases should almost always be discussed, and treatment planned, in a multidisciplinary setting.

There are other options for women who have had a chest wall recurrence after mastectomy with radiation. Hyperthermia (in the temperature range from $104°$ F to $113°$ F [$40°$ C to $45°$ C]) has been shown to be cytotoxic. Initially, it was thought that the combination of radiation and hyperthermia would decrease local recurrence rates because the therapies are complementary, working through different mechanisms. Unfortunately, randomized trials failed to demonstrate any added benefit to hyperthermia, although these trials varied greatly in terms of both treatment plans and patient eligibility. For patients who have already had postmastectomy radiation, combined hyperthermia and radiation (with a decreased dose of radiation) remains an option, although reported local control rates vary.

Another approach being examined is photodynamic therapy (PDT). This uses a photosensitizing agent that is taken up by both normal and malignant tissue but is rapidly cleared from nonmalignant cells. Once accumulated in malignant tissue, the tumors are exposed to a laser light (the wavelength depends on the agent used), which induces a phototoxic reaction. This leads to selective necrosis of the tumor. PDT has been successfully used to treat cancers of the skin, bronchi, and esophagus but its use is limited by the depth to which the light penetrates. Several small series of PDT for chest wall recurrences have been reported with minimal toxicity, although the optimal agents and doses (of both agent and light) are still being worked out.

Management of the Axilla after Local Recurrence

As with primary breast cancer, a local recurrence may be associated with disease in the regional lymph nodes. This could either represent spread from the recurrent tumor or residual disease not diagnosed at the time of primary treatment. The approach to restaging the axilla has changed considerably over the past decade with the advent of SLN biopsy. Before SLN biopsy, almost all women who experienced an IBTR had already undergone an ALND. Today, however, many women with recurrences will have never undergone an ALND, having had a negative SLN biopsy at the time of their initial lumpectomy.

When faced with a local recurrence requiring surgical therapy, the surgeon must decide how to approach the regional lymph nodes (Fig. 21–1). This approach will depend on how the patient was initially treated and what adjuvant treatments are planned after surgery; thus the need for repeat axillary staging in the face

of a local recurrence requires a multidisciplinary approach. Factors to consider include the previous axillary surgery (none versus SLN biopsy versus ALND), the initial stage of disease and likelihood of distant metastases, and the impact of identifying regional disease on adjuvant therapy decisions. It should go without saying that any patient with a local recurrence should have a thorough physical examination and possibly an ultrasound of the axilla, with FNAB of any clinically suspicious lymph nodes.

For the patient with an IBTR who has already undergone a complete ALND and has no clinical evidence of regional disease, simple mastectomy alone is sufficient. SLN biopsy may be attempted in this situation, and although there may be drainage to a residual axillary node, there is a high likelihood of aberrant drainage patterns, with the lymphoscintigraphy showing uptake in the supraclavicular, internal mammary nodes (IMN), or contralateral axillary nodes (Fig. 21–2). The surgeon must decide what the benefit to the patient would be in going after these sentinel nodes, either on preventing further recurrence or adjuvant therapy decisions.

For the woman with an invasive recurrence after BCT for ductal carcinoma in situ (DCIS), SLN biopsy is recommended at the time of mastectomy. For the woman with an IBTR who did not undergo ALND, such as the woman with a

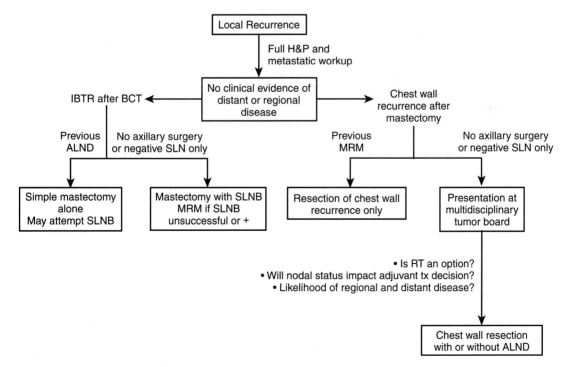

Figure 21–1. Management of lymph nodes in the face of a local recurrence.

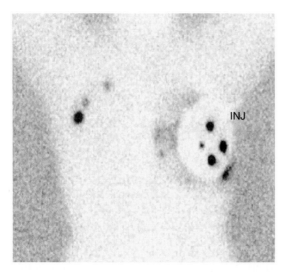

Figure 21-2. Lymphoscintigraphy showing uptake in the contralateral axilla in a patient who had previous ipsilateral axillary surgery.

negative SLN, repeat axillary staging with lymphatic mapping and SLN biopsy is still a reasonable option. Several studies have demonstrated the feasibility of SLN biopsy in patients who have had prior breast surgery including BCT. This includes women who have undergone prior axillary surgery, including a previous SLN biopsy. The surgeon should plan ahead of time what will occur if the lymphatic mapping is unsuccessful. Although less common than with a previous ALND, patients with previous SLN biopsy may have aberrant axillary drainage. Again, when planning on remapping a patient with a local recurrence, the surgeon must be prepared to chase the SLN to more unusual locations, with the decision how to proceed based on how the information will affect further treatment.

For the patient who presents with a chest wall recurrence after a modified radical mastectomy (MRM), with no clinical evidence of regional recurrence, he or she does not require any specific addressing of the axilla. However, patients who have the axillary nodes intact (either no SLN was performed, or the SLN was negative) are a more difficult situation. With no intact breast, SLN biopsy is not feasible. Therefore, these patients face two choices. The first is to only address the chest wall recurrence, ignoring the axilla. The second is to perform an ALND at the time of the resection of the chest wall recurrence. The surgeon must balance the potential in leaving behind resectable nodal disease against the fact that many patients may harbor distant disease and that radiation

or systemic therapy may handle microscopic regional disease. Again, this decision must be made in a multidisciplinary setting, taking into account how treatment might change if an ALND is performed. If the patient will be receiving chest wall radiation therapy, the axillary basin will likely be included, so ALND might not be needed (and the combination of radiation therapy and ALND carries a high risk of lymphedema). For patients who have had postmastectomy radiation but have an intact axilla (a relatively small population as positive nodes are the most common reason for postmastectomy radiation therapy), an ALND should be performed. Whether the finding of regional disease would impact the medical oncologist's decision to offer systemic therapy should also be taken into consideration.

Regional Recurrence

In addition to local recurrences, patients may present with regional recurrences, either isolated or in conjunction with an in-breast or chest wall recurrence. Regional nodal recurrences are relatively rare, occurring in only 1% to 3% of cases. There was some concern that this may increase with the use of SLN; however, early reports suggest a similarly low regional recurrence rate for patients with a negative SLN who do not undergo ALND. Most regional recurrences are detected on routine physical examination, although occasionally they are detected on surveillance imaging. The presence of a palpable mass in the axilla or supraclavicular fossa should be considered recurrence until proven otherwise. In some cases, patients may present new onset lymphedema, pain in the arm and shoulder, or increasing sensory or motor loss in the arm or hand. These latter symptoms are often the result of brachial plexus involvement. These symptoms may also be caused by cervical spine metastases. CT, MRI, and bone scan can help make the diagnosis and should be considered in any patient with new onset pain, paralysis, paresthesias, or lymphedema, even in the absence of palpable disease.

Internal mammary recurrences often present as a deep, fixed mass in an intercostal space at the ipsilateral sternal border. These often first present with pain and tenderness, without a noticeable mass. It may be difficult to differentiate from a chest wall recurrence or sternal metastasis. Also in the differential of parasternal pain are costochondritis (Tietze syndrome), neuroma, or radiation-induced sarcoma. Persistent pain should prompt a CT, bone scan, or MRI to make the diagnosis.

The first step in the approach to regional recurrence, as with local recurrence, is to rule out distant disease. In addition to a complete history and physical, patients should have a CT of the chest/abdomen/pelvis and a bone scan. Again, PET scans have also been used in this situation or when the results of the CT or bone scan are equivocal.

If there is no evidence of distant disease, the patient should still be approached with curative intent, although the likelihood of cure changes with the location of the regional disease. Isolated axillary recurrences are most amenable to treatment and are associated with the best long-term survival. Patients with disease in other nodal regions are highly likely to develop distant metastases, and they have a poor outcome.

Treatment of Axillary Recurrence

As with local recurrence, the management paradigms for regional recurrence are in a state of flux given the changes in locoregional management (SLN biopsy, postmastectomy radiation). If there is no evidence of distant disease and the recurrence is surgically resectable, then this should be the initial approach. For patients who had a previous SLN biopsy but the axillary nodes are intact, resection involves a complete ALND. For patients who had a previous ALND, resection is still recommended, although this may be more technically challenging. The surgeon should make every attempt to resect the entire area of recurrent disease. In a previously operated on axilla, this may be difficult and require resection of muscle or sacrifice of axillary structures such as the thoracodorsal or long thoracic nerve. MRI may be helpful in planning surgery and determining the necessary extent. If the axillary recurrence seems difficult to resect, or unresectable (chest wall involvement, brachial plexus involvement), preoperative therapy should be considered to improve the likelihood of complete resection. Intraoperatively, the surgeon must assess the adequacy of the original ALND. In many cases of an axillary recurrence after ALND, it becomes apparent that only a superficial clearance or level I only dissection was performed. In this case, a formal level I and II dissection should be performed.

If patients are unresectable, even after systemic therapy, radiation is used, although the ability of radiation to control gross regional disease is limited, and this is primarily palliative. If the disease is resected, the question

remains as to whether postoperative radiation therapy should be used. Factors to be weighed include the previous use of radiation therapy (it is important to know the exact fields used if the patient had previous BCT), the nature of the recurrence, and the surgery performed. It is important to remember that the combination of surgery and radiation to the axilla carries high risks of brachial plexus injury and chronic lymphedema, but so does uncontrolled disease within the axilla.

If the patient had an ALND for a regional recurrence after a negative SLN, then surgery alone may be satisfactory if the recurrence is limited and the resection complete. For patients at a high risk of a second regional recurrence (multiple involved nodes, extracapsular extension), and no history of radiation to the axillary basin, radiation therapy should be strongly considered. Radiation should also be used after resection in patients with no history of axillary radiation and a regional recurrence after an ALND. A more difficult situation is the patient who has had axillary radiation. Limited field reirradiation may be considered if the disease can not be completely resected.

Management of Supraclavicular Recurrence

Patients with an isolated supraclavicular recurrence have worse outcomes than patients with axillary recurrences, with a high rate of distant disease. There has been extensive discussion as to whether or not this should be considered a regional recurrence or systemic disease, with little published data to help guide treatment decisions. Multimodality therapy is the rule, and with an aggressive approach, a small fraction of patients with an isolated supraclavicular recurrence may be cured. The sequence of therapy has not been established. Systemic therapy is typically performed first. The patient should then be restaged. If there is still no evidence of distant disease, surgery and radiation therapy should be considered. Again, the decision needs to be based on whether the field has been previously radiated, the feasibility of resection, and the likelihood of a second supraclavicular recurrence after surgery (Fig. 21–3).

Use of Systemic Therapy after Locoregional Recurrence

The use of systemic therapy in patients who have had a locoregional recurrence but have

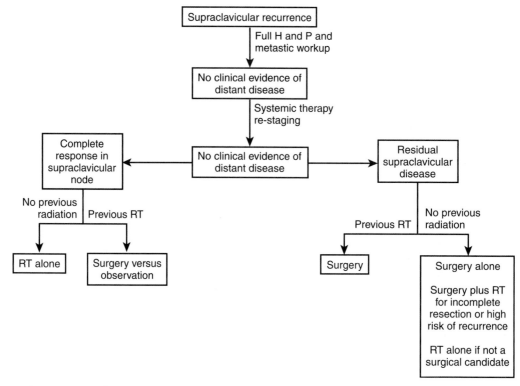

Figure 21–3. Approach to the patient with a supraclavicular recurrence.

no evidence of distant disease remains an unanswered question. Because there is a high risk of distant recurrence among any patient who suffers an in-breast, chest wall or regional recurrence, it is usually recommended, especially considering the large and expanding list of agents. However, there is little data documenting the benefit, if any, on survival. A Cochrane review of systemic therapy in women with a locoregional recurrence of breast cancer concluded that there was insufficient evidence to support this practice. For this reason, randomized trials are ongoing. The International Breast Cancer Study Group (IBCSG) is conducting a trial in which patients undergoing surgery for locally or locoregionally recurrent breast cancer are randomly assigned to chemotherapy (with the regimen chosen at the discretion of the investigator) or no chemotherapy. Patients with hormone-receptor-positive tumors also receive hormone therapy, and the use of trastuzumab (Herceptin) is optional for women with Her2-positive tumors. Patients with resected disease should be strongly encouraged to participate in this trial.

Whether the recurrent disease is to be initially resected or not, it is imperative for the surgeon to obtain enough tissue to perform ER, PR, and Her-2-neu staining on. This information will help guide systemic therapy decisions. It is not sufficient to rely upon the ER/PR/Her-2 neu status of the primary tumor because the recurrence may be quite different. Even when the tumor was originally ER/PR negative, the recurrence may be ER/PR positive (although this is not common). If the diagnosis of recurrence was made by FNAB, and systemic therapy before resection is a consideration, a core biopsy or excisional biopsy should be performed. If the disease is resectable, then immunohistochemistry (IHC) staining can be performed on the specimen.

For women who are not participating in the randomized trial, systemic therapy should be considered. For women who are ER/PR positive, hormonal therapy is typically recommended. An aromatase inhibitor (AI) is often used in postmenopausal women, particularly if they have already had treatment with tamoxifen, but also if she has not had any adjuvant hormonal therapy. A selective estrogen receptor modulator (SERM) should be used in women who recurred within 1 year of treatment with an AI or in premenopausal women. An alternative approach for premenopausal women is ovarian suppression/ablation.

Whether chemotherapy should be added to hormonal therapy in women who are ER/PR positive is unclear, and a thorough discussion of the known and unknown risks and benefits must be discussed with the patient. A stronger argument for chemotherapy can be made in the patient whose recurrence is not hormone responsive.

The success of trastuzumab in conjunction with doxorubicin and taxane-based chemotherapy in the adjuvant setting for patients expressing Her-2 neu strongly suggests that women with locoregional recurrences who are Her-2/neu positive and did not previously receive trastuzumab, should be treated.

As previously discussed, in some cases of an isolated regional recurrence, induction systemic therapy should be considered. These include cases in which resection would be difficult or in which the likelihood of distant recurrence is extremely high. Examples include the large chest wall or axillary recurrence where adjacent structures may need to be resected to obtain negative margins or the isolated supraclavicular recurrence. The need to present these patients in a multidisciplinary setting before proceeding with surgical therapy can not be overemphasized.

Surgery in Stage IV Disease

Unfortunately, many patients will recur not with local or regional disease, but with metastatic disease. When patients present with metastatic disease, the goals of therapy shift from cure to palliation. Patients with metastatic breast cancer are unlikely to be cured. Goals of therapy shift to symptom control, improved quality of life, and prolongation of survival. This approach centers almost exclusively on systemic therapy, with surgery and radiation reserved for rare situations in which they can provide palliation (such as surgery for an enlarging or ulcerating mass or radiation for bone metastases).

There is, however, some evidence that surgical resection of metastatic disease may play a role in the treatment of breast cancer. A subset of stage IV patients has limited systemic tumor burden or biologically indolent disease. Although complete remissions are rare, approximately 5% to 10% of patients with stage IV disease will survive over 5 years, and 2% to 5% may be cured of their disease. These patients tend to be younger and healthier with limited metastatic disease. In this situation, there may be a benefit to multimodality therapy, including surgery, not only to prevent complications (which may postpone the need for more toxic systemic therapy) but also to improve progression-free survival.

Although there are multiple articles suggesting that surgery of stage IV disease may prolong survival, it is imperative to remember that these are exclusively retrospective reviews and observational studies, which all suffer from tremendous selection bias. There are no randomized trials showing resection of metastatic disease improves survival, and it is unlikely there ever will be as the number of eligible patients would be small, and few patients agree to be randomized between surgery and no surgery. Care must be taken when interpreting this data and applying it to individual patients.

Patient Selection for Surgery

When faced with a patient with potentially resectable stage IV disease, a careful assessment of the patient's medical condition, the extent and biology of the cancer, and the feasibility and risks of complete resection is necessary. Many surgeons would approach these patients with the idea of "looking for a reason not to operate." In other words, a thorough search for metastatic disease should be undertaken to be sure they do not have additional disease elsewhere. This may include not only CT scan and bone scan, but also PET scan. Although the role of PET scanning in the diagnostic evaluation of breast cancer is evolving, this represents one situation in which it may be of significant benefit. PET scanning appears to be more sensitive than other imaging modalities for the detection of distant metastatic disease (with the exception of brain secondary to the high background activity of gray matter).

In many cases it is important not to proceed with or exclude surgery based on imaging studies alone. Pulmonary nodules on CT may be granulomatous disease. A solitary pulmonary nodule may be a primary lung cancer rather than a metastatic breast cancer, especially in a smoker. An adnexal mass on a CT in a woman with breast cancer is more likely to be of nonbreast origin than a breast cancer metastasis. These may be benign or primary ovarian cancers. Although breast cancer is the second most common cancer to metastasize to the adrenal gland (lung is the first), many newly diagnosed adrenal masses may be hyperplasia, fatty involvement, or nonfunctioning adenomas. Even an intracranial lesion may represent a meningioma. FNAB, core-needle, or open biopsy may be necessary to avoid misdiagnosis. PET

BOX 21–6 FACTORS WHEN CONSIDERING RESECTION OF STAGE IV DISEASE

- Patient age
- Comorbidities
- Ability to tolerate resection
- Likelihood of complete resection
- Single-organ versus multiple-organ disease
- Solitary versus multiple lesions
- Disease-free interval
- Estrogen receptor/progesterone receptor (ER/PR) status
- Human epidermal growth factor receptor 2 (Her-2/neu) status
- Options for postsurgical systemic therapy

scans also have a significant false-positive rate, and suspicious areas should be worked up with more focused imaging and possible biopsy.

Once a thorough workup has been completed, several factors must be weighed when considering whether resection is reasonable (Box 21–6). The most significant issue is the performance status of the patient and an estimation of the relative risks of a planned operation. Patients with significant medical comorbidities should be not be considered ideal candidates for resection given the high rates of postoperative morbidity and mortality. Patients evaluated for lung resection should have a complete pulmonary evaluation, whereas those being considered for liver resection should have relatively preserved liver function.

The best candidates for surgery are those with single organ involvement. The overwhelming majority of studies examining metastasectomy for breast cancer are limited to patients with disease limited to one organ. Most oncologists consider the presence of disease outside one organ to be a contraindication to surgery. There are some reports of resection in the presence of additional disease, such as hepatic resection in the face of both liver and bone disease, the argument being that metastatic bone disease is more indolent and has a more prolonged natural history. However, this situation should be limited to patients who have well-controlled or stable disease.

Even better than single-organ disease are patients with only one metastatic focus. Solitary metastases appear to have a better outcome after surgery than multiple metastases.

For example, patients undergoing resection of a single lung metastasis appear to have a longer survival than patients undergoing resection of two or more lesions. This may be related to biology but may also be representative of the ability to achieve a compete resection. This is particularly true in the setting of hepatic metastases, in which the ability to achieve a complete resection while retaining a sufficient volume of functional liver and the location of the lesions are probably more important considerations. Bilobar disease or location close to the porta hepatis is usually considered a contraindication to resection. Complete resection appears to be associated with a significantly better outcome than incomplete in most series.

An important factor to consider is disease-free survival (DFS). The interval between the diagnosis of the primary breast cancer and the development of distant disease is an important prognostic indicator for any patient with metastatic breast cancer, reflective of the underlying biology of the disease. A longer disease-free interval (DFI) is associated with a better outcome after resection of all forms of metastatic disease. What remains unclear is whether their prolonged survival is secondary to the surgery or whether they have more indolent disease and would have survived just as long without surgical intervention.

Another consideration is the postsurgery systemic therapy options for the patient. Although there is no clear evidence suggesting a benefit to continuing systemic therapy after metastasectomy, this is a frequent strategy and is supported by some retrospective series. Many series suggest that ER positivity is associated with a better outcome after surgery of stage IV disease, most likely as a result of the benefit of ongoing endocrine therapy.

Resection of Specific Metastatic Sites

Lung Metastases

From 10% to 25% of patients with breast cancer that develop metastatic disease will have disease that is limited to the lung. In many cases, this will represent bilateral disease, precluding resection. However, for the patient with a solitary pulmonary nodule, resection should be strongly considered. One reason is that more than 50% of single solid pulmonary nodules in patients with a history of breast cancer will be other types of tumors, such as primary lung cancer, which may be amenable to curative resection. Beyond that, there is the potential for long-term survival. Pulmonary metastasectomy provides an opportunity for long-term survival in patients with stage IV breast cancer. In retrospective series, 5-year survival rates range from 31% to 80%, and median survival durations are between 42 and 79 months. In the largest series of 467 patients derived from the International Registry of Lung Metastases, survival rates were 38% and 20% after 5 and 15 years, respectively. Long-term benefit from resection has also been suggested in two nonrandomized series comparing surgically treated patients with those treated by other means. However, in the absence of randomized trials, it is difficult to know for certain if these results are better than could have been achieved without surgery and whether the results are secondary to selection bias. Patients may have not been recommended surgery because of poor prognostic signs (i.e., multiple metastases, short DFI) or low performance status. Even for patients with more than one nodule, resection may be feasible. Based on the data from the International Registry of Lung Metastases, the prognosis of patients with pulmonary metastases after pulmonary metastasectomy can be stratified into four groups (Table 21–3).

Liver Metastases

The liver is involved in over one half of patients with metastatic breast cancer, but it is rare to find isolated liver disease (5% to 12% of stage IV patients) and liver involvement is a poor prognostic sign. With modern chemotherapy, the median survival for patients with liver only metastatic disease is approximately 22 to 27 months. Although the resection of liver metastases from colon cancer is common, the resection of breast cancer metastases to the liver is less common and more controversial. However, for patients who are appropriately selected, liver resection may prolong survival to a greater extent than standard nonsurgical therapies. In retrospective series, 5-year survival rates for resectable patients range from 18% to 59%. Although the absence of randomized trials makes it difficult to know with certainty that these outcomes are better than can be achieved with systemic therapy alone, the reported long-term survival rates among selected patients seem higher than can be achieved with chemotherapy alone.

The ideal candidate (albeit rare) has a solitary metastasis, no evidence of extrahepatic metastatic disease, normal liver function, a good performance status, and a long DFI after treatment of the primary tumor. An essential part of the workup in patients who are considered for hepatectomy is precise imaging of the liver with either helical CT or MRI and full staging to rule out distant disease, possibly with the use of PET scanning. If multiple nodules can be resected, it may still be a consideration, but bilobar disease should be considered a contraindication to resection. Initial laparoscopic exploration may spare unresectable patients the morbidity of a laparotomy because up to one half of patients even considered for resection are discovered to have diffuse liver lesions or peritoneal dissemination at the time of laparotomy.

Because of the limited number of patients with isolated liver metastases who are candidates for resection, other forms of liver-directed therapy have been explored. The majority of these are ablative techniques that were introduced for the treatment of unresectable primary hepatocellular cancer or colorectal metastases, including percutaneous ethanol injection, cryotherapy, radiofrequency ablation (RFA), and

TABLE 21–3 • *International Registry of Lung Metastases Stratification of Patients Undergoing Pulmonary Metastasectomy*						
	Resection	Disease-Free Survival (Months)	Number of Metastases	5-Year Survival Rate (%)	10-Year Survival Rate (%)	Median Survival (Months)
Group I	Complete	≥36	Solitary	50	26	59
Group II	Complete	<36	Solitary	35	21	36
Group III	Complete	<36	Multiple	13	13	2
Group IV	Incomplete	—	—	18	—	25

interstitial laser therapy. Because of its ease of delivery and efficacy, RFA has evolved into the treatment of choice for the ablation of metastatic tumors involving the liver, including breast cancer; it has largely replaced cryosurgical ablation. RFA entails the local application of radiofrequency thermal energy to a lesion, in which a high frequency alternating current moves from the tip of an electrode into the tissue surrounding that electrode. As the ions within the tissue attempt to follow the change in the direction of the alternating current, their movement results in frictional heating of the tissue. As the temperature within the tissue becomes elevated beyond 140° F (60° C), cells begin to die, resulting in a region of necrosis surrounding the electrode. Another potential use for RFA is in patients who appear to have isolated, potentially resectable liver metastases as a temporizing maneuver while awaiting interval reevaluation to ensure the absence of extrahepatic disease.

Brain Metastases

Although 10% to 16% of women with stage IV breast cancer have brain involvement, making it the second most common cause of brain metastases, like liver metastases, brain metastases typically occur late in the course of the disease and are rarely isolated. Brain metastases are associated with a poor prognosis, with a median survival (untreated) of only 1 to 2 months. Whole brain radiation therapy (WBRT) provides effective but brief palliation (symptoms return within months) and increases median survival to 4 to 6 months. Systemic chemotherapy may provide similar benefits.

In the one third of patients with brain metastases who have no evidence of extracranial disease, a small subset will have solitary brain metastases, and these patients may be amenable to treatment. Surgical resection is associated with improved outcomes relative to WBRT alone and can provide rapid and more durable symptom palliation. Uncontrolled series suggest median survival durations of 16 to 37 months can be achieved in highly selected patients. Thus, surgical resection should be considered in selected patients with solitary metastases without extracranial disease. Surgery should only rarely be considered in patients with more than one brain metastasis, except possibly if one large symptomatic lesion predominates.

Over the last decade, stereotactic radiosurgery (SRS) has emerged as an appealing alternative to resection in patients with a limited number of cerebral metastases. SRS combines the principle of stereotactic localization to achieve accurate targeting with multiple convergent radiation beams of equal intensity to deliver a high radiation dose to a well-defined area within the brain. SRS has been used as a primary treatment for single or multiple lesions, as a means of administering a local "boost" to a brain metastasis after WBRT and also for salvage therapy in patients who recur following surgery or WBRT. Whether or not the results with SRS are better than can be achieved with resection is difficult to ascertain. Although there is no question that SRS represents a reasonable alternative to surgery for patients who are not surgical candidates (because of location, comorbidity), a randomized trial directly comparing both treatments has not been conducted. In the absence of data from randomized trials, the choice of SRS over surgery in patients with solitary lesions is typically based on the size and accessibility of the lesion, presence or absence of symptoms, and the patient's functional status. Because the risk of neurotoxicity and local failure is higher with larger lesions, SRS is best reserved for lesions with a diameter of 3 cm or less. Surgery offers the best potential for immediate decompression of large solitary symptomatic lesions, whereas for smaller asymptomatic lesions, it is reasonable to consider either surgery or SRS.

Bone Metastases

Bone is the most common site of metastatic involvement in breast cancer, and in comparison to other sites of spread, is typically characterized by an indolent course and good response to endocrine maneuvers. In approximately 20% of cases, bone metastases are solitary, and in such cases, radiation therapy can provide effective pain relief and prevent fracture. RFA has also been used to treat painful individual bone. Given the relative effectiveness of systemic therapy and radiation or RFA, there is a limited role for resection as a curative option for the majority of bone metastases. Surgery is used for the palliative treatment of epidural spinal cord or nerve compression syndromes and to reduce or prevent bone metastasis-associated fractures. One exception in which a curative resection of a bone metastases may be indicated is in the sternum.

For the rare situation where bone involvement is limited to the sternum, potentially curative surgical resection may be considered.

Isolated sternal involvement may be metastatic disease, but it may also represent locoregional recurrence from the breast or internal mammary nodes. Also, possibly because there is no communication with the paravertebral venous plexus through which cancer cells can spread to other bones, sternal metastases may remain solitary for a long time. Sternal resection can provide optimal local control, palliate thoracic pain, prevent the complications associated with progressive sternal disease, and may be associated with prolonged relapse-free survival.

Breast Surgery in the Face of Stage IV Disease

Approximately 3% of women with newly diagnosed breast cancer have metastatic disease at the time of presentation. Until recently, the general rule was that there was no indication for breast surgery in this setting unless it was needed for palliative purposes. This was based on the idea that once metastatic disease is present, aggressive local therapy would have no impact on outcome. Other than a biopsy to confirm the diagnosis and perform immunohistochemical staining, the breast tumor was left in place and monitored as a measure of response to therapy.

Several retrospective reviews have raised the possibility that breast surgery in the presence of known metatstatic disease may improve survival. These range from single institution reviews to large database studies. Across these studies, a consistent improvement in survival is seen in the women who had complete resection of their primary tumor. This holds even when the analysis is adjusted for age, nature of the metastatic disease and the use of systemic therapy. Several biologic theories have been proposed, including the idea that surgery prevents continued dissemination of disease from the primary, increases immune recognition or removed growth factors produced by the primary that influence distant metastases. However, there are other explanations for this as well. It is possible that many of the patients who had excellent outcomes after surgery in the face of stage IV disease were actually incorrectly classified (e.g. a CT showing what were thought to be pulmonary metastases were actually benign). The more likely explanation is that these retrospective studies reflect a significant selection bias. Patients who are younger, healthier and have more controllable disease are selected for surgery while patients expected to have a lower survival are not offered surgery. Many patients receive chemotherapy first in this setting, and so surgery may be reserved for those with a good response to systemic therapy.

Only a randomized trial will answer whether routine resection of the primary tumor in the face of metastatic disease can impact survival, and while this trial faces significant hurdles, it is being planned. Until then, when faced with this situation, the surgeon must weigh several factors in deciding whether to offer the stage IV patient primary breast surgery. These include their age and co-morbidities, the surgery that would be necessary for control (lumpectomy vs. mastectomy), the predicted response to systemic therapy (size, grade, nodal status, ER, PR and Her-2/neu status) or the demonstrated response to systemic therapy, the number and sites of the metastases (single vs. multiple, bone-only vs. visceral), and the palliative benefit of resection. Primary breast surgery may be appropriate in selected patients with metastatic disease.

Principles of Systemic Therapy for Metastatic Breast Cancer

Although a subset of patients with stage IV breast cancer may benefit from surgery, this reflects a small number of patients even when a liberal use of surgery in stage IV disease is applied. The management of metastatic breast cancer is primarily systemic and is not considered curative. The goals of treating patients with stage IV cancer are to prolong survival, particularly symptom-free survival, thus improving quality of life (Box 21–7). The goal of the medical oncologist is to balance the symptoms caused by the cancer versus the symptoms caused by the systemic therapies. This is complex because the natural history of advanced breast cancer can be quite prolonged and treatment may involve multiple regimens of chemotherapy, which are constantly adjusted based on tumor response and patient symptoms.

BOX 21–7 GOALS OF SYSTEMIC THERAPY IN STAGE IV DISEASE

- Prolong survival
- Alleviate symptoms
- Prevent tumor-related complications
- Improve quality of life

When patients are first diagnosed with stage IV breast cancer, a thorough staging must be performed to delineate the extent of disease, and a detailed history and physical examination are performed looking to evaluate the patient's present symptoms and quality of life. A biopsy of a metastatic lesion should be considered not only to document true stage IV disease (as compared with a false-positive study) but also to see if the cancer is hormone-receptor positive and Her-2/neu positive. The decision to initiate therapy is then based on both the history and the tumor biology. Patients with minimal symptoms and hormone sensitive tumors are usually begun on endocrine therapy. There is no survival advantage to starting chemotherapy or combined chemotherapy/endocrine therapy at this point as compared with endocrine therapy alone.

For patients who have hormone-receptor-negative disease or have tumors that are refractory to hormonal therapy, chemotherapy is considered. This is not mandatory because patients with minimal symptoms may be observed. However, patients with tumor-related symptoms or have a heavy tumor burden (particularly visceral disease) are given chemotherapy. Patients with significant symptoms or in visceral crisis are started on chemotherapy in combination with endocrine therapy if they are hormone sensitive. Patients overexpressing Her-2/neu are generally started on Herceptin.

The likelihood of responding to chemotherapy depends on several factors, including the tumor biology, the DFI since initial treatment, whether adjuvant chemotherapy was used and what agents, the number of regimens they have already received for their stage IV disease, and the sites of the disease. When the disease progresses in the face of treatment, the regimen is typically changed. Sometimes, patients who have had extended periods of response or stable disease may be taken off therapy ("chemo holiday"). The likelihood of response and duration of response tends to be greatest with first-line chemotherapy and decreases with each subsequent line of treatment.

The median survival for patients with stage IV breast cancer is typically 2 to 3 years but this is widely variable and a large number of patients (as high as 20%) may live for many years. Although there is no randomized data comparing chemotherapy to no treatment, the retrospective data would suggest that survival is prolonged in patients being treated because patients who respond tend to live longer than those who do not. However, although survival may be prolonged, it is important that patients understand that cure is highly unlikely.

At some point, the cancer will no longer respond to treatment and the side effects of the therapy start to outweigh the benefits. Participation in clinical trials of new agents remains an option at this point and is generally strongly encouraged, although patients should be counseled that these trials are unlikely to significantly alter the course of the disease. Eventually, and this point is different for all patients, purely palliative or "best supportive care" may be the most appropriate choice.

Suggested Readings

1. Clemons M, Danson S, Hamilton T, et al. Locoregionally recurrent breast cancer: incidence, risk factors and survival. Cancer Treat Rev 2001;27:67–82.
2. Easson AM, McCready DR. Management of local recurrence of breast cancer. Expert Rev Anticancer Ther 2004;4(2):219–226.
3. Newman EA, Cimmino VM, Sabel MS, et al. Lymphatic mapping and sentinel lymph node biopsy for patients with local recurrence after breast-conservation therapy. Ann Surg Oncol 2006;13(1):52–57
4. Wright FC, Walker J, Law L, et al. Outcomes after localized axillary node recurrence in breast cancer. Ann Surg Oncol 2003;10:1054–1058.

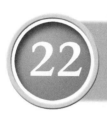

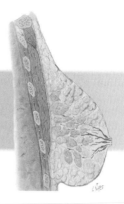

Breast Cancer in Special Populations

Breast Cancer in Special Populations: Key Points

- Understand the incidence and risk factors for male breast cancer.
- Know the surgical and adjuvant treatment for male breast cancer.
- Describe your approach to the patient who is pregnant presenting with breast cancer.
- Know when pregnancy is and is not a contraindication to imaging, surgery and anesthesia, radiation therapy, chemotherapy, or hormonal therapy.
- Understand how age may impact decisions in breast cancer treatment.
- Know the disparities that exist between African American and Anglo American women and the possible explanations.
- Understand the differences in presentation, histology, and stage of breast cancer among African Americans compared with Anglo Americans.

Male Breast Cancer

Although breast cancer is the most common malignancy among women, it is extremely rare among men. In 2008, there were an estimated 1990 new cases of male breast cancer, which represents only 1% of all breast cancer cases and 450 deaths. Male breast cancer shares many of the same characteristics with female breast cancer, although there are some stark differences. The median age of onset of male breast cancer is 66, approximately 10 years older than for females. Several risk factors have been identified for breast cancer in men (Box 22–1). Many of these are related to alterations in estrogen/androgen balance because androgens appear to have a protective effect on breast tissue by inhibiting cell proliferation. However, the relationship between hormones and male breast cancer is not clear because men with breast cancer do not exhibit abnormalities in peripherally detectable hormone levels. In addition, other conditions that result in increased estrogen, such as obesity, thyroid disease, marijuana use, or exogenous estrogen use do not seem to increase the risk of breast cancer.

A family history of breast cancer is present in approximately 15% to 20% of cases. Breast cancer gene (BRCA) 2 mutations are associated with a 6% lifetime risk of male breast cancer, which might not sound high compared to the risk in females, but represents a 100-fold higher risk compared to the general population. BRCA2 mutations are responsible for between 5% and 15% of male breast cancers. BRCA1 mutations do not have as significant a role. Male breast cancers in BRCA2 carriers may exhibit a more

BOX 22–1 RISK FACTORS FOR MALE BREAST CANCER

Gynecomastia or previous benign breast disease
Jewish ancestry
Family history of breast cancer
Previous chest wall irradiation
Testicular disease (orchitis, cryptorchidism, congenital inguinal hernia, infertility, orchiectomy, injury)
Liver disease (cirrhosis, alcoholic liver disease, schistosomiasis)
Klinefelter syndrome
Prolactinoma
Breast cancer gene (BRCA) 2 mutation
Cowden syndrome (PTEN mutation)

aggressive phenotype, with higher grade and overexpression of human epidermal growth factor receptor 2 (Her-2/neu). A mutation in the tumor suppressor gene PTEN, which is associated with Cowden syndrome, or the mismatch repair gene hMLH1 have also been reported in patients with male breast cancer, although whether or not there is a causal relationship remains unclear.

Clinical Presentation and Workup

The typical presentation of male breast cancer is that of a painless, firm subareolar mass. Less commonly, it may present as a mass in the upper, outer quadrant. Because there is minimal breast tissue, the nipple is commonly involved (ulceration, retraction) although nipple discharge is rare. The mass may be fixed to the overlying skin or underlying muscle. The differential diagnosis would include gynecomastia, infection (abscess), or a nonbreast primary such as sarcoma.

Mammogram is helpful, being abnormal in 80% to 90% of cases, and can help differentiation between gynecomastia and breast cancer. However, false-negatives do occur and so a tissue diagnosis is warranted for any suspicious mass in the breast. This should be either a core biopsy or open biopsy because fine-needle aspiration (FNA) can be inaccurate. Invasive ductal carcinoma represents more than 90% of cases; invasive lobular is rare. Ductal carcinoma in situ (DCIS) is also rare in men. Over 90% of male breast cancers express estrogen receptor (ER) and progesterone receptor (PR). The her-2/neu protooncogene is less likely to be overexpressed in men than in women. Staging workup is similar to that of female breast cancer. A full history and physical should be performed looking for signs or symptoms of metastatic disease. Ultrasound of the breast and axilla are often performed because sentinel lymph node (SLN) biopsy can be avoided if an ultrasound-guided FNA can document nodal metastases preoperatively. Computed tomography (CT) scan and bone scan should be obtained if the patient has signs or symptoms suggestive of metastatic disease.

Treatment

Localized male breast cancer is treated by mastectomy. Radical mastectomy should not be necessary unless there is extensive chest wall involvement. Given the lack of breast tissue and central location of the tumors, breast-conserving therapy (BCT) is not typically considered. Radiation is typically not recommended after mastectomy, although recommendations have been made to use postmastectomy radiation therapy for the same indications you would use in women (locally advanced disease or multiple positive axillary nodes) to decrease the likelihood of locoregional recurrence.

The management of the axilla has changed with the advent of SLN biopsy. Although modified radical mastectomy has been the standard, SLN has been shown to be successful in men as well and may spare the morbidity of axillary lymph node dissection (ALND) for patients who are node negative. Patients with a positive sentinel node should have a complete lymph node dissection. As with female breast cancer, the number of positive nodes correlates with survival. Patients with histologically negative nodes have a 10-year disease-specific survival between 77% and 84%. This drops to around 50% with one to three positive nodes and 14% to 24% for four or more positive nodes (Table 22–1).

Adjuvant Systemic Therapy

The recommendation for adjuvant therapy is based largely on the benefits seen in women and small retrospective reports (compared to historical controls) because breast cancer in men is too uncommon to perform randomized trials. Because the majority of cases are hormone-receptor positive, 5 years of adjuvant tamoxifen is frequently recommended. However, men have more difficulty than women tolerating the side effects and may not last the full 5 years (Box 22–2). Chemotherapy is also typically recommended for men at high risk of recurrence as it is in women, although chemotherapy

BOX 22–2 SIDE EFFECTS OF TAMOXIFEN IN MEN

Decreased libido
Weight gain
Hot flashes
Mood alteration
Depression

appears to be used less often in men when compared stage by stage. The indications are the same as for women, node-positive disease or tumor size greater than 1 cm. Chemotherapy should also be considered for men with hormone-receptor-negative disease. Her-2/neu and p53 expression have been associated with poor prognosis and may push toward more aggressive systemic therapy. The choice of agents is also similar to women, with anthracycline-based chemotherapy for patients who are node negative, and anthracyclines and taxanes for patients who are node positive.

With adequate therapy, the 5-year survival by American Joint Committee on Cancer (AJCC) tumor stage is between 80% and 100% for stage I disease, 65% to 80% for stage II disease, 25% to 60% for stage III disease, and between 0% and 25% for stage IV disease. Although in the past breast cancer was considered more aggressive in men than in women, the most recent data suggests that when matched for stage and grade, there is not a significant difference in outcome between genders.

In patients with metastatic disease, if they are still receptor positive, hormone therapy should be considered the first-line treatment with systemic chemotherapy reserved for second-line treatment. Hormone therapy can be medical (tamoxifen, megestrol acetate, androgens, steroids) or surgical (orchiectomy, adrenalectomy,

TABLE 22–1 • *Disease-Specific and Overall Survival Rates in Male Breast Cancer From 1,986 Patients in the Surveillance, Epidemiology and End Results Database, 1988–2001*				
	Stage I	**Stage II**	**Stage III**	**Stage IV**
Disease-specific survival (%)				
5 year	96	88	60	23
10 year	93	74	44	21
Overall survival (%)				
5 year	78	66	39	14
10 year	55	39	21	5

From Giordano SH. A review of the diagnosis and management of male breast cancer. The Oncologist 2005;10:471-479.

date of delivery will be important pieces of information in planning therapy. Amniocentesis may be necessary to determine pulmonary maturity.

When pregnant women are diagnosed with breast cancer, one option is to terminate the pregnancy. However, breast cancer can be successfully treated during pregnancy, and early termination does not improve the outcome of the breast cancer.

Surgery can be performed safely in pregnant women when planned with both anesthesiology and obstetrics (Box 22–3). Therefore, there is no contraindication to performing a modified radical mastectomy (MRM) in a pregnant woman. However, pregnant women are often just as motivated to conserve the breast and avoid ALND as nonpregnant women. Unfortunately, radiation therapy to the breast, an important component of BCT, is contraindicated during pregnancy. The risk to the fetus is high because it cannot be adequately shielded. If a woman wishes to pursue breast conservation, she has several options.

If the cancer is detected in the third trimester, or the late second trimester, she may undergo lumpectomy and defer the radiation until after delivery. If, based on the stage of the cancer, she will require systemic chemotherapy, this will delay the implementation of radiation therapy up to 6 months. This may allow women in the first or second trimester to opt for breast conservation. Neoadjuvant chemotherapy can also be considered when appropriate. This results in a catch 22 because women who have smaller cancers early in the pregnancy will more often require mastectomy because they do not require adjuvant chemotherapy and thus would have an unacceptable delay between lumpectomy and radiation. Women in this situation may consider this option; however, they may be exposing themselves to a higher local recurrence rate.

Pregnant women who are clinically node negative may undergo SLN biopsy for axillary staging. The procedure should be done with radiolabelled colloid only and not isosulfan blue dye secondary to the risk of allergic reaction. The radiolabelled colloids are associated with a minimal dose of radiation exposure to the fetus as a result of the rapid uptake in the maternal reticuloendothelial system.

Although there are increased risks, adjuvant chemotherapy can be administered to pregnant women with breast cancer (Box 22–4). Potential agents include cyclophosphamide, doxorubicin, and 5-Fluorouracil (5-FU). Methotrexate is contraindicated. Chemotherapy should not be administered during the first trimester because there is an increased risk of abortion and malformations. Beyond the first

---

BOX 22–3 ANESTHETIC CONCERNS IN THE PREGNANT PATIENT

Altered physiology of pregnancy
- Increased blood volume with physiologic anemia
- Increased heart rate and cardiac output
- Elevated diaphragm, decreased functional residual capacity
- Increased oxygen consumption
- Decreased partial pressure of carbon dioxide (pCO_2), decreased buffer base capacity, and normal acid-base balance (pH)
- Increased fibrinogen and platelet count

Prolonged gastric emptying and increased risk of aspiration
- Use of oral noncolloidal antacids and Reglan
- Rapid sequence induction with cricoid pressure
- Hypotension resulting from aortocaval compression
- Left lateral tilt with 15-degree wedge under right hip

Maternal hyperventilation and fetal acidosis
- Monitor fetal heart rate, avoid hyperventilation, and maintain normal pH

Risk of preterm labor

BOX 22–4 RISKS OF CHEMOTHERAPY ON THE FETUS AND NEONATE

Immediate risks
Spontaneous abortion
Teratogenesis
Premature birth or low birth weight

Possible complications secondary to in utero exposure
Carcinogenesis
Sterility
Delayed physical or mental growth
Mutation

trimester, chemotherapy does not appear to increase the risk of fetal abnormalities. The optimal timing would have chemotherapy conclude 4 weeks before delivery, so that decreased blood counts do not lead to bleeding or infectious complications. However, a careful discussion needs to be held with the patient regarding the risks and benefits of adjuvant chemotherapy. Adjuvant chemotherapy may be associated with intrauterine growth restriction and prematurity. In addition, there is little long-term data on children exposed to chemotherapy in utero. Endocrine therapy, particularly tamoxifen, is contraindicated during pregnancy. Postpartum tamoxifen can be considered for use in hormone-receptor-positive tumors.

Breast Cancer in Older Patients

The current median age at diagnosis for breast cancer is 61, and most of the women who die of breast cancer are over the age of 65. As the population grows and ages, new breast cancer cases increase as the incidence of breast cancer rises with age. It is therefore not surprising that an individual surgeon's practice will continue to see an increasing percentage of breast cancer patients in their 70s and 80s. It is therefore important to understand how to approach the elderly woman with breast cancer, knowing when age should factor into surgical decision making and when it should not.

When compared to their younger counterparts, breast cancers in older women tend to have different biologic characteristics. Breast cancers in older women are more often of a lower grade, are ER/PR positive, and associated with a decreased expression of poor prognostic markers such as Her-2/neu. They are also less likely to involve the regional nodes. Despite the fact that older women are often treated less aggressively, their prognosis is good. In a study of tumor biology and outcome from the Surveillance, Epidemiology and End Results (SEER) database, women over 70 with node-negative tumors had an 8-year overall survival rate comparable to an age-matched population without breast cancer. Women with node-positive tumors had only a modest decrease in overall survival. This is despite the fact that older women had lower rates of surgery, radiation, and chemotherapy than younger patients. Although this would imply that breast cancers in older women have a more indolent course,

that statement is certainly controversial and could lead to undertreatment of the elderly population, resulting in excessive local, regional, and distant recurrence.

Certainly, when looking at the older population as a whole, there is a decreased overall survival and an increased risk of death from causes other than breast cancer, and this must be taken into account when reviewing treatment options. However, the clinician must also take into account that overall patients are living longer, thus a healthy older patient may have a longer period to develop recurrence than just 10 years ago. It is therefore not correct to say that simply because a patient is over 70 or 75 it is reasonable to offer less aggressive therapies. Instead, when facing an individual elderly patient with breast cancer, their chronologic age should be secondary, and their physiologic age should be examined. This would include looking at their functional status, comorbidities, and life expectancy. In this manner, the risks and benefits of surgery and adjuvant therapy can be more accurately weighed. There are several tools that may be useful in this situation. The Eastern Cooperative Oncology Group (ECOG) and Karnofsky performance scales are often used to identify patients with decreased functional status and hence worse outcomes with therapy (Tables 22–2 and 22–3). The comprehensive geriatric assessment (CGA) is a structured evaluation of elderly patients on multiple levels including physical and functional status, comorbidities, nutritional status, and

TABLE 22–2 • Eastern Cooperative Oncology Group (ECOG) Performance Status Criteria

Grade	Status
0	Fully active, able to carry on all predisease performance without restriction
1	Restricted in physically strenuous activity but ambulatory and able to carry out work of a light or sedentary nature (e.g., light housework, office work)
2	Ambulatory and capable of all self-care but unable to carry out any work activities; up and about more than 50% of waking hours
3	Capable of only limited self-care; confined to bed or chair more than 50% of waking hours
4	Completely disabled; cannot carry on any self-care; totally confined to bed or chair
5	Dead

TABLE 22-3 • *Karnofsky Performance Status*

Grade	Karnofsky Scale
100	Normal, no complaints; no evidence of disease
90	Able to carry on normal activity; minor signs or symptoms of disease
80	Normal activity with effort; some signs or symptoms of disease
70	Cares for self but unable to carry on normal activity or to do active work
60	Requires occasional assistance but is able to care for most personal needs
50	Requires considerable assistance and frequent medical care
40	Disabled; requires special care and assistance
30	Severely disabled; hospitalization is indicated, although death is not imminent
20	Very ill; hospitalization and active supportive care are necessary
10	Moribund
0	Dead

geriatric syndromes such as dementia or depression. It may also be useful to assess these patients in a multidisciplinary or tumor board setting, to gain the input of medical oncologists and radiation oncologists before planning surgical therapy.

If your assessment of the elderly patients reveals a healthy woman with minimal functional limitations, then the surgical options are no different than the younger patient. Primary surgery can be either mastectomy or BCT. Morbidity and mortality rates of mastectomy in older patients are comparable to younger patients, although there is clearly some selection bias. It is important to remember that age is *not* a contraindication to BCT. Although some studies demonstrate that older women have lower rates of breast conservation, when older women are presented with both options they are just as likely to prefer breast conservation as younger women. To assume an older woman cares less about body image and the psychosocial implications of mastectomy would be incorrect, and surgeons should offer the two surgical options in the same manner as they would a younger woman.

For elderly women with larger primary tumors who still desire breast conservation, neoadjuvant therapy also remains an option.

If there is a concern regarding neoadjuvant chemotherapy in this population, an alternative approach might be neoadjuvant hormonal therapy. In older patients who are hormone-receptor positive, neoadjuvant hormonal therapy with tamoxifen, anastrozole, or letrozole have been reported to have clinical response rates similar to those seen for chemotherapy.

The same recommendation should be made for axillary evaluation. It has been suggested that because older women are less likely to be node positive and have decreased overall survival, that axillary evaluation with SLN biopsy may not be necessary. However, knowing whether an elderly patient is node positive or node negative may significantly change recommendations for adjuvant therapy, and SLN biopsy has few side effects in older women. This is an example in which the multidisciplinary approach is quite useful because the medical oncologist can weigh in on whether systemic therapy might change with the information gleaned from a SLN biopsy.

A more controversial issue is the management of the elderly patient with the positive SLN. Although the standard of care is a complete ALND, the overall survival benefit of the complete ALND is unknown for all patients with breast cancer, let alone older patients, and older women tend to have worse quality of life scores and difficulties with function after ALND. However, even in the absence of an overall survival benefit, there may be a benefit to regional control. Predictive models and nomograms can help assess an individual woman's risk of harboring additional disease in the nonsentinel lymph nodes, and this information can be used for a balanced discussion with the patient regarding the relative pros and cons of completing the ALND in the elderly patient with breast cancer who is SLN positive.

Another area of discussion is whether radiation is a necessary adjunct to lumpectomy among older women. Radiation therapy is well tolerated in elderly patients, and there is no doubt that radiation will decrease in-breast recurrences after lumpectomy and chest wall recurrences after mastectomy. Overall, the decreased local recurrence rates associated with radiation will impact overall survival (see Chapter 15), although most of these trials had upper age cutoffs. Therefore, there has been some question to the benefit of radiation therapy in the elderly population. Two randomized studies addressed this issue. In a randomized trial of radiation therapy compared to no radiation therapy in 796 patients over the age of 50, radiation had no impact on overall survival but did decrease local recurrence rates from 7.7% to 0.6% ($p < 0.001$). In a study limited to women who were hormone-receptor positive over the age of 70, radiation decreased locoregional recurrence from 4% to 1% ($p < 0.001$) but again had no impact on distant disease-free or overall survival. It may, therefore, be reasonable to offer lumpectomy alone to a subset of older women, omitting radiation therapy. This decision should be based on multiple factors including the woman's life expectancy, functional status, ability to go through radiation, tumor size, hormonal status, and lymph node status. Again, the tumor board approach is particularly helpful and may impact the surgical decision making if lumpectomy alone is a consideration.

When faced with an elderly patient with moderate to significant comorbidities, it can sometimes be difficult to judge how aggressive to be in managing their breast cancer. In patients who are not good candidates for surgery, hormonal therapy alone is often used if the patient is hormone-receptor positive. In randomized trials of primary endocrine therapy versus surgery, overall survival is similar, however, locoregional control is significantly worse. Even among patients with advancing age and comorbidities, both lumpectomy and mastectomy are well tolerated and many patients treated with hormone therapy alone will ultimately require surgery for local control. They may end up being worse candidates for surgery when that time comes. Therefore, endocrine therapy alone should be reserved for patients with significant comorbidities for whom surgery would carry excessively high risks.

Finally, the most controversial aspect of breast cancer care among the elderly is the use of systemic adjuvant therapy. The benefits of adjuvant therapy for breast-cancer-specific prognosis must be weighed against the treatment related toxicity and the nonbreast-cancer prognosis. Clinical trial data is limited as many prospective, randomized trials failed to accrue significant numbers of elderly patients. The Early Breast Cancer Trialists' Collaborative Group (EBCTCG) has performed a meta-analysis on a large number of clinical trials, allowing for analysis of small subsets including the elderly, and much of the basis for systemic therapy in the elderly comes from this data.

For hormone-receptor-positive tumors, selective estrogen receptor modulators (SERMs) and aromatase inhibitors (AIs) clearly reduce recurrence and mortality and are well tolerated in the elderly population. Unless the patient has an extremely good-prognosis tumor or significant comorbidity that precludes it, hormonal therapy should be strongly considered. Tamoxifen can reduce breast cancer mortality by 31% in postmenopausal women, regardless of age, and the side effects (vasomotor symptoms, endometrial cancer, thromboembolic disease) are infrequent and do not significantly contribute to the likelihood of dying of nonbreast cancer causes. AIs are slightly better than tamoxifen, improving disease free survival by 3% to 5%. This effect was most pronounced in women over 64 years of age. For women who took 5 years of tamoxifen, the addition of letrozole improved overall survival in patients who were node positive. For women who took 2 to 3 years of tamoxifen, switching to an AI, as opposed to staying on tamoxifen for the full 5 years, improved disease-free survival. Therefore postmenopausal women should have an AI as part of their hormonal therapy, although which agent and when to introduce it is less clear. The major complication of the AIs is musculoskeletal complications, including osteoporotic fractures. These women should undergo baseline and yearly bone densitometry.

Adjuvant chemotherapy decisions are more difficult because there is a smaller benefit and more side effects to consider. This includes the addition of chemotherapy to hormonal therapy in patients who are hormone-receptor positive and the systemic options for patients who are hormone-receptor negative. Even if a benefit is present, the side effects of chemotherapy can be more significant in older women. Myelosuppression and neutropenic infections increase with age. Age is a known risk factor for anthracycline-associated cardiac toxicity, and age is associated with higher rates of cardiomyopathy in women treated with chemotherapy. An increased mortality rate secondary to chemotherapy has been reported in older women, which may offset some of the benefit. It is hard to truly study this, even prospectively, because of the selection bias in entering older women onto clinical trials (as a result of both strict entry criteria and physician bias). The EBCTCG overview is limited by the small number of women over 70 in the clinical trials and the lack of data regarding newer agents. However, it seems unlikely that elderly women with node-negative disease would benefit from adjuvant chemotherapy. Several randomized trials, including National Surgical and Adjuvant Breast Project (NSABP) data, show a decreasing impact of adjuvant chemotherapy with age among node-negative patients. A more significant impact of chemotherapy is seen among patients who are node positive. Trastuzumab may be a good choice in Her-2/neu-positive tumors among elderly patients with good baseline cardiac function, although Her-2/neu overexpression decreases with age. A more detailed discussion of systemic therapy in the elderly population is beyond the scope of this textbook; however, the complexity of these decisions underscore the importance of axillary staging among older patients and argues against the routine avoidance of SLN biopsy among women over a certain age. As with so many situations in breast cancer, a multidisciplinary approach is mandated.

Breast Cancer among African American Women

Although the treatment of breast cancer among African American women is identical to that of Anglo American women, there are several differences in disease presentation and outcome that are important to recognize. Breast cancer incidence among African American women is lower than that of Anglo American women. Despite this, the mortality rates are paradoxically higher. This is partly explained by the more advanced stage at which African American women tend to present; however, the reasons for this are not completely clear.

It might be immediately assumed that the advanced stage at presentation, and the increased mortality, can be attributed to socioeconomic factors and barriers to screening and early diagnosis. Although this certainly plays a part, there also appear to be some biologic differences between breast cancer in the African American population and their Anglo counterparts. Some evidence for this comes from the association of age and breast cancer development. Although breast cancer risk increases as a function of age for both groups, African American women have a higher incidence of breast cancer under the age of 45 than do Anglo women. These rates tend to equalize around the fifth decade. Over the age of 50, incidence rates for Anglo women surpasses those of African American women, resulting in a higher lifetime risk. Whereas 20% of Anglo patients with breast cancer are younger

than 50 years of age, this number rises to 30% to 40% for African American patients with breast cancer.

This may represent a difference in the biology of the disease or may be related to a difference in risk factors. As previously described, there is a short-term increased risk of breast cancer in the postpartum period with premenopausal women. The higher prevalence of early childbearing among African American women may increase the incidence below age 50 and ultimately decrease the risk of breast cancer later in life. Another potential explanation is in differences in diet and other environmental factors.

There may also be genetic factors at play. Breast cancer among women in the Ghanaian and Nigerian populations of western Africa (who share a common ancestry with present generation African American) have similarities to that of African American women (younger age of onset, higher rate of ER-negative disease). This suggests the possible contribution of founder effects.

Breast cancer among African American women is a more aggressive disease, with higher rates of adverse prognostic factors such as hormone-receptor negativity, stage at presentation, and aneuploid tumors. This not only suggests a more aggressive disease, but it also limits therapeutic options. African American cancers are more likely to be node positive, even when correcting for age and tumor size. This, in part, contributes to the decreased survival, but does not completely explain it. Among patients in the Detroit SEER-based tumor registry, even after adjusting for age, tumor size, nodal status, and hormone-receptor status, there was a significantly elevated mortality risk for young African American women compared to Anglo American women. This suggests that beyond more aggressive disease, socioeconomic status may impact treatment as well as screening. Poverty, lack of insurance, restricted access to health care, and possibly discriminatory practices within the health care system may not only prevent African American women from being diagnosed earlier, but also limit treatment options. Does socioeconomic status completely explain these disparities? It does not appear so. A meta-analysis of 14 studies looking at the difference in survival between African American and Anglo American women showed that even when socioeconomic status is controlled for, race is still an independent and significant predictor of mortality risk. Data from clinical trials also supports this finding. Therefore, it appears that the more aggressive disease and worse outcome seen among African American women compared with Anglo American women is the result of several factors. These include inherent genetic differences between the two populations, differences in risk factors impacting the biology of the disease, and disparities in screening and delivery of treatment.

Breast Cancer among Other Ethnicities

The Hispanic American community is the most rapidly growing minority in the United States, and breast cancer among Hispanic American women has some similarities to the African American population. As with African American women, socioeconomic disadvantages also play a significant role, with poverty and lack of insurance providing barriers to screening and treatment. Compared with non-Hispanic women, Hispanic Americans appear to have a younger age distribution and lower survival rate. There is significantly less research in this area, and it is difficult to fully evaluate the epidemiology of breast cancer in Hispanic American women because of the diversity within the population. Hispanic Americans originate from Mexico, Puerto Rico, Cuba, Central America, South America, Spain, and Portugal, each with different genetic, cultural, and dietary backgrounds.

Breast cancer among the Asian American population provides interesting data regarding the causes of breast cancer. Historically, breast cancer incidence has been low among women who originate or reside from an Asian country. Studies of Asian women who moved to the United States demonstrate a strong environmental cause of breast cancer because the risk of breast cancer increases with the length of time spent in the United States and number of generations who have lived here. Thus, an Asian woman who moves to the United States has a higher risk than a woman who lives in an Asian country, and an Asian woman born in the United States has an even higher risk, nearly approximating that of a non-Asian woman born in the United States. Similarly, breast cancer rates in Asia have increased as countries have adopted westernized cultural practices. These data have prompted multiple searches for the reproductive, dietary or cultural practices thought to account for these trends, with limited success. Epidemiologic studies among Asian Americans women is also hampered by the heterogeneity of the population, which may include women from Japan, China, Korea,

Hawaii, the Philippines, India, Pakistan, and other countries, again all with different backgrounds, diets, and cultures.

Suggested Readings

1. Anderson WF, Althuis MD, Brinton LA, et al. Is male breast cancer similar or different than female breast cancer? Breast Cancer Res Treat 2004;83:77.
2. Barnes DM, Newman LA. Pregnancy-associated breast cancer: a literature review. Surg Clin North Am 2007;87(2):417–430
3. Bradley CJ, Given CW, Roberts C. Race, socioeconomic status, and breast cancer treatment and survival. J Natl Cancer Inst 2002;94:490.
4. Chakravarthy A, Kim CR. Post-mastectomy radiation in male breast cancer. Radiother Oncol 2002;65:99.
5. Cimmino VM, Degnim AC, Sabel MS, et al. Efficacy of sentinel lymph node biopsy in male breast cancer. J Surg Oncol 2004;86(2):74–77.
6. Giordano SH. A review of the diagnosis and management of male breast cancer. The Oncologist 2005;10:471–479.
7. Hughes KS, Schnaper L, Berry D, et al. Lumpectomy plus tamoxifen with and without irradiation in women 70 years of age or older with early breast cancer. N Engl J Med 2004;31(10):971–977.
8. Jones BA, Patterson EA, Calvocoressi L. Mammography screening in African American women: evaluating the research. Cancer 2003;97(1 Suppl):258–272.
9. Keleher AJ, Theriault RL, Gwyn KM, et al. Multidisciplinary management of breast cancer concurrent with pregnancy. J Am Coll Surg 2002;194:54–64.
10. Lambe M, Hsieh C, Trichopoulos D, et al. Transient increase in the risk of breast cancer after giving birth. N Engl J Med 1994;331:5–9.
11. Leslie KK, Lange CA. Breast cancer and pregnancy. Obstet Gynecol Clin North Am 2005;32(4):547–558.
12. Liede, A, Karlan, BY, Narod, SA. Cancer risks for male carriers of germline mutations in BRCA1 or BRCA2: a review of the literature. J Clin Oncol 2004;22:735.
13. Mabuchi, K, Bross, DS, Kessler, II. Risk factors for male breast cancer. J Natl Cancer Inst 1985;74:371.
14. Newman LA. Breast cancer in African-American women. Oncologist 2005;10:1–14.
15. Newman LA, Martin IK. Disparities in breast cancer. Curr Prob Cancer 31(3):134–156, 200
16. Ottini L, Masala G, D'Amico C, et al. BRCA1 and BRCA2 mutation status and tumor characteristics in male breast cancer: a population-based study in Italy. Cancer Res 2003;63:342.
17. Palmer JR, Wise LA, Horton NJ, et al. Dual effect of parity on breast cancer risk in African-American women. J Natl Cancer Inst 2003;95:478.
18. Ribeiro G, Swindell R, Harris M, et al. A review of the management of male breast carcinoma based on an analysis of 420 treated cases. The Breast 1996;5:141.
19. Rugh HS. Management of breast cancer diagnosed during pregnancy. Curr Treat Options Oncol 2003;4:165–173.
20. Vetto J, Schmidt W, Pommier R, et al. Accurate and cost effective evaluation of breast masses in males. Am J Surg 1998;175:383.
21. Woo JC, Yu T, Hurd TC. Breast cancer in pregnancy: a literature review. Arch Surg 2003;138:91–98.

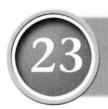

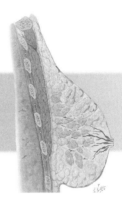

Other Tumors of the Breast

PHYLLODES TUMORS

FIBROMATOSIS OF THE BREAST

SARCOMA
Angiosarcoma of the Breast

LYMPHOMA

METASTASES TO THE BREAST

Other Tumors of the Breast: Key Points

- Know the difference in presentation between a phyllodes tumor and a fibroadenoma.
- Describe the surgical treatment of phyllodes tumor.
- Describe the surgical treatment of fibromatosis of the breast.
- Understand the risk factors for sarcoma, including those specific to breast cancer therapy.
- Describe the clinical presentation of angiosarcoma of the breast.
- Know the multidisciplinary treatment of soft tissue sarcoma.
- Be familiar with the clinical presentation and management of breast lymphoma.

Phyllodes Tumors

Phyllodes tumors encompass an unusual spectrum of fibroepithelial tumors of the breast that exhibit a range of clinical behavior. Overall they represent less than 1% of all breast neoplasms. Although the median age is 45, they have been described both in adolescents and elderly patients. This is an older age distribution than with fibroadenoma; so a fibroadenoma-like mass in older patients should raise a concern for phyllodes. Patients with Li-Fraumeni

syndrome have a higher risk of phyllodes tumors. They have also been described in men who have gynecomastia.

Phyllodes tumors most commonly present as a palpable mass in the breast. Because they often have a biphasic growth phase, patients may seek medical attention for a mass that has been stable for a long period of time but recently started to enlarge. The lesions can get quite large, with phyllodes tumors over 20 cm having been reported, although even extremely large tumors can still be benign histologically.

BOX 23–1 FEATURES SUSPICIOUS
FOR PHYLLODES TUMOR VERSUS
FIBROADENOMA

- Rapid growth
- Greater than 3 cm
- Sudden increase in growth of a long-standing breast mass
- Fibroadenoma-like mass in patient old than 35 years of age
- Rounded borders or lobulated appearance on mammogram
- Cystic area within solid mass on ultrasound
- Hypercellular stromal fragments on fine-needle aspiration
- Indeterminate features on fine-needle aspiration or core-needle biopsy

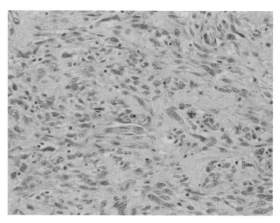

Figure 23–1. Histology of phyllodes tumor. Phyllodes tumors are differentiated from fibroadenomas by the expanded and increased cellularity of the stromal component. The distinction between benign, borderline, and malignant is based on stromal cellularity, cytologic atypia, mitoses, and necrosis. (Image courtesy of Dr. Maria Braman, Department of Pathology, University of Michigan).

On examination, the masses are similar to fibroadenomas; mobile, round, smooth, and well-defined margins (Box 23–1). Even with malignant phyllodes tumors, signs associated with malignancy such as skin or nipple retraction or bloody nipple discharge are rare. Lymph node involvement is also quite rare, although some patients may have palpable adenopathy.

The workup is similar to any new or enlarging breast mass, including mammogram, ultrasound, and biopsy. The biggest difficulty is differentiating these tumors from fibroadenoma. Not only do they feel like fibroadenomas, but on imaging they also have radiographic findings that mimic fibroadenomas (oval or round, solid, hypoechoic, well-circumscribed masses). On ultrasound, there may be coarse microcalcifications present or a cystic area within the solid mass.

Histologically, phyllodes tumors are characterized by both epithelial and stromal elements. It is the stroma, however, that is truly distinguishing. Clonal analysis reveals that the epithelial component is polyclonal, whereas the stromal component is monoclonal, demonstrating that the stroma is the neoplastic component of the tumor. Under the microscope these tumors contain elongated ductal elements and papillary protrusions of connective tissue lined by epithelium that produce the classic leaflike appearance (Fig. 23–1). The stromal overgrowth and hypercellularity distinguish these lesions from fibroadenomas.

Unfortunately, fine-needle aspiration (FNA) carries a high rate of false-negative results for diagnosing phyllodes tumors because they have a heterogeneous composition. Core-needle biopsy is much more accurate, although still may be hampered by sampling error. This presents a clinical problem because many of these patients will present with what appears to be a fibroadenoma, for which FNA (combined with clinical and radiologic evaluation and an experienced cytopathologist) is a useful tool. Clinicians should lean toward core-needle biopsy if they suspect a higher likelihood of a phyllodes tumor. This would include any long-standing mass that suddenly gets larger, a mass greater than 3 cm in size or a fibroadenoma-like mass in a patient over the age of 35. Also any radiographic findings not consistent with fibroadenoma, such as cystic areas within a solid mass, should prompt a core-needle biopsy. If an FNA was performed and there were either hypercellular stromal fragments or other indeterminate findings, either a core or excisional biopsy should be performed.

Phyllodes tumors are characterized as benign, borderline, or malignant based on their histologic appearance. Increased cellular atypia, mitotic activity, stromal overgrowth, and tumor necrosis are associated with malignant potential. One of the most important features is the tumor margin; whether it is circumscribed or infiltrative. Over half of phyllodes tumors are benign, whereas about one quarter are malignant. Surprisingly, there is slightly less correlation with outcome and histologic features. Benign tumors can recur and even spread and malignant lesions can have indolent courses. Because of this, some authors have suggested approaching all phyllodes tumors as though they have some malignant potential. It is important to keep in mind that overall, phyllodes tumors have a favorable prognosis.

Once a diagnosis of phyllodes tumor is made, surgical excision is indicated. The standard recommendation is a wide excision with 1-cm margins. The 1-cm margin is recommended because there may be microscopic projections of tumor extending into the pseudocapsule of compressed breast tissue that surround these lesions. Often these are simply enucleated because they are suspected to be fibroadenomas. This is clearly inadequate and reexcision is recommended. The data is less clear when a phyllodes tumor is diagnosed after a negative, but narrow, margin excision. For borderline or malignant tumors, reexcision is clearly indicated. For clearly benign phyllodes tumors, this is less clear. However, given the difficulties in pathologic classification and the potential of even benign lesions to recur, a reexcision is reasonable. In cases where tumor size precludes breast conservation, simple mastectomy is indicated. Sentinel lymph node (SLN) biopsy or routine axillary dissection is not indicated because lymph node metastases occur in less than 5% of patients. Axillary lymph node dissection (ALND) should be performed in patients with confirmed pathologic nodes.

The role of adjuvant radiation therapy is controversial. There is no prospective randomized data to base decisions on. It does not appear indicated when a 1-cm margin has been obtained and unlikely to be of benefit when a clearly benign phyllodes tumor has been excised with negative margins. It should be considered in situations in which negative margins cannot be obtained. The role of adjuvant chemotherapy is clearer—there is no role. Hormone-receptor expression on the stromal component is rare and so there is no role for measuring these or treating with hormonal therapy. Although malignant phyllodes tumors have a risk of distant recurrence, chemotherapy has limited efficacy and so probably provides little benefit in the adjuvant setting.

The most common type of recurrence is local, occurring in approximately 15% of patients. Most local recurrences are within 2 years, are usually the same histology (although transformation to more aggressive subtypes has been reported), and in most cases, are not associated with distant recurrence. Treatment should be reexcision with 1-cm margins if possible. Some authors have argued for radiation after reexcision of a recurrent phyllodes because patients with one local recurrence have a higher risk of further episodes of recurrence. However, this is a controversial recommendation. If a reexcision with 1-cm margins is not possible, mastectomy is indicated.

Overall, approximately 5% to 10% of patients with phyllodes tumors will develop distant disease. This is higher for malignant phyllodes tumors, closer to 20%. The metastases are composed of only the stromal elements, with no epithelial component. Average survival of patients with metastatic phyllodes tumors is less than 2 years. Chemotherapy is indicated, although multiple single and combination regimens have been used with varying success and responses are generally of short duration. The National Comprehensive Cancer Network (NCCN) recommends that the treatment of metastatic phyllodes tumors follow the guidelines for metastatic soft tissue sarcoma.

Fibromatosis of the Breast

Fibromatosis of the breast is similar to fibromatosis in other sites, such as desmoid tumors of the abdominal wall. Although they do not metastasize, these lesions have a high propensity for local recurrence and possibly local invasion. Fibromatosis is characterized by a nonencapsulated proliferation of spindle cells. Fibromatosis of the breast will often present like invasive cancer with a palpable mass that may have associated skin retraction or chest wall fixation. Imaging will also appear consistent with invasive breast cancer. However, on pathology, these lesions demonstrate interlacing bundles of spindle-shaped cells surrounded by collagen, with minimal if any cytologic atypia. The proliferation surrounds the ducts and lobules without destroying them.

The treatment of fibromatosis is wide excision with careful assessment of the margins to assure complete resection. Otherwise local recurrence is highly likely. Radiation therapy may be considered if complete excision is not possible, but the goal should be widely negative margins whenever possible. Low levels of estrogen receptor (ER) and progesterone receptor (PR) expression have been described, as has response to tamoxifen, and so this should be considered when excision is not possible.

Sarcoma

Sarcomas are malignant tumors of mesenchymal tissue. They can occur anywhere in the body, including in the breast, although this is quite rare, accounting for less than 1% of breast malignancies. There are several risk factors that have been identified for sarcoma. Genetic conditions may predispose to sarcoma including Li-Fraumeni syndrome, Gardner syndrome, or neurofibromatosis type 1. There are also environmental exposures that have been linked to sarcoma. Vinyl chloride, arsenic compounds, and herbicides are some of the agents that have been implicated. Several viruses have also been associated with sarcoma such as the human immunodeficiency virus (HIV).

There are two risk factors for sarcoma that are particularly worrisome for the development of breast sarcoma. The first of these is ionizing radiation. The risk of postirradiation sarcoma increases with the dose of radiation used (it is rarely seen with doses less than 40 Gy). The average latency period for sarcomas after radiation is approximately 5 to 12 years (shorter for angiosarcomas than other histologies). Fortunately, the risk of secondary sarcoma in women who undergo radiation for breast-conserving therapy (BCT) is quite small. The cumulative incidences of radiation induced sarcoma are approximately 0.2% at 10 years and 0.78% at 30 years.

Another risk factor for sarcoma is chronic edema, which can of course be a complication of breast therapy. Angiosarcomas of the arm or breast in women with chronic lymphedema after breast cancer treatment is known as Stewart-Treves syndrome.

Breast sarcomas usually present as a large, painless, firm mass within the breast, a presentation similar to fibroadenomas or adenocarcinoma. They rarely have any overlying skin or nipple changes. Angiosarcomas of the breast may have some color changes in the overlying skin, either a bluish tint or erythema. Sarcomas often grow faster than epithelial breast cancer and so may be larger in size when diagnosed. On mammography, calcifications, spiculations, and other signs associated with breast cancer are rarely present. Thus, these lesions may be mistaken for benign tumors.

The diagnosis will come down to the biopsy. Common subtypes within the breast include fibrosarcoma, angiosarcoma, malignant fibrous histiocytoma (MFH), myxofibrosarcoma, and leiomyosarcoma. Outside of angiosarcoma, which has a much worse prognosis, the histologic subtype is not a significant prognostic factor. Coreneedle biopsy is often adequate, but sometimes sarcomas have necrotic centers and the coreneedle biopsy will not retrieve enough viable tissue to make a diagnosis. In this case an excisional or incisional biopsy may be indicated. This may also be needed to differentiate a primary breast sarcoma from a metaplastic carcinoma. The latter is diagnosed because of associated invasive carcinoma or in situ disease.

Once the diagnosis is made, staging should include a computed tomography (CT) scan of the chest to rule out lung metastases (the most common site of spread from sarcoma) and serve as a baseline for future follow-up. A magnetic resonance imaging (MRI) of the breast may also be useful in planning surgical therapy. As is often recommended with breast cancer, patients diagnosed with sarcoma should be referred to a multidisciplinary sarcoma center. Because sarcoma is a rarer disease than breast cancer, there are less institutions with experience treating sarcoma, and experience is critically important given the complexities of sarcoma management. The use of radiation therapy and chemotherapy is more controversial for sarcoma, as is the use of preoperative versus postoperative therapy.

The most important component of sarcoma therapy is surgery, and this will primarily consist of mastectomy, although wide local excision with negative margins may be acceptable for some patients (small, low-grade tumors). When appropriate, wide local excision has been shown to have equal outcomes to mastectomy, as along as negative surgical margins are obtained. As sarcomas rarely spread to the regional nodes, SLN biopsy or ALND is not routinely recommended. Some histologic subtypes do have higher incidences of regional spread and may justify SLN biopsy. These include breast liposarcomas, carcinosarcomas, synovial sarcomas, epithelioid sarcomas, and possibly rhabdomyosarcomas (although these subtypes are quite rare within the breast). In some cases, a simple mastectomy may not be adequate because skin or muscle involvement may require a more radical excision. The benefit of radiation is controversial for breast sarcoma, but given the benefit for extremity soft tissue sarcoma, is generally recommended for patients with high-grade tumors, tumors greater than 2 cm or for those in whom positive margins can not be obtained. Chemotherapy is more controversial. A thorough review of the pathology and a treatment plan devised by a tumor board consisting of medical, radiation, and surgical oncologists with experience in sarcoma is paramount to successful treatment.

Angiosarcoma of the Breast

Sarcomas are extremely heterogeneous, but angiosarcomas deserve special mention because they may be associated with therapies that are specific to breast cancer; they are the most common type of breast sarcoma in many series; and they may present differently than other types of sarcoma. Angiosarcomas of the breast are categorized as primary or secondary, with secondary angiosarcomas occurring in the face of breast lymphedema or radiation therapy. Although primary angiosarcomas typically occur in the second to fourth decade of life, secondary angiosarcomas occur after breast cancer treatment and thus are usually diagnosed in women over 50.

As with other sarcomas, angiosarcomas may often present as a superficial, palpable, painless mass. However, there may be a blue or purple discoloration and more than one mass. Some patients may present with complaints of ecchymosis, but there is no history of trauma. Diffuse breast enlargement may be present. Any woman who underwent breast or chest wall radiation and now presents with a new mass or discoloration in the irradiated field must prompt suspicion and biopsy. Angiosarcomas may often extend well beyond what is apparent clinically. Wide excision is rarely adequate, and most patients will require a mastectomy or a more radical resection including a wider area of skin or concomitant chest wall resection. Once diagnosed, MRI should be obtained to help delineate the extent of the tumor, although MRI can underestimate this as well. Radiation therapy is recommended as an adjunct to surgery, but many of these patients have already had radiation. It is important to review the dose and fields of the previous radiation. Chemotherapy is controversial, but given the extremely poor prognosis, often recommended. These are aggressive tumors with an extremely poor outcome. They metastasize early to the lung, liver, and also to the contralateral breast, bones, and skin. The median survival from the time of diagnosis is about 15 months. Future therapies may include vascular-targeting therapies such as antiangiogenesis agents or tyrosine kinase inhibitors. As with all sarcomas, timely referral to a center specializing in sarcoma is strongly recommended.

Lymphoma

Lymphoma of the breast is quite rare, making up less than 0.5% of breast malignancies. Breast lymphomas can either be primary or secondary. Secondary breast lymphoma is more readily recognized because the patients have evidence of concurrent widespread disease. Patients with primary breast lymphoma have no evidence of widespread disease beyond the breast, although axillary lymph nodes or bone marrow may be involved. The clinical and radiologic presentation of primary breast lymphoma is nonspecific, and there is little to suggest lymphoma as compared with other breast malignancies. Most present as a painless mass in the breast, although there may be some thickening of the skin or pain, and they tend to be more rapidly growing than typical breast cancers. Enlarged axillary lymph nodes may also be present. The classic "B" symptoms of lymphoma (fever, weight loss, night sweats) are only rarely present. Mammography and ultrasound are nonspecific. Thus the diagnosis comes down to the biopsy, which will also require flow cytometry. Therefore an FNA or core-needle biopsy might suggest the diagnosis, but an excisional (or incisional) biopsy is usually needed to obtain adequate tissue for staining and flow cytometry.

Most breast lymphomas are of B-cell origin. Primary breast lymphomas tend to be large cell tumors, whereas secondary breast lymphomas are more commonly diffuse small cell tumors. Hodgkin lymphoma and T-cell lymphomas of the breast have been described.

Once diagnosed, the next step should be CT staging of the neck, chest, abdomen, and pelvis and bone marrow biopsy. If the disease is widespread or felt to be secondary lymphoma, systemic therapy is initiated. For cases of primary breast lymphoma, the treatment is guided by the grade and subtype of the disease. Low-grade tumors may be treated by local excision alone, or with radiation therapy. High-grade tumors should also be treated with chemotherapy. There is no indication for radical surgery, such as mastectomy or ALND because the prognosis is similar to lymphomas at other sites and mostly dependent on systemic therapy. These patients are best seen and evaluated at a multidisciplinary lymphoma clinic.

Metastases to the Breast

The breast is an unusual place for other cancers to metastasize to. The most common primary tumors that have been described to spread to breast tissue include lymphomas, lung cancer, melanoma, renal cell carcinoma, and ovarian cancer. Other types that have been described include prostate, thyroid, rectal, gastroesophageal, cervical, vaginal, or pancreatic cancer. Although many patients will have a history of a previous cancer, some will present synchronously and the breast metastasis may be the first sign of disease. As with many of these unusual tumor types, there is little that might suggest metastases rather than a new primary breast cancer, with the exception that sometimes there may be multiple lesions, including bilateral masses. Ultimately the diagnosis will come down to the biopsy and may require an excisional biopsy if core-needle biopsy does not allow for an accurate diagnosis. Treatment is obviously dependent on the primary cancer, and breast surgery is rarely indicated unless the patient needs palliation of a large or ulcerating tumor.

Suggested Readings

1. Aviles A, Delgado S, Nambo MJ, et al. Primary breast lymphoma: results of a controlled clinical trial. Oncology. 2005;69(3):256–260.
2. Ben Hassouna J, Damak T, Gamoudi A, et al. Phyllodes tumors of the breast: a case series of 106 patients. Am J Surg 2006;192:141–147.
3. Chan WH, Cheng SP, Tzen CY, et al. Surgical treatment of phyllodes tumors of the breast: retrospective review of 172 cases. J Surg Oncol 2005;185–194.
4. Jacklin RK, Ridgway PF, Ziprin P, et al. Optimizing preoperative diagnosis in phyllodes tumor of the breast. J Clin Path 2006;59(5):454–459.
5. Kirova YM, Vilcoq JR, Asselain B, et al. Radiation-induced sarcoma after radiotherapy for breast carcinoma: a large-scale single institution review. Cancer 2005;104(4):856–863.
6. Lee AH. The histological diagnosis of metastases to the breast from extramammary malignancies. J Clin Path 2007;60(12):1333–1341.
7. Lin Y, Guo XM, Shen KW, et al. Primary breast lymphoma: long-term treatment outcome and prognosis. Leuk Lymphoma 2006;47(10):2102–2109.
8. Mason HS, Johari V, March DE, et al. Primary breast lymphoma: radiologic and pathologic findings. Breast J 2005;11(6):495–496.
9. Mermershtain W, Cohen AD, Kortez M, et al. Cutaneous angiosarcoma of the breast after lumpectomy, axillary lymph node dissection and radiotherapy for primary breast cancer: case report and review of the literature. Am J Clin Oncol 2002;25(6):597–598.
10. Thomas T, Lorino C, Ferrara JJ. Fibromatosis of the breast: a case report and literature review. J Surg Oncol 1987;35(1):70–74.
11. Tiwary SK, Singh MK, Prasad R, et al. Primary angiosarcoma of the breast. Surgery 2007;141(6):821–822.
12. Williams SA, Ehlers RA 2nd, Hunt KK, et al. Metastases to the breast from nonbreast solid neoplasms: presentation and determinants of survival. Cancer. 2007;110(4):731–737.

Subject Index

Note: Page numbers followed by '*f*' denotes figures; '*t*' denotes tables; '*b*' denotes boxes.